Discourse Analysis in Adults With and Without Communication Disorders

A Resource for Clinicians and Researchers

Discourse Analysis in Adults With and Without Communication Disorders

A Resource for Clinicians and Researchers

Carl A. Coelho, PhD, CCC-SLP, BC-ANCDS
Leora R. Cherney, PhD, CCC-SLP, BC-ANCDS
Barbara B. Shadden, PhD, CCC-SLP, BC-ANCDS

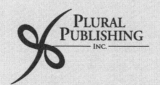

PLURAL
PUBLISHING
INC.

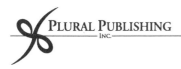

5521 Ruffin Road
San Diego, CA 92123

Email: information@pluralpublishing.com
Website: https://www.pluralpublishing.com

Typeset in 10.5/13 Minion Pro by Flanagan's Publishing Services, Inc.
Printed in the United States of America by McNaughton & Gunn, Inc.

Library of Congress Cataloging-in-Publication Data:
Names: Coelho, Carl A., editor. | Cherney, Leora Reiff, editor. | Shadden,
   Barbara B. (Barbara Bennett), editor.
Title: Discourse analysis in adults with and without communication
   disorders : a resource for clinicians and researchers / [edited by] Carl
   Coelho, Leora R. Cherney, Barbara B. Shadden.
Description: San Diego, CA : Plural Publishing, Inc., 2022. | Includes
   bibliographical references and index.
Identifiers: LCCN 2022019113 (print) | LCCN 2022019114 (ebook) | ISBN
   9781635503753 (paperback) | ISBN 1635503752 (paperback) | ISBN
   9781635503760 (ebook)
Subjects: MESH: Communication Disorders--diagnosis | Communication | Adult
   Aging--physiology
Classification: LCC RC423 (print) | LCC RC423 (ebook) | NLM WL 340.2|
   DDC 616.85/5--dc23/eng/20220523
LC record available at https://lccn.loc.gov/2022019113
LC ebook record available at https://lccn.loc.gov/2022019114

Contents

Preface   *ix*

Acknowledgments   *xi*

About the Editors   *xiii*

Contributors   *xv*

1 Discourse Analysis in Adults With and Without Communication   1
Disorders: An Overview
Carl A. Coelho, Barbara B. Shadden, and Leora R. Cherney

Section I. Discourse and Typical Aging   9
Heather Harris Wright, Topic Chair

2 Cognitive and Linguistic Characteristics of Narrative Discourse   15
Production in Healthy Aging
Andrea Marini

3 Discourse Processing in Older Adults: Considering Discourse   33
Elicitation Tasks
Stephen Kintz and Hana Kim

4 Conversation and Typical Aging   51
Marion Leaman and Aviva Lerman

Section II. Discourse in Aphasia   67
Mary Boyle, Topic Chair

5 Analyzing Linguistic Features of Discourse in People With Aphasia   73
Lucy Bryant

6 Weaving Research Evidence and Clinical Expertise Together in   93
Discourse Analysis of Spoken Personal Narratives in Aphasia
Lucy Dipper and Madeline Cruice

7 Clinical Application of Conversation Analysis in Aphasia   109
Jamie H. Azios and Nina Simmons-Mackie

8 Cross-Cultural Perspectives on Conversational Assessment and   131
Treatment in Aphasia: Learnings From a First Nations Context
Elizabeth Armstrong, Tara Lewis, Alice Robins, Ian Malcolm,
and Natalie Ciccone

**Section III. Discourse of People With Cognitive   149
Communication Disorders**
Leanne Togher, Topic Chair

9 Discourse Assessment Across the Recovery Continuum of   155
Traumatic Brain Injury
Elise Elbourn, Joanne Steel, and Elizabeth Spencer

10 Assessing Conversation After Traumatic Brain Injury   173
Louise C. Keegan, Nicholas Behn, Emma Power, Susan Howell,
and Rachael Rietdijk

11 Assessing Discourse in People With Right Hemisphere Disorders   193
Melissa D. Stockbridge, Jamila Minga, Alexandra Zezinka Durfee,
and Melissa Johnson

12 Using Technology and Telepractice to Evaluate Discourse After   211
Traumatic Brain Injury
Rachael Rietdijk and Peter Meulenbroek

**Section IV. Discourse of People Living With   229
Neurodegenerative Disorders**
J. B. Orange, Topic Chair

13 Clinical Implications of Discourse Analysis for Individuals With   235
Primary Progressive Aphasia
Sarah Grace Dalton, H. Isabel Hubbard, and Jessica D. Richardson

14 What Discourse Analysis Reveals About Conversation and   253
Language Processing in the Context of Dementia of the
Alzheimer's Type
Jackie Guendouzi

15 Multilevel Discourse Analysis in Parkinson's Disease and
Related Disorders   269
Katharine Aveni and Angela Roberts

16 Discourse in ALS: Interplay of Language, Motor, and   289
Executive Factors
Sharon Ash and Sanjana Shellikeri

**Section V. Discourse Databases for Use With Clinical   309
Populations**
Carl A. Coelho, Co-editor

17 Discourse Databases for Use With Clinical Populations   311
Davida Fromm and Brian MacWhinney

Index   *329*

Preface

In the early 1980s, Carl Coelho was working as a speech-language pathologist in an acute rehabilitation hospital. There were 40 beds devoted to stroke rehabilitation and 20 beds for traumatic brain injury (TBI). It was a great environment to learn about adult neuro disorders. During this period, he became interested in the cognitive communication behavior of patients with TBI and struggled with how best to characterize their deficits. Fortunately, Carl worked close to the University of Connecticut, where he had completed his doctorate, and remained in contact with two of his mentors, Betty Liles and Robert Duffy. When they would meet, he often described patients he worked with. During one of these conversations, Betty suggested that he should make recordings of their narrative discourse. With her assistance, Carl began to analyze discourse samples from the TBI patients, which shed new light on the nature of their disrupted communication.

At about the same time, Leora Cherney was pondering how best to address the communication impairments of right hemisphere stroke patients she was seeing daily in the rehabilitation facility where she was working. She was struck by the relative paucity of information that these patients conveyed in the context of fluent, often verbose, language production. In some ways, this was not unlike the communication of patients with early dementia of the Alzheimer's type (DAT). So, for her doctoral dissertation, Leora decided to compare the discourse of these two groups of patients to

begin to tease out the contribution of right hemisphere lesions to the language of DAT.

Meanwhile, Barbara Shadden was facing a different challenge. After moving to the University of Arkansas to pursue her research about the experience of living with aphasia, she discovered that access to individuals with aphasia was quite limited. There was, however, a large population of older residents, many retirees from other parts of the country. Barbara soon found herself fascinated by the limited information available about communication in typically aging adults. She began searching for ways to assess language in a more functional manner, particularly discourse in all its forms. Early research outcomes underscored the heterogeneity of discourse skills in her subjects, and the complex interaction of factors such as tasks, elicitation methods, cognitive challenges, and personal relevance. One intriguing finding was that the discourse of some of the outliers in these typically aging adults looked a lot like the communication of those with conditions such as dementia and right hemisphere disorders. It was quite clear that few discourse assessment clinical tools and measures were available to speech-language pathologists and that normative data were limited.

So how did we come together? Over the next years, other researchers were also studying the discourse of persons with acquired language disorders. More publications were appearing in research journals, but the clinical value of discourse analysis was not appreciated. There was a well-established

Education and Training Department at the Rehabilitation Institute of Chicago, where Leora was working. Aware of the gap in knowledge regarding discourse analysis, she sought out the opportunity to organize a 2-day workshop with the support of Don Olson, the Director of Education and Training. Leora and Barbara had already met at a conference where Barbara was presenting on discourse in the elderly. To complement their expertise, they invited Carl to join them, rounding out their experience with discourse in various neurologic patient populations to include TBI. The initial workshop in 1992 was so successful that, over the next 4 years, it was repeated several times not only in Chicago, but also in Dallas and San Francisco. The workshops focused on the clinical application of discourse analysis for adults with acquired language disorders. Subsequently, Don encouraged the three of us to write a book. The discourse manual was published in 1998 and became informally known as the "Green Book." It became a popular resource for many clinicians and researchers interested in discourse assessment.

In the past several years, interest in the use of discourse analysis has grown immensely and is now considered by clinicians to be a standard component of assessment batteries for acquired language disorders in adults. Still, there is a need for clinicians and researchers to have access, in one place, to information about discourse assessment methods and their application to various neurologic populations. This book confirms the widespread use of discourse analysis by clinicians and researchers, illustrates the myriad of analyses that are now being used, and focuses on what might be most helpful for the clinician, depending on their caseload. The book is organized into four topic areas: aging, aphasia, cognitive communication disorders, and neurodegenerative disorders. There is also a chapter on discourse resources. We are grateful to the topic chairs of each section: Heather Harris Wright, Mary Boyle, Leanne Togher, and J. B. Orange. The topic chairs have brought together an international group of authors who are experts in their fields and provide up-to-date information about each topic.

As indicated, we have known each other for more than 30 years. Each of us has had satisfying, independent careers. Our shared interest in discourse brought us together initially and now this second discourse book brings the trio together again. We work well together and have a great deal of mutual respect. We have enjoyed the process of creating this book and hope that you find it useful in your clinical practice and research endeavors.

Carl Coelho
Leora Cherney
Barbara Shadden

Acknowledgments

I would like to thank the colleagues I worked with in clinical settings for sharing their hunches about how communication unravels after an acquired brain injury. Those discussions were the basis for many of the questions I have sought to answer in my research. I was also fortunate to have mentors at the University of Arizona and the University of Connecticut who encouraged me to look beyond test scores and disordered behavior, and to focus instead on the individual with the disorder. That perspective reinforced the notion for me that there is no substitute for clinical experience particularly in the classroom. I am grateful for the many patients I had the opportunity to work with and learn from.

Finally, I want to acknowledge my wife, Elaine, for her constant support and endless patience. You are the best.

—Carl Coelho

I am deeply appreciative of the many opportunities that have been afforded to me over the years to learn and grow professionally. The chance to write the original 1998 discourse book is one such example, and it has been a joy to connect again with Carl and Barbara.

I am indebted to the many role models, mentors, colleagues, and collaborators who have shared their wisdom and experiences with me—sometimes unaware of the impact that they have made. I am also grateful to the patients and family members who have been the inspiration for the work that I do.

I would like to recognize my family, especially my husband, Marc, for their continued patience and understanding. Finally, I would like to acknowledge and thank my mother, who is now in her mid-90s and with whom I am lucky enough to share daily meaningful conversations. She is my biggest supporter.

—Leora Cherney

Acknowledgments are tough to write, because so many people make a difference in one's life. A big thank you to Carl and Leora, my collaborators in our collective efforts to highlight the importance of discourse analysis. They wouldn't let me say no to being part of this project, and it has been a great journey. The three of us are clinicians at heart, and I want to acknowledge how much I have learned from my clients and their family members over the years. They are the reason I know discourse matters. I am also grateful to my students for being generous in trying out new ideas and new techniques. Finally, to Pat, Marilyn, and Angela: a simple thank you for being there.

—Barbara Shadden

About the Editors

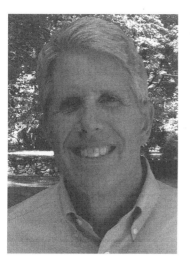

Carl A. Coelho, PhD, CCC-SLP, BC-ANCDS, is professor emeritus and former head of the Department of Speech, Language, and Hearing Sciences at the University of Connecticut, where he also served as director of the Cognitive Science Program. Prior to beginning his academic career, he worked 18 years as a clinician and department director of speech-language pathology and audiology in rehabilitation hospitals. Dr. Coelho spent the next 27 years developing coursework and teaching about the management of communication disorders. He is past-president of the Academy of Neurologic Communication Disorders and Sciences and recipient of Honors of the Academy. Dr. Coelho also served as the vice president of the National Aphasia Association. His research on cognitive communication disorders in adults with acquired brain injuries has been published in more than 100 journal articles and chapters. Dr. Coelho is a Fellow of the American Speech-Language-Hearing Association and has received Distinguished Alumnus Awards from the University of Arizona and the University of Connecticut

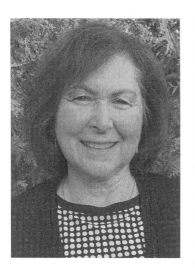

Leora R. Cherney, PhD, CCC-SLP, BC-ANCDS, is the scientific chair of Think and Speak at the Shirley Ryan AbilityLab (formerly the Rehabilitation Institute of Chicago) and professor in both the Department of Physical Medicine and Rehabilitation and the Department of Communication Sciences and Disorders at Northwestern University. She has 40 years of clinical and research experience in adult neurologic communication disorders. She is the founder and director of SRALab's Center for Aphasia Research and Treatment, which conducts cutting-edge research and offers both an intensive comprehensive aphasia program (ICAP) and weekly aphasia community groups. Her innovative research has explored factors to enhance aphasia treatment outcomes for behavioral, pharmacological, and neuromodulatory interventions. Dr. Cherney has authored more than 100 journal publications and five books. She has received numerous prestigious awards, including:

Honors of the Association of both the Illinois and the American Speech-Language-Hearing Association; Honors of the Academy of Neurologic Communication Disorders and Sciences; the American Congress of Rehabilitation Medicine (ACRM) and National Stroke Association Excellence in Post-Acute Stroke Award; and the ACRM Women in Rehabilitation Science Award.

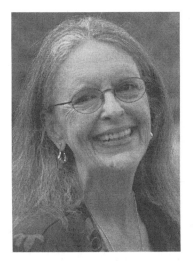

Barbara B. Shadden, PhD, CCC-SLP, BC-ANCDS, is university professor emerita in the Program in Communication Disorders and former director of that program and co-director of the Office for Studies on Aging at the University of Arkansas. She has published and presented on topics in aging, aphasia, and other neurogenic disorders, and discourse, including five textbooks and numerous refereed articles, invited journal articles, and book chapters, as well as more than 150 major presentations. She has also served on the editorial board of two journals; as editor of three journal issues; and as reviewer for seven journals, three publishers, and three funding agencies. Dr. Shadden has served in leadership roles in a number of professional organizations, including Aphasia Access, and her recognitions include: ASHA Fellow; Honors of the Association, Academy of Neurologic Communication Sciences and Disorders; University of Arkansas Alumni Distinguished Teaching Award; and Honors of the Association of Council of Academic Programs in Communication Sciences and Disorders.

Contributors

Topic Chairs

Mary Boyle, PhD, CCC-SLP, BC-ANCDS
Professor
Department of Communication Sciences
  and Disorders
Montclair State University
Bloomfield, New Jersey
Topic Chair for Aphasia (Section II)

J. B. Orange, PhD
Professor
School of Communication Sciences and
  Disorders
Scientific Director
Canadian Centre for Activity and Aging
Western University
London, Ontario, Canada
*Topic Chair for Neurodegenerative Disorders
  (Section IV)*

Leanne Togher, PhD
Professor
Communication Disorders Following TBI
NHMRC Elizabeth Blackburn Senior
  Research Fellow
Director
Communication Sciences
School of Health Sciences
University of Sydney
Sydney, New South Wales, Australia
*Topic Chair for Cognitive Communication
  Disorders (Section III)*

Heather Harris Wright, PhD, CCC-SLP
Professor
Communication Sciences and Disorders
Associate Dean for Research

College of Allied Health Sciences and
  College of Nursing
East Carolina University
Greenville, North Carolina
Topic Chair for Typical Aging (Section I)

Contributors

Elizabeth Armstrong, PhD
Foundation Chair in Speech Pathology
School of Medical and Health Sciences
Edith Cowan University
Perth, Western Australia, Australia
Chapter 8

Sharon Ash, PhD
Research Specialist
Penn Frontotemporal Degeneration
  Center
Department of Neurology
University of Pennsylvania
Philadelphia, Pennsylvania
Chapter 16

Katharine Aveni, BA
Doctoral Student
Department of Communication Sciences
  and Disorders
Northwestern University
Evanston, Illinois
Chapter 15

Jamie H. Azios, PhD, CCC-SLP
Associate Professor
Department of Speech and Hearing Sciences
Lamar University
Beaumont, Texas
Chapter 7

Nicholas Behn, PhD
Lecturer
Division of Language and Communication
   Science
City, University of London
London, United Kingdom
Chapter 10

Lucy Bryant, PhD
Lecturer
Speech Pathology
University of Technology Sydney
Sydney, New South Wales, Australia
Chapter 5

Natalie Ciccone, PhD, CPSP
Professor and Associate Dean
School of Medical and Health Sciences
Edith Cowan University
Joondalup, Western Australia, Australia
Chapter 8

Madeline Cruice, PhD
Reader
Division of Language and Communication
   Science
City, University of London
London, United Kingdom
Chapter 6

Sarah Grace Dalton, PhD, CCC-SLP
Assistant Professor
Department of Speech Pathology and
   Audiology
Marquette University
Milwaukee, Wisconsin
Chapter 13

Lucy Dipper, PhD
Reader
Division of Language and Communication
   Science
City, University of London
London, United Kingdom
Chapter 6

Alexandra Zezinka Durfee, PhD
Postdoctoral Research Fellow
Department of Neurology
Johns Hopkins University School of
   Medicine
Baltimore, Maryland
Chapter 11

Elise Elbourn, PhD
Lecturer
Speech Pathology
School of Health Sciences
University of Sydney
Sydney, New South Wales, Australia
Chapter 9

Davida Fromm, PhD
Research Faculty
Department of Psychology
Carnegie Mellon University
Pittsburgh, Pennsylvania
Chapter 17

Jackie Guendouzi, PhD
Professor
Speech Pathology
Department of Health and Human Sciences
Southeastern Louisiana University
Hammond, Louisiana
Chapter 14

Susan Howell, PhD
Speech and Language Therapist
Clinical Research Fellow
University College London
London, United Kingdom
Chapter 10

H. Isabel Hubbard, PhD, CCC-SLP
Project Manager
Department of Speech and Hearing
   Sciences
University of New Mexico
Albuquerque, New Mexico
Chapter 13

Melissa Johnson, PhD
Associate Professor
Communication Sciences and Disorders
	Department
Nazareth College
Rochester, New York
Chapter 11

**Louise C. Keegan, PhD, CCC-SLP,
BC-ANCDS**
Associate Professor and Program Director
Speech-Language Pathology
Moravian University
Bethlehem, Pennsylvania
Chapter 10

Hana Kim, PhD
Postdoctoral Research Fellow
Department of Neurology
Johns Hopkins University School of Medicine
Baltimore, Maryland
Chapter 3

Stephen Kintz, PhD
Assistant Professor
Communication Sciences and Disorders
University of Arkansas
Little Rock, Arkansas
Chapter 3

Marion C. Leaman, PhD
Assistant Professor
Department of Hearing and Speech
University of Kansas Medical Center
Kansas City, Kansas
Chapter 4

Aviva Lerman, PhD
Adjunct Professor
Program of Communication Disorders
Hadassah Academic College
Jerusalem, Israel
Chapter 4

Tara Lewis, BSp
Senior Advisor

Aboriginal and Torres Strait Islander
	Strategy and Practice
Speech Pathology Australia
Senior Lecturer
Australian Catholic University
Brisbane, Queensland, Australia
Chapter 8

Brian MacWhinney, PhD
Professor
Department of Psychology
Carnegie Mellon University
Pittsburgh, Pennsylvania
Chapter 17

Ian Malcolm, PhD
Emeritus Professor
Applied Linguistics
Edith Cowan University
Mt. Lawley, Western Australia, Australia
Chapter 8

Andrea Marini, PhD
Associate Professor
Cognitive Science Department
University of Udine
Udine, Italy
Chapter 2

Peter A. Meulenbroek, PhD, CCC-SLP
Assistant Professor
Communication Sciences and Disorders
University of Kentucky
Lexington, Kentucky
Chapter 12

Jamila Minga, PhD, CCC-SLP
Assistant Professor
Communication Sciences
Department of Head and Neck Surgery
Department of Neurology, Stroke, and
	Vascular Neurosciences
Duke University School of Medicine
Durham, North Carolina
Chapter 11

Emma Power, PhD
Associate Professor
Speech Pathology
Allied Health and Rehabilitation Science
University of Technology Sydney
Ultimo, New South Wales, Australia
Chapter 10

Jessica D. Richardson, PhD, CCC-SLP
Associate Professor
Department of Speech and Hearing
    Sciences
University of New Mexico
Albuquerque, New Mexico
Chapter 13

Rachael Rietdijk, PhD
Postdoctoral Research Fellow
Speech Pathology
Sydney School of Health Sciences
University of Sydney
Sydney, New South Wales, Australia
Chapters 10 and 12

Angela C. Roberts, MA-SLP, PhD
Canadian Research Chair
School of Communication Sciences and
    Disorders
Department of Computer Science
Western University
London, Ontario, Canada
Chapter 15

Alice Robins, MSpPath
Speech Pathologist
Monash Medical Center
Melbourne, Victoria, Australia
Chapter 8

Sanjana Shellikeri, PhD
Postdoctoral Researcher

Penn Frontotemporal Degeneration
    Center
Department of Neurology
University of Pennsylvania
Philadelphia, Pennsylvania
Chapter 16

**Nina Simmons-Mackie, PhD, CCC-SLP,
BC-ANCDS**
Professor Emeritus
Communication Sciences and Disorders
    Department
Southeastern Louisiana University
Hammond, Louisiana
Chapter 7

Elizabeth Spencer, PhD
Senior Lecturer
Speech Pathology
School of Health Sciences
College of Health, Medicine, and Wellbeing
University of Newcastle
Callaghan, New South Wales, Australia
Chapter 9

Joanne Steel, PhD
Lecturer
Speech Pathology
School of Health Sciences
College of Health, Medicine, and Wellbeing
University of Newcastle
Callaghan, New South Wales, Australia
Chapter 9

Melissa D. Stockbridge, PhD, CCC-SLP
Research Associate
Department of Neurology
Johns Hopkins University School of
    Medicine
Baltimore, Maryland
Chapter 11

1 Discourse Analysis in Adults With and Without Communication Disorders: An Overview

Carl A. Coelho, Barbara B. Shadden, and Leora R. Cherney

Introduction and Rationale

We, the editors of this new book on discourse analysis, have been actively engaged in clinical care and research in the areas of aging, aphasia, traumatic brain injury, right hemisphere disorders, and other neurological communication disorders for more than 40 years. Together, we authored a book in 1998 entitled *Analyzing Discourse in Communicatively Impaired Adults,* otherwise known by some as the "Green Book." This book was organized around various discourse assessment approaches with only a brief annotated bibliography about discourse in different clinical populations. At the time, the literature on discourse in various clinical groups was rather limited. The book was well received and, although it has been out of print for many years, it continues to be a popular resource for clinicians and researchers interested in examining discourse in adults with acquired communication disorders.

Interest in discourse analysis has grown dramatically in recent years, as reflected by the steady increase in research publica-tions and clinical applications. For example, new resources on discourse assessment and treatment include a textbook (Kong, 2016) and two special journal issues devoted exclusively to discourse in adult populations in the journals *Topics in Language Disorders* (Fromm, 2021) and *Seminars in Speech and Language* (Richardson, 2020). Among the topics addressed were: the selection of discourse outcome measures to assess clinical change, development of new discourse measures, use of nontranscription-based discourse measures, a systematic review of discourse interventions, and prediction of cognitive impairment in acquired neurogenic disorders using discourse production.

Consistent with this trend, clinical researchers globally have begun to identify common areas of interest and needs related to the applications of discourse analysis in adult populations with acquired brain injuries. For example, one such working group is addressing "the lack of standardization in methodology, analysis, and reporting" of discourse assessment in aphasia (Stark et al., 2021, p. 4367). In other words, clinicians and researchers are not only utilizing discourse analysis to better understand the communication changes and disorders in new populations but are also striving to develop comprehensive discourse protocols with clear reporting guidelines (Stark et al., 2022). At the same time, clinicians and researchers can make use of advances in technology to facilitate the collection and analysis of discourse, resulting in richer data. With this in mind, we felt a new textbook organized around clinical populations and reviewing progress in the use of discourse analysis was timely.

The New Book

To accomplish this goal, we recruited four internationally renowned clinical researchers from the United States, Australia, and Canada, each with many years of experience using discourse analyses, to serve as topic chairs. These individuals, Drs. Heather Harris Wright, Mary Boyle, Leanne Togher, and J. B. Orange, coordinated the selection of discourse analysis topics across four population groups: (I) aging, (II) aphasia, (III) cognitive communication disorders (i.e., traumatic brain injury [TBI] and right hemisphere disorders [RHD]), and (IV) neurodegenerative diseases (i.e., primary progressive aphasia, dementia of the Alzheimer's type, Parkinson's disease, and amyotrophic lateral sclerosis). Each topic chair recruited experienced clinical researchers who are leaders in discourse research worldwide. The chapters identify the most important discourse genres, measures, and analyses for each population and illustrate their clinical value for the management of communication differences and disorders.

Definitions

In the new book, our definitions of pragmatics and discourse remain unchanged. Dis-

course is considered the most natural unit of language (Kemmerer, 2015). In our original 1998 discourse book, we defined discourse as "continuous stretches of language that convey a message" (Cherney, Shadden, & Coelho, 1998, p. 2). Discourse may be oral or written and involves both comprehension and production, with rules specific to the speaker and the listener. While the unit of discourse is typically longer than a word, in some instances, a word alone may express a message, as in aphasia. Therefore, a word may also be considered as discourse (Ulatowska, Allard, & Chapman, 1990).

There are several types of discourse, such as narrative, procedural, descriptive, persuasive, and conversational. Each serves a different function and has different characteristics. However, successful communication through any discourse genre requires complex interactions among linguistic, cognitive, and social elements that are each sensitive to even mild disruption (Cherney et al., 1998). Discourse may be considered a point of intersection between language and cognition (Ylvisaker, Szekeres, & Feeney, 2008), framed within social action and interaction (van Dijk, 1980) in which the speaker's intent and the communicative situation play a major role. As clinicians and researchers, choices must be made as to what type or genre of discourse is of interest and what specific measures are appropriate to the research question or clinical activity being targeted.

Caveats

We are aware that there is not 100% consensus across all definitions of discourse. There is a multitude of discourse analyses that may be classified in different ways. One common approach is to divide discourse behaviors and measures into microstructural, macrostructural, or superstructural levels. There is not always agreement about the components of each of these levels, and some measures may cross these structural boundaries.

Microstructural analyses involve word and sentential levels of discourse and may include word choice, syntactic complexity and diversity, semantic structure, and verbal disruptions. The microstructural level also includes linking meaning within and across sentences as measured by cohesion ties. However, because cohesive links support the complex construction of meaning in the discourse as a whole, cohesion has been described as "sitting at the intersection of micro- and macrostructure" (see Chapter 15).

Macrostructural elements relate to the broader meaning(s) of discourse. For example, macrostructural analyses can examine the central theme or the gist of discourse by rating global coherence (Wright et al., 2014) or exploring main concepts and themes. Cohesion is not the only discourse behavior that crosses structural boundaries. Various measures of informational content may overlap these boundaries between micro- and macrostructure. Information analyses may even include superstructural elements that examine the structure, schema, and/or organization of different discourse genres. Van Dijk (1980) describes superstructure as global form in contrast to macrostructure as global meaning. Examples of superstructure include story grammar for narratives and the order of essential steps in a procedure.

It should be noted that some writers refer to micro- and macrostructural analyses as *micro-* and *macrolinguistic*. Typically, the focus on *linguistic* reflects an author's theoretical background. In this book, the terms microstructure and macrosructure are used most commonly, reflecting our focus on analyzing discourse elements. We believe the terms can be used interchangeably in this context. The different perspectives of the chapter authors in this book are reflected in their respective chapters.

It is important to remember that discourse is one element within the area of pragmatics. Pragmatics has been defined as the set of rules that govern the use of language in context (Bates, 1976) or the study of the relationships between language and the contexts in which language is used (Davis, 1986). There are three aspects of the communicative situation that determine the social appropriateness of language: the extralinguistic, paralinguistic, and linguistic contexts (Cherney et al., 1998). All of these influence discourse and need to be considered. Some of the chapters in the new book focus more specifically on the linguistic context, whereas other chapters address more broadly the extralinguistic (e.g., physical or temporal setting; communication partner) and paralinguistic (e.g., intonation, pauses) components of pragmatics.

Some other considerations influenced how this book was developed. It will be immediately apparent that most of the chapters are focused on the analysis of discourse production and not discourse comprehension. We acknowledge that comprehension is a critical component of functional communication. We did not intentionally exclude any chapters on discourse comprehension. Rather, the chapters that appear in the book reflect the current research on discourse in adult populations. Future research on discourse should also target discourse comprehension. Similarly, all of the chapters report on studies of spoken discourse with little on written discourse. More insight into the written narratives of adults with and without acquired neurologic communication disorders would be useful.

The title of the book also clearly indicates that its focus is on discourse assessment and its implications for treatment, rather than directly addressing specific interventions. This focus reflects two factors.

One is the expanding research on discourse across multiple disciplines that requires us to be selective about what we can include in a text. The other is the need to understand the nature of discourse in neurotypical and disordered populations and methods to assess and analyze discourse behaviors. This is necessary before identifying the best treatments to achieve optimal functional communication outcomes.

An additional topic that is not addressed broadly in the area of discourse analysis pertains to the measurement of reliability of discourse measures. A number of discourse papers have been published without considering the reliability of the discourse measure. This is an important issue if we intend to move discourse research forward. There are two primary objectives for increasing the reliability of discourse measures. One objective is to increase replicability of findings on promising analyses across research labs. The second is to encourage clinicians to consistently use reliable discourse analyses that are recognized by external agencies (e.g., insurance companies) as meaningful functional outcomes. Whether researchers are collecting data from 50 participants or a clinician is sampling discourse of a single individual, reliability is important. Researchers and clinicians should have more comprehensive protocols for examining inter- and intrajudge reliability that should be reported in publications. Many of the chapters in this book address the reliability of the measures that they describe.

Overview of Book Chapters

The book is organized into four topic sections pertaining to adult populations: aging, aphasia, cognitive communication disorders, and neurodegenerative diseases. Each topic section consists of three or four chapters that focus on the use of discourse analysis to assess adults from each population. The book concludes with a chapter that crosses disorders and provides discourse analysis resources including TalkBank. The topic sections are summarized briefly.

Aging

This first section was coordinated by Dr. Wright, who has studied language in normal aging for many years. The chapters in this section describe how normal aging impacts cognition and language and how those, albeit subtle, changes may alter some aspects of discourse production. These findings are important for clinicians who are called upon to evaluate and treat older individuals with suspected communication disorders. Clinicians must determine whether certain communication patterns are differences or deficits, and can use discourse to help make this differentiation.

Aphasia

Dr. Boyle, who has worked as a clinician and clinical researcher in aphasia throughout her career, oversaw the four chapters in the section on aphasia. The chapters in this section discuss discourse in aphasia from a variety of perspectives, including the analyses of words, sentences, narratives, and conversation. The final chapter in this section (Chapter 8) presents a powerful argument for the consideration of cross-cultural differences when interpreting discourse performance of individuals with aphasia. Many clinicians ignore or are not prepared to factor such information into their diagnostic summaries. Cross-cultural differences should be considered when interacting with our clients and their significant others regardless of their communication disorder. Therefore, this chapter is relevant for clinicians and researchers working with all clinical populations.

Cognitive Communication Disorders

The four chapters in this section were organized by Dr. Togher, who has a long history of clinical research in TBI. Discourse analysis is an important component of any assessment battery for cognitive communication disorders secondary to acquired brain injuries. Chapters in this section address the use of discourse measures to monitor recovery in TBI and the assessment of conversation in TBI. A chapter about RHD addresses the current status of discourse management in this population. A final chapter on the use of technology for discourse analysis and telehealth is presented. This is an important topic for clinicians who may be interested in adding discourse analysis to their assessment battery but do not feel they can invest the time.

Neurodegenerative Diseases

Dr. Orange, a longtime clinical researcher in neurodegenerative diseases, facilitated the chapters for this section. The communication disorders of four distinct populations are characterized through the use of discourse analysis: primary progressive aphasia (PPA), dementia of the Alzheimer's type, Parkinson's disease (PD), and amyotrophic lateral sclerosis (ALS). The authors offer insights into each condition, including the cognitive communication disorders present in PD and ALS. The use of discourse analysis emphasizes that these two diseases are not exclusively characterized by their neuromotor symptomology.

Data Sharing

The book includes an important final chapter on TalkBank, described by the authors as "the primary discourse databases currently available for adult populations with and without spoken communication disorders" (see Chapter 17). This resource includes discourse protocols and free access to numerous video-recorded and transcribed discourse samples for researchers working in areas such as aphasia, TBI, RHD, and dementia. Training materials on discourse analysis methods are also available on Talk-Bank's website. In addition, the chapter identifies other discourse databases available to researchers and clinicians.

Companion Website

A virtual companion website that includes supplemental materials from many of the chapters is available. This website is a dynamic resource that will be regularly updated. Examples of content include specific details on elicitation tasks, numerous discourse measures, case examples with analyzed transcripts, and other related resources.

Summary

This book builds upon the foundation established decades ago in *Analyzing Discourse in Communicatively Impaired Adults*. At that time, discourse analysis was being utilized by a much smaller group of clinicians and researchers as they studied individuals with aphasia or cognitive communication disorders. Our new book demonstrates that discourse can be analyzed in hundreds of ways and is being applied to many more adult populations. For example, discourse can be used to differentiate normal aging from communication disorders and to better understand the inherent nature of many communication disorders.

While the field of discourse analysis has expanded and continues to grow, a major challenge remains. Specifically, how do we get more clinicians to begin using these assessments to increase their insight of their clients' communication disorders? A big factor in their hesitation is likely the substantial investment of time required for collecting and analyzing discourse samples. Although many clinicians appreciate the information gained from discourse analysis, they do not feel they can devote the time in a busy day to learning and using such analyses. More research focused on the development of time-saving analysis procedures is critical. A variety of such techniques are being trialed in various research centers, as mentioned in many of the chapters. Clinicians are responsible for familiarizing themselves with the nature of discourse deficits in the populations they serve and with the various approaches to discourse assessment and treatment. We hope this book assists clinicians with this learning process.

As we reflect on the 17 chapters in this new book, we are impressed with the breadth and depth of content generated by the diverse group of authors. The chapters illustrate how the study of discourse has grown. They underscore the importance of considering discourse in any clinical population and highlight promising new avenues of investigation. We are grateful to the topic chairs and chapter authors for their contributions. In particular, it is heartening that many of the authors are relatively young researchers who have interest and expertise in discourse analysis. If this trend continues, the field of discourse analysis is in good hands.

References

Bates, E. (1976). *Language in context.* Academic Press.

Cherney, L. R. (1998). Pragmatics in discourse: An introduction. In L. R. Cherney, B. B. Shadden, & C. A. Coelho (Eds.), *Analyzing discourse in communicatively impaired adults* (pp. 1–7). Aspen Publishers.

Cherney, L. R., Shadden, B. B., & Coelho, C. A. (Eds.). (1998). *Analyzing discourse in communicatively impaired adults.* Aspen Publishers.

Davis, G. A. (1986). Pragmatics and treatment. In R. Chapey (Ed.), *Language intervention strategies in adult aphasia* (2nd ed.). Williams & Wilkins.

Fromm, D. (Ed.). (2021). Advances in discourse analysis related to neurogenic disorders [Special issue]. *Topics in Language Disorders, 41*(1), 2–4. https://doi.org/10.1097/TLD.00000000 00000239

Kemmerer, D. (2015). *Cognitive neuroscience of language.* Psychology Press.

Kong, A. P. H. (2016). *Analysis of neurogenic disordered discourse production.* Routledge.

Richardson, J. D. (Ed.). (2020). Advances in discourse assessment and treatment [Special issue]. *Seminars in Speech and Language, 41*(1), 1–124. https://www.thieme-connect. de/products/ejournals/issue/10.1055/s-009- 45430

Stark, B. C., Bryant, L., Themistocleous, C., den Ouden, D-B., & Roberts, A. C. (2022). Best practice guidelines for reporting spoken discourse in aphasia and neurogenic communication disorders, *Aphasiology,* https://doi.org/ 10.1080/02687038.2022.2039372

Stark, B. C., Dutta, M., Murray, L. L., Fromm, D., Bryant, L., Harmon, T. G. . . . Roberts, A. C. (2021). Spoken discourse assessment and analysis in aphasia: An international survey of current practices. *Journal of Speech, Language, and Hearing Research, 64*(11), 4366– 4389. https://doi.org/10.1044/2021_JSLHR- 20-00708

Ulatowska, H. K., Allard, L., & Chapman, S. B. (1990). Narrative and procedural discourse in aphasia. In Y. Joanette & H. H. Brownell (Eds.), *Discourse ability and brain damage: Theoretical and empirical perspectives* (pp. 180–198). Springer-Verlag.

van Dijk, T. A. (1980). *Macrostructures: An interdisciplinary study of global structures in discourse, interaction, and cognition.* Lawrence Erlbaum Associates.

Wright, H. H., Koutsoftas, A. D., Capiloutis, G. J., & Fergadiotis, G. (2014). Global coherence in younger and older adults: Influence of cognitive processes and discourse type. *Aging, Neuropsychology and Cognition, 21*(2), 174–196. https://doi.org/10.1080/13825585 .2013.794894

Ylvisaker, M., Szekeres, S. F., & Feeney, T. (2008). Communication disorders associated with traumatic brain injury. In R. Chapey (Ed.), *Language intervention strategies in aphasia and related neurogenic communication disorders* (5th ed). Lippincott Williams & Wilkins.

SECTION I
Discourse and Typical Aging

Heather Harris Wright, Topic Chair

Introduction

Age-related changes in language and cognitive functions have been extensively researched over the past half-century, with a more recent focus on these functions and their interaction at the discourse level. As a result, the study of discourse has spanned many disciplines, including linguistics, psychology, gerontology, and communication sciences. Discourse is considered the most complex form of language and, for discourse to be successful, it requires combining units of information in a coherent manner to convey a meaningful message. Therefore, a major objective of discourse is coherence. Coherence is how units of discourse connect, make sense, or hang together (Glosser, 1993; Ulatowska & Olness, 2004).

To account for the structure of discourse and involvement of cognitive processes, several models of discourse have been developed (e.g., Chafe, 1994; Kintsch, 1998; Kintsch & van Dijk, 1978; Labov, 1972; Mandler, 1984; van Dijk, 1997). The structure of the various models is dependent on the type of information conveyed, which is often driven by a specific discourse genre of interest, such as conversation, expository, procedural, or narrative. Conversation is the exchange of information among two or more individuals. Expository discourse can take many forms, such as a discourse conveying factual and informative information or a persuasive discourse with the purpose of swaying the listener's opinion. Procedural discourse is an account of the steps involved in an activity or routine, such as making a pot of coffee or planting a flower in a garden. Narrative discourse includes a description of events unfolding over time or space and typically includes a beginning and an ending; different forms of narrative discourse can include picture descriptions, recounting personal events, and stories such as story retelling and story generation.

Models or frameworks of discourse have taken several forms, considering various components of discourse. For example, Kintsch and van Dijk's (1978) integrative discourse model considers all components of discourse from the smallest linguistic unit (i.e., phoneme) to the organization of concept units (e.g., sequence of steps for making coffee). Longacre's (1996) discourse framework is organized around the different discourse types. He classifies discourse by its underlying knowledge structure, which includes linguistic characteristics (e.g., tense markers) and how utterances connect to one another. According to Longacre, it is these underlying knowledge structures that differentiate discourse genres. Most frameworks, however, consider discourse at the structural or organization level, which is when coherence is apparent (for other models, see Chafe, 1994; Glosser, 1993; Labov, 1992).

Kintsch and van Dijk (1978) completed the seminal work in discourse, and their model serves as the foundation for much of the research in this area. They describe discourse structure as requiring four levels of representation. Unique to this model is that all discourse genres are considered. The first level (*surface*) includes traditional linguistic units such as phonemes and morphemes as well as word combinations that lead to the utterances. It is at this level where adults with aphasia often have significant difficulties. A surface-level impairment is apparent because the person has obvious difficulties retrieving words and producing language. The second level (*semantic*) represents the concepts expressed and the links between them. A *microproposition* is the smallest semantic unit and is typically a verb or preposition plus noun. A breakdown or impairment at this level results in a lack of connectedness, fragmented micropropositions, or missing or vague arguments. The third level (*situational*) encompasses the relationships among concepts that represent the situations and/or events depicted. Impairment at this level could include missing concepts, tangential productions, or an incomplete story due to missing elements. The fourth level (*structural*) is the organization of the concept units, represented as sequential and/or temporal. At this level, the structure of the discourse is identified (e.g., the schema for a story or script for a procedure). Impairments at this level could include omission of schema elements or steps within a script, and/or misordering of elements or steps.

The basis of integrative discourse models, like that of Kintsch and van Dijk, is that several cognitive operations are involved at each level of representation. Within the literature, cognitive aging is an expansive field of study that involves understanding how cognitive changes normally occur across the adult lifespan. For the chapters in this section, what is relevant is how age-related changes in cognitive function contribute to age-related changes in discourse. Understanding normal changes in discourse production is critical for determining pathological as well as exceptional changes (Burke & MacKay, 1997; Craik & Salthouse, 2007). The most common cognitive functions implicated as contributors are memory ability, such as reduced working memory capacity and reduced ability to acquire new information, and attention, specifically reduced selective attention abilities.

The Chapters in This Section

Marini's chapter (Chapter 2) starts the section with a comprehensive discussion of cognitive and linguistic characteristics of narrative discourse production in healthy aging. He begins with an overview of the microlinguistic and macrolinguistic organization of discourse production followed by the cognitive processes focused on discourse planning—specifically attention, memory, and executive functions. With an understanding of the linguistic characteristics and interaction between cognition and language processes in narrative discourse planning, Marini next explores age-related effects on cognitive skills. These age-related effects are typically evident in adults aged 70 and older, and they influence narrative discourse production in different ways. Older adults have a lifetime of experience in generating narratives, so they also may develop strategies to accommodate for age-related changes in cognitive skills. For example, the mental lexicon continues to grow with age. Yet, older individuals produce shorter and less complex utterances, possibly to accommodate for reduced attention and working memory skills. Further, age-related effects are evident in macrolinguistic skills. Older adults tend to produce more verbose and less cohesive and coherently organized narrative discourses, but as age increases, so does interindividual variability in macrolinguistic skills. Marini's chapter highlights the microlinguistic and macrolinguistic skills that decline with age, age-related changes in cognitive processes that contribute to the declines, and those skills that tend to be more age resistant until much later in life, supporting the complex interplay among age, cognition, and linguistic skills in narrative discourse production.

Kintz and Kim's chapter (Chapter 3) continues and expands the discussion of age-related changes in language function by considering the different discourse-elicitation tasks used in research and clinical settings. They begin by overviewing the different discourse genres, the general cognitive and linguistic skills each requires, and examples of elicitation tasks to generate them. Each discourse genre has been investigated in the aging population, but to varying degrees. Kintz and Kim review more commonly measured language skills, such as productive vocabulary, syntactic structure, cohesion, and coherence. They explore how age affects performance across the different types of discourse. For example, lexical diversity is a method for quantifying productive vocabulary and tends to be relatively stable across the adult life span well into the 70s; however, production of diverse vocabulary varies depending on the discourse elicitation task. Procedural discourse tasks tend to elicit the least lexically diverse samples, whereas conversations have the most diverse samples, regardless of

age. Marini noted that syntactic complexity declines with age in narrative discourse; however, this finding is not uniform across all discourse genres. Age-related changes in syntactic complexity are not consistently evident in expository or conversation discourses, and Kintz and Kim discuss factors that contribute to variable performance.

In general, cohesion and coherence decline as a function of age. Older adults tend to produce fewer cohesive ties and more cohesive errors; they have greater difficulty maintaining discourse coherence. However, inconsistencies in performance exist. For example, elicitation tasks using pictorial stimuli tend to result in more cohesion errors but better maintenance of coherence than nonpictorial discourse elicitation tasks, which result in fewer cohesive errors but greater aging effects on measures of coherence. Kintz and Kim overview the different demands of these tasks and the interplay among task demands, age, and these language processes. Chapter 3 highlights how age influences discourse performance and how its influence depends on the discourse type and task used to elicit the discourse sample.

For the final chapter (Chapter 4) in this section, Leaman and Lerman review conversation and typical aging. Conversation is the most common form of discourse used in everyday communication, and it is critical for maintaining social relationships. Conversation is also the least studied discourse genre in typical and clinical populations. The authors begin their chapter discussing factors that can influence conversation, such as partner relationship, location and purpose of the conversation, and interpersonal and cultural expectations. These factors also contribute to the heterogeneity of conversation and the challenges in studying it. Unique to the conversation genre and different from all others is the fact that other discourse genres are often embedded in conversation. However, the frequency of this has not been investigated. Leaman and Lerman overview foundational information about sensory functions, including hearing and vision, cognition, and bilingualism, that contribute to conversational interactions in older adults. In exploring language abilities in conversation, aging is associated with an increase in tip-of-tongue experiences, slower rate of speech, more dysfluencies, fillers and silent pauses, and reduced efficiency in conversation exchanges. Leaman and Lerman conclude Chapter 4 with an overview of clinical applications, including recently developed measures specific for conversation to measure efficiency and word retrieval abilities.

Conclusions

In summary, several factors that influence discourse performance in typical aging can impact clinical populations. Findings consistently demonstrate changes in discourse ability in adults over 65. These changes are critical for clinical populations as many of our patients with acquired neurogenic communication disorders (e.g., aphasia, dementia) are older. For example, older adults produce significantly less informative discourse and have more difficulty providing coherent discourse but may also produce more lexically diverse discourse compared to younger adults. Episodic memory ability significantly predicts informativeness in older adults' picture description samples, whereas memory and attention influence maintenance of global coherence. Type of discourse elicitation task, linguistic measures used, and cognitive functions may all influence performance. It is essential to understand when changes in performance are age related (e.g., fewer cohesive ties with pictorial stimuli) during evaluation of clinical populations to appropriately diagnose impairment and develop a treatment plan. Each chapter summarizes aging effects on discourse and offers insights on how to apply findings from the aging literature to clinical populations.

References

Ash, S., Moore, P., Antani, S., McCawley, G., Work, M., & Grossman, M. (2006). Trying to tell a tale: Discourse impairments in progressive aphasia and frontotemporal dementia. *Neurology, 66*(9), 1405–1413. https://doi.org/10.1212/01.wnl.0000210435.72614.38

Burke, D. M., & MacKay, D. G. (1997). Memory, language, and ageing. *Philosophical Transactions of the Royal Society of London–Series B: Biological Sciences, 352,* 1845–1856. https://doi.org/10.1098/rstb.1997.0170

Chafe, W. L. (1994). *Discourse, consciousness, and time: The flow and displacement of conscious experience in speaking and writing.* University of Chicago Press.

Craik, F. I. M., & Salthouse, T. A. (Eds.). (2007). *The handbook of aging and cognition* (3rd ed.). Psychology Press. https://doi.org/10.4324/9780203837665

Glosser, G. (1993). Discourse production patterns in neurologically impaired and aged populations. In H. H. Brownell & Y. Joanette (Eds.), *Narrative discourse in neurologically impaired and normal aging adults* (pp. 191–211). Singular Publishing.

Gordon, P. C. (1993). Computational and psychological models of discourse. In H. Brownell & Y. Joanette (Eds.), *Narrative discourse in normal aging and neurologically impaired adults* (pp. 23–46). Singular Publishing. https://doi.org/10.1093/oxfordhb/9780199772391.013.14

Jørgensen, M., & Phillips, L. (2002). *Discourse analysis as theory and method*. Sage. https://doi.org/10.4135/9781849208871

Juncos-Rabadán, O., Pereiro, A. X., & Rodríguez, M. S. (2005). Narrative speech in aging: Quantity, information content, and cohesion. *Brain and Language, 95*(3), 423–434. https://doi.org/10.1016/j.bandl.2005.04.001

Kintsch, W. (1998). *Comprehension: A paradigm for cognition*. Cambridge University Press.

Kintsch, W., & van Dijk, T. (1978). Toward a model of text comprehension and production. *Psychological Review, 85*(5), 363–394. https://doi.org/10.1037/0033-295X.85.5.363

Labov, W. (1972). *Language in the inner city: Studies in the Black English vernacular*. University of Pennsylvania Press.

Longacre, R. E. (1996). *The grammar of discourse* (2nd ed.). Plenum Press.

Mandler, J. M. (1984). *Stories, scripts, and scenes: Aspects of schema story*. Erlbaum.

Marini, A., Boewe, A., Caltagirone, C., & Carlomagno, S. (2005). Age-related differences in the production of textual descriptions. *Journal of Psycholinguistic Research, 34*(5), 439–463. https://doi.org/10.1007/s10936-005-6203-z

Mozeiko, J., Le, K., Coelho, C., Krueger, F., & Grafman, J. (2011). The relationship of story grammar and executive function following TBI. *Aphasiology, 25*(6–7) 826–835. https://doi.org/10.1080/02687038.2010.543983

Rogalski, Y., Altmann, L. P., Plummer D'Amato, P., Behrman, A. L., & Mariske, M. (2010). Discourse coherence and cognition after stroke: A dual task study. *Journal of Communication Disorders, 43*(3), 212–224. https://doi.org/10.1016/j.jcomdis.2010.02.001

Ska, B., Scherer, L. C., Flôres, O. C., Oliveira, C. R. D., Netto, T. M., & Fonseca, R. P. (2009). Theoretical, behavioral and neuroimage evidence on discourse processing aging. *Psychology and Neuroscience, 2*(2), 101–109. http://doi.org/10.3922/j.psns.2009.2.002

Ulatowska, H. K., & Olness, G. S. (2004). Discourse. In R. D. Kent (Ed.), *The MIT encyclopedia of communication disorders* (pp. 300–302). The MIT Press.

van Dijk, T. A. (Ed.). (1997). *Discourse as structure and process*. Sage.

Wright, H. H., Capilouto, G. J., Srinivasan, C., & Fergadiotis, G. (2011). Story processing ability in cognitively healthy younger and older adults. *Journal of Speech, Language, and Hearing Research, 54*(3), 900–917. https://doi.org/10.1044/1092-4388(2010/09-0253)

Wright, H. H., Koutsoftas, A., Capilouto, G. J., & Fergadiotis, G. (2014). Global coherence in younger and older adults: Influence of cognitive processes and discourse type. *Aging, Neuropsychology, and Cognition, 21*(2), 174–196. https://doi.org/10.1080/13825585.2013.794894

2 Cognitive and Linguistic Characteristics of Narrative Discourse Production in Healthy Aging

Andrea Marini

Introduction

Human communication relies on a wide range of skills. Among these, the ability to convey complex meanings through discourse is of crucial importance. For this reason, over the past 40 years, growing attention has been dedicated to the analysis of the linguistic and cognitive characteristics of both discourse processing and production (e.g., Gernsbacher, 1990; Kintsch & van Dijk, 1978). Such developments have triggered an increasing interest in the field of the neuropsychology of language, targeting how language is processed above the sentence level in daily communicative interactions in persons with healthy aging or in individuals with communicative impairments related to neurodevelopmental disorders, acquired brain lesions, or neurodegenerative diseases (e.g., Le et al., 2012).

The terms *healthy*, *typical*, and *normal* aging are often used interchangeably. Regardless of terminology, the study of discourse across the life span, along with associated cognitive and linguistic processes, is at the core of eliciting, measuring, interpreting, and managing discourse behaviors in adults with neurological challenges. Understanding the range of typical discourse behaviors allows for development of norms and discourse profiles that can differentiate typically from atypically aging adults and further distinguish the various neurological conditions that affect discourse.

This chapter focuses primarily on narrative production and aging. It outlines the characteristics of the linguistic system and provides a model of discourse production that highlights the interaction between cognition and language. The rest of the chapter addresses the issue of how changes in healthy aging affect the cognitive skills that allow for efficient discourse processing, contributing to reduced discourse production abilities.

A Sketch of the Organization of the Linguistic System

Language develops rapidly in early infancy and during childhood, reaches a quite stable level during adulthood (Marini et al., 2005), and declines gradually in the elderly (Thornton & Light, 2006). Just as linguistic development is triggered by cognitive development, linguistic decline is a consequence of the intrinsic deterioration of both linguistic systems and general cognitive abilities (Marini & Andreetta, 2016). Indeed, language processing relies on a complex interplay between linguistic skills and other cognitive abilities (including memory, attention, executive functions, and perception) and is basically organized around micro- and macrolinguistic dimensions of processing (e.g., Marini et al., 2011).

Microlinguistic processes allow for organizing phonemes into morphological sequences and words and for determining the syntactic context required by each word to generate well-formed sentences. Two core systems are engaged at this level. The first is involved in lexical processing: It allows for the identification of lexical concepts; selection of the target words in the mental lexicon; and access to their morphosyntactic, morphological, phonological, syllabic, and phonetic information (Levelt, 1989). The morphosyntactic information associated with words is then used by a second core system that allows for the computation of hierarchical structures generated by a basic recursive combinatorial operation that Chomsky (1995) labeled "Merge." For example, this cognitive operation might generate the noun phrase *the car* by merging the words [*the*] and [*car*]. This new sequence might then be merged with a verb [*watch* [*the car*]] to form a verb phrase. The recursive application of the same merging operation leads to sentence generation (Friederici et al., 2017).

During a communicative interaction, macrolinguistic processes allow for the generation/identification of a communicative intention as well as for the contextualization of meanings created through microlinguistic processes. Macrolinguistic processes include the ability to organize the propositions conveyed by sentences through cohesive and coherent ties that help generate a story's mental model (i.e., a mental construction of a narrative; Johnson-Laird, 1983) or scenario (i.e., through a process of scene construction; Buckner & Carroll, 2007).

The interplay between cognitive and linguistic skills is particularly evident when examining narrative (story) production. The cognitive-linguistic connections involved in narrative planning and production are summarized in Table 2–1 and described in the following text. Broader definitions of the core cognitive processes are available on the companion website.

Discourse Planning

Discourse production begins with the need to generate a communicative intention and a structure or mental depiction of the contents of what must be conveyed (i.e., a mental model or scenario). In a narrative, this mental model provides a foundation for developing the story structure (Gernsbacher, 1990). At all stages of discourse preparation, multiple cognitive processes are involved, including sustained attention throughout, working memory, long-term declarative memory, and executive functions (e.g., Marini et al., 2019; Mozeiko et al., 2011).

Attention is needed to keep the cognitive resources focused on discourse planning (sustained attention); avoiding distraction coming from other sources of information (selective attention); and distributing the available cognitive resources to the different stages of discourse planning, sentence conceptualization, and the subsequent stages of

Table 2–1. A Description of the Role Played by Executive Functions, Attention, Theory of Mind, Long-Term and Working Memory, and Motor Planning and Control in Different Stages of Discourse Planning and Sentence Production

Stage of Discourse Production	Cognitive Functions Involved in Discourse Production and Their Roles
Discourse planning and conceptual preparation of single sentences	Executive functions • Planning: needed to organize discourse contents and structure and to generate mental models and scenarios according to the communicative intention • Monitoring: constant control of the development of story structure and organization • Inhibitory control: inhibition of potentially irrelevant information • Updating: continuous updating of what to say next depending on what has been already communicated (depends on working memory) • Shifting: the ability to shift between strategies to select new episodes while discourse unfolds and its foundations are laid Attention • Sustained: keeping the cognitive resources focused on discourse planning • Selective: avoid distractions derived from other sources of information • Divided: distribute the available cognitive resources to phases of discourse planning, conceptual preparation, and message production Working memory • Episodic buffer: needed to host the propositions that will later be produced through the subsequent stages of message production Long-term declarative memory • Semantic: crucial to select the target scripts and access to other knowledge such as story grammar structures. It also contains the lexical concepts that will be eventually activated. • Episodic: needed to remember the events in the story to be produced and organize them Theory of Mind • Needed to calibrate what the speaker wants to convey according to the expectations and knowledge of his/her interlocutors
Lexical selection	Executive functions • Monitoring the selection process • Inhibiting the activation of wrong lexical nodes (i.e., semantic competitors such as "cat" instead of "dog") triggered via semantic priming Attention • Sustained: keeping the cognitive resources focused on the selection of the target lexical entry • Selective: avoid distractions derived from other sources of information • Divided: distribute the available cognitive resources to the lexical selection phase while planning additional computations needed for discourse and sentence generation

continues

Table 2–1. *continued*	
Stage of Discourse Production	***Cognitive Functions Involved in Discourse Production and Their Roles***
Lexical selection *continued*	Working memory • Phonological working memory: keep the lexical concept active until needed Long-term declarative memory • Semantic: repository of lexical items in the mental lexicon Long-term nondeclarative memory • Semantic priming: process not under the direct control of the speaker that raises the activation levels of semantically related words facilitating their selection
Lemma activation and grammatical processing	Executive functions • Planning: organize the sentence to be produced • Monitoring: constant control of the generation of the sentence • Inhibitory control: inhibition of potentially irrelevant information and the activation of wrong morphosyntactic information Attention • Sustained: keeping the cognitive resources focused on the construction of the target sentence • Selective: avoid distractions derived from other sources of information • Divided: distribute the available cognitive resources to phases of lexical access, articulation, and grammatical construction Working memory • Phonological working memory: keep all lexical information active until needed while generating the sentence • Episodic buffer: needed to keep track of the information already introduced in preceding sentences to establish efficient cohesion and local coherence ties among them Long-term declarative memory • Semantic: repository where the morphosyntactic information related to the selected lemma is stored Long-term nondeclarative memory • Procedural memory: needed to perform routine processes such as Merge that are not under the direct control of the speaker
Lexical access	Executive functions • Monitoring: constant control of the access procedure • Inhibitory control: inhibition of potentially irrelevant information Attention • Sustained: keeping the cognitive resources focused on the access to all morphological, syllabic, and phonetic information stored in the selected lexical entry in the mental lexicon • Selective: avoid distractions derived from other sources of information • Divided: distribute the available cognitive resources to phases of lexical access, articulation, and grammatical construction

Table 2–1. *continued*	
Stage of Discourse Production	***Cognitive Functions Involved in Discourse Production and Their Roles***
Lexical access *continued*	Working memory • Phonological working memory: necessary to keep all lexical information active until needed to produce it while generating the sentence Long-term declarative memory • Semantic: repository where morphological, syllabic, and phonetic information pertaining to the selected lexical entry are stored in the mental lexicon
Articulation	Motor planning and control • Needed to utter the selected words in the generated sentences Working memory • Phonological working memory: necessary to keep all lexical information active until needed to utter it Long-term nondeclarative memory • Procedural memory: needed to perform the routine movements of the phonetic apparatus that are not under the direct control of the speaker

its production (divided attention). Working memory is needed to keep active the propositions that will be later produced (phonological working memory). An important role in this stage is also played by long-term declarative memory (both semantic and episodic), which allows the speaker to retrieve information about how that specific discourse should be organized (e.g., its story grammar with elements such as introduction, scenario, characters, time frame, episodes [Haberlandt et al., 1980] and the relevant scripts [Schank & Abelson, 1977]).

According to Mozeiko et al. (2011), efficient discourse processing also requires executive functions: the ability to *inhibit* the production of irrelevant pieces of information such as off-topic comments and derailments, *update* incoming information with what has been previously communicated through working memory, and *shift*

between strategies to select new episodes or new informative words. Additional executive skills include the ability to *monitor* the ongoing communicative process and *plan* the efficient organization of the message. In this preliminary stage, the speaker also needs to pay attention to the interlocutors' expectations by generating a theory of their mind (Theory of Mind, or ToM) while considering both linguistic (i.e., what has already been said) and extralinguistic (e.g., information about the place and time in which the conversation takes place) context.

Conceptual Preparation and Lexical Selection

Once the story structure has been generated, the speaker must organize it in sequences that form the macrostructure of the discourse to be produced. This macrostructure will then be converted into single propositions forming the microstructure of discourse (e.g., Kintsch & van Dijk, 1978). These propositions will be generated through a process of conceptual preparation and eventually produced through stages of lexical selection, access, and articulation (e.g., Indefrey & Levelt, 2000). The stage of conceptual preparation allows for the activation in long-term semantic memory of the target lexical concept (i.e., a concept "for which there is a lexical item in the mental lexicon," Levelt, 2001, p. 13464) that best fits with the communicative intention of the speaker. The activated lexical concept triggers a process of lexical selection where the semantic information contained in the lexical concept is spread to lemmas in a component of long-term semantic memory known as the *mental lexicon* (Roelofs, 1992).

Discourse planning and conceptual preparation rely on other cognitive skills as well, as shown in Table 2–1. Pivotal are the abilities to keep the cognitive resources focused on the selection of the target lexical item (sustained attention), ignoring distracting stimuli (selective attention), and distributing the available cognitive resources among the different processes that are taking place at the same time (divided attention). It is also necessary to maintain the selected lexical concept in phonological working memory, monitor the selection process, and inhibit the activation of potential lexical competitors that, if not correctly blocked, may lead to the production of semantic errors (for example, a semantic paraphasia such as *table* instead of *chair*). The selected lexical item and all the information contained in it (i.e., semantic, morphosyntactic, morphological, phonological, and phonetic) are stored in the mental lexicon. To produce the intended sentence, it is necessary to have access to such information.

Lexical Access and Grammatical Processing

In the process of lexical access, the first available information regards its grammatical category (e.g., name, verb), gender (e.g., male or female), and the morphosyntactic valences necessary for grammatical encoding (i.e., the generation of the sentence). Overall, the selected word with such morphosyntactic information is labelled *lemma*. Once the lemma has been activated, its morphosyntactic information likely interacts with the Merge function (i.e., the aforementioned basic recursive combinatorial operation hypothesized by Chomsky, 1995) to trigger sentence generation and placement of the selected lemma in the correct position in the sentence.

Lemma activation and grammatical processing are also characterized by a complex interaction between different cognitive skills (again, see Table 2–1). In this case, executive functions are needed to plan the sentence, monitor its generation, and inhibit the potential activation of wrong morphosyntactic information. Furthermore, attention is required to keep the cognitive resources focused on the construction of the target sentence (sustained attention), avoid distraction (selective attention), and distribute the available resources to the different phases under elaboration. During the stage of sentence generation, working memory plays a double role. Phonological working memory keeps all lexical information active until needed while generating the sentence; the episodic buffer is involved in keeping track of all the information already introduced in previous sentences to establish efficient cohesion and local coherence ties among them. Both long-term declarative and nondeclarative memories are involved in such processes. Semantic memory is the repository where the morphosyntactic information related to the selected lemma is stored; procedural memory is required to perform highly automatized and routine processes such as Merge that are not under the direct control of the speaker.

Lexical Access and Articulation

Through a phase of morphological encoding, the word's morphemes become available and the activation is spread to the word's phonological code with a speed dependent on the word's frequency (stage of phonological encoding). This phonological information must then be combined into syllables (stage of syllabification), which receive a stress pattern resulting in a phonological word. Finally, a process of phonetic encoding will convert the retrieved phonemes into abstract articulatory representations (i.e., the articulatory score). Different cognitive skills such as focused, divided, and selective attention, executive functions, working memory, and long-term declarative memory play important roles during the process of lexical access.

The articulatory scores will eventually be produced during the stage of articulation. In this last stage of discourse production, motor planning and control produce the selected words in the generated sentences, working memory keeps all lexical information active until needed, and long-term nondeclarative procedural memory enables the performance of routine movements of the articulators that are not under the conscious control of the speaker.

Age-Related Effects on Cognitive Skills Required for Efficient Discourse Production

To different degrees, aging affects most of the cognitive functions required to generate a narrative discourse (Harada et al., 2013), including aspects of memory (Baghel et al., 2017). Adults aged 70 or older are usually characterized by having reduced working memory capacity and efficiency (e.g., Mattay et al., 2006), especially when task demands are high (for example, when decisions must be made among distractor and target stimuli; e.g., Sander et al., 2012). Aging also affects long-term declarative semantic and episodic memory (Rönnlund et al., 2005), whereas long-term nondeclarative memory (e.g., procedural) appears not to be significantly affected (Lezak et al., 2012).

Memory decline may be related to reduced inhibitory control, attention, and speed of information processing (Glisky, 2007). Indeed, older individuals are characterized by having slower information processing speed (Cohen et al., 2019). Consequently, they are slower to respond on cognitive tasks (e.g., Salthouse, 1996). Nonetheless, even when such slowing has been controlled in the analyses, older individuals tend to have persistent difficulties on tasks when compared with younger participants. One possibility is that such difficulties may stem from another widely observed characteristic of older individuals, their deficient inhibitory control (e.g., Hasher et al., 1999). This difficulty is likely related to their reduced efficiency in several cognitive tasks, including those assessing working memory and language processing. Inhibition plays a major role in many stages of language production, from discourse planning to lexical selection and access. Consequently, older adults frequently have reduced discourse production efficiency. Growing evidence suggests that difficulties in inhibitory control and processing speed may be associated with deficient executive control (i.e., planning and monitoring skills affect other abilities such as attention and working memory), determined by age-induced alterations in the prefrontal cortex and in dopamine levels (e.g., Gazzaley, 2012). A growing body of evidence collected over the past 20 years suggests that healthy aging affects both cognitive and affective ToM (Ruitenberg et al., 2020).

Another cognitive system that plays a relevant role in message production is attention (Drag & Bieliauskas, 2010). Several investigations have assessed age-related effects on the ability to keep the attention focused on the task at hand for a prolonged period (sustained attention) while inhibiting irrelevant stimuli (selective attention) and dividing the available cognitive resources among different tasks (divided attention). Nonetheless, the available evidence suggests a major interindividual heterogeneity, with some individuals having adequate levels of both sustained and selective attention while others support a more varied picture (e.g., Zanto & Gazzaley, 2019). Overall, it seems that the efficiency in sustained attention does not change markedly until 50 to 69 years of age (e.g., Carriere et al., 2010) but shows a significant deterioration after the age of 70 (e.g., Mani et al., 2005). Interestingly, there is evidence suggesting that older adults may have adequate performance on cognitive tasks assessing sustained attention levels at the expense of response times (Thomson & Hasher, 2017), suggesting the adoption of a strategy to cope with increasing task demands that may contribute to the reduced speech rate observed in par-

ticipants over 75 years of age in previous studies (e.g., Frau et al., 2021).

Age-Related Effects on Macrolinguistic Skills

Aging effects on macrolinguistic organization may not always be detrimental. As older adults have more experience in generating stories, they tend to have higher abilities in the construction of a text (e.g., James et al., 1998). For example, their written diaries and personal narratives may include more embedded episodes than those produced by younger individuals (e.g., Kemper, 1990). However, several investigations showed that the abilities to plan, monitor, and organize narratives decline with age (Pistono et al., 2017). Indeed, the stories produced by older persons are also generally characterized by augmented verbosity (Gold & Arbuckle, 1995) and reduced cohesive and coherent organization (see Ellis et al., 2016, for a review). Relevant changes include increased errors of cohesion and local coherence (i.e., the ability to relate the utterances through adequate linguistic and conceptual ties; Kemper et al., 1990; Nippold et al., 2014).

A gradual decrease in discourse informativeness (often defined by a lower density of words or propositions expressing content relevant to the story) is also generally reported. For example, Frau et al. (2021) have shown that healthy adults aged between 76 and 86 produced speech samples characterized by significantly more errors of local coherence than younger adults aged 20 to 40 years. Similarly, in Marini et al. (2005), the narrative speech samples produced by persons in their 70s and 80s contained more errors of both local (i.e., missing or ambiguous referents and topic shifts) and global (i.e., tangential utterances and semantically erroneous formulations) coherence than those of adults in their 20s and 30s. The absence of a significant difference between the oldest group's performance and that of the middle-aged suggests that the production of local coherence errors is a gradual side effect of aging, which is likely to have started already when people enter their 50s.

Aging also weakens global coherence (for example, the ability to semantically relate remote utterances within a given discourse). Typical errors of global coherence may include the production of utterances that are fillers, repetitions, tangential, or semantically unrelated to the gist of the story at hand. When older adults are involved in spontaneous conversation, they produce more off-topic speech than younger individuals (e.g., Wills et al., 2012). Therefore, the narrative discourse of older people is often perceived as vague and incoherent.

The narrative weaknesses observed in the elderly might not depend entirely on a linguistic disturbance *per se* (Marini & Andreetta, 2016). As shown in Table 2–1, phases of discourse planning and conceptual preparation rely on an extensive cognitive network that is particularly affected by aging (e.g., Pistono et al., 2017) and includes working memory, long-term declarative memory, attention, ToM, and executive skills such as inhibitory control. According to the *inhibition deficit hypothesis* (Hasher & Zacks, 1988), in the elderly, the ability to suppress irrelevant pieces of information and focus on the mainstream of a narrative might be weakened because of a declined ability to monitor the process of message production. This might eventually trigger the introduction of extraneous comments and derailments while generating a story.

Some studies have delineated the potential interconnections between declines in attention and augmented off-topic verbosity in narrative production tasks (Arbuckle & Gold, 1993; Trunk & Abrams, 2009). For example, Arbuckle and Gold (1993) analyzed attentional skills and off-topic verbosity in biographical recounts produced by a large sample of 196 adults aged 61 to 90. Attentional measures included a test tapping into shifting attention (i.e., Trail Making Test, or TMT; Reitan, 1992) and one measuring inhibition and perseveration (i.e., Wisconsin Card-Sorting Test, or WCST; Berg, 1948). Age had a significant impact on both attention skills and production of off-topic speech. Furthermore, the performance on the WCST predicted participants' off-topic verbosity; this finding clearly supports the inhibition deficit hypothesis.

In a second study, James et al. (1998) asked younger and older adults to recount personal events and perform a picture description task. The older group produced more off-topic speech only when producing personal narratives but not while performing the picture description task. As autobiographical recounts might trigger the activation of several irrelevant topics that a well-functioning cognitive system should inhibit in the phase of message planning, the authors considered this result as an indirect support to the inhibition deficit hypothesis. Interestingly, Wright et al. (2014) found no relationship among measures of long-term declarative episodic memory and attention and the ability to maintain global coherence in personal recounts of a group of young adults aged 20 to 39 years. However, a relationship was found in a group of older adults aged 70 to 87 years, suggesting that the influence of cognitive skills on macrolinguistic processing may differ across the life span.

Healthy aging does not affect macrolinguistic processing in all individuals in the same way. With age, the interindividual variability increases. This means that, in theory, a specific ability might be preserved in one person but weakened in another. For example, Obler et al. (1994) reported a marked increase in variability with age in narrative length. Similarly, in Marini et al. (2005), the group of participants in their late 70s to mid-80s showed a relevant intragroup variation in almost all measures assessing microlinguistic, macrolinguistic, and informative aspects of discourse production. However, this variability was significantly lower in levels of syntactic complexity, degree of global coherence, and a measure of thematic informativeness. This suggests that the abilities to organize a narrative discourse following rules of global coherence, extract the expected concepts from the story, and even build syntactically well-formed sentences (i.e., a microlinguistic skill) were consistently affected in the group of individuals in their mid-70s to early 80s.

Age-Related Effects on Microlinguistic Skills

Once the story structure has been generated and organized, the speaker needs to verbalize it through phases of lexical selection, access, and articulation as well as through grammatical processing (see model on the companion website).

Lexical Selection and Access

Several studies have shown that older people might experience word-finding difficulties (Albert et al., 2009; Connor et al., 2004). Nonetheless, a major feature of lexical knowledge is that words are stored in the mental lexicon and hosted in semantic memory. A characteristic of the mental lexicon is that it is incremental. For this reason, older adults usually have larger vocabularies than younger individuals (Thornton &

Light, 2006), at least until they enter their 80s and 90s (Lindenberger & Baltes, 1997). Nonetheless, many investigations suggest that lexical retrieval efficiency begins to weaken around the age of 50 and deteriorates significantly in people in their 70s (Connor et al., 2004; Kemper et al., 1990). Frequency of tip of the tongue (ToT) states (Segaert et al., 2018), especially for proper names, increases with aging (e.g., James, 2004). Furthermore, older individuals often achieve lower scores on tasks assessing naming and verbal fluency (e.g., MacKay et al., 2002). Nonetheless, other investigations failed to detect any age-related difference on naming tasks (e.g., Goulet et al., 1994). Different factors may account for such heterogeneity in results. Indeed, in naming tasks, a critical variable is the frequency level of the selected items to be named. In some experiments, such items might have been too easy or too difficult, leading to potential floor or ceiling effects.

Another confounding variable is the criterion according to which specific age groups have been selected, with some studies including younger participants aged 18 to 65 years and older ones from 59 to 85 years old (see also Verhaegen & Poncelet, 2012). Overall, a mild decrease in naming performance can be seen already in participants in their 50s (e.g., Connor et al., 2004), with significant declines approximately after the age of 70 (Verhaegen & Poncelet, 2012). Difficulties in lexical processing may result in increased production of semantic paraphasias, hesitations, and false starts that may reduce speech rates (Kavé & Goral, 2017).

In line with this hypothesis, on a narrative production task, semantic paraphasias (reflecting a problem in lexical section) were almost nonexistent in people aged 20 to 74 years of age but significantly increased in individuals aged from 75 onward (Marini et al., 2005). Frau et al. (2021) reported a gradual increase in the production of semantic errors in a cohort of Italian-speaking healthy adults across three age groups (young adults ranging from 20 to 40 years, older adults ranging from 65 to 75 years, and senior adults ranging from 76 to 86 years), supporting the hypothesis that the process of lexical selection is affected by the process of aging. These results are consistent with earlier works in which older participants were found slower and less accurate in retrieving appropriate nouns or definitions in tasks involving picture naming and description (e.g., Au et al., 1995).

Overall, then, studies assessing ToT states, naming skills, and lexical selection and access in healthy aging show that the ability to retrieve words from memory begins to weaken slightly after the age of 50 but significantly deteriorates only in people in their 70s onward (Marini & Andreetta, 2016). Furthermore, they suggest this pattern does not reflect a deterioration in lexical knowledge but does indicate a potential weakening in the stages of lexical selection and access (see model on the companion website), likely related to the weakening of the cognitive skills required to perform such processes. Indeed, as previously noted, these two stages of lexical production rely not only on the linguistic information stored in the mental lexicon; they also need the appropriate functioning of other cognitive skills such as sustained and selective attention, inhibitory control, and working memory that are known to be significantly affected by aging.

Alternatively, it has been proposed that age-related changes in lexical retrieval stem from weakened connections among lexical-semantic and phonological representations in the mental lexicon that might eventually lead to more lexical retrieval difficulties in the elderly (Transmission Deficit Hypothesis; e.g., Burke & Shafto, 2004). Together

with the above-mentioned cognitive difficulties, the weakening of such connections might contribute to the lexical difficulties discussed so far.

Grammatical Skills

Grammatical skills gradually decline with age (Rabaglia & Salthouse, 2011). Older individuals tend to produce sentences that are shorter and less complex than younger people's (e.g., Glosser & Deser, 1992; Kemper & Sumner, 2001; Shadden, 1997). Recent findings apparently suggest that aging does not directly affect pure grammatical skills (e.g., the Merge function). Indeed, such abilities are largely based on long-term nondeclarative procedural memory that is not affected by healthy aging. Rather, the reduced grammatical abilities observed in the elderly likely stem from a reduced efficiency in the processes of lexical selection and, most importantly, access needed to generate accurate sentences. For example, investigating the effects of aging on different processes involved in fluent sentence production in two experiments, Hardy et al. (2020) showed that aging weakens the lexical, but not the syntactic, processes involved in sentence production. Indeed, older individuals have more difficulties in lexical retrieval (for example, in the selection of appropriate function words; Heller & Dobbs, 1993) and in the generation of adequate subject-verb agreement links between words (Thornton et al., 2004). In line with this hypothesis, in Marini et al. (2005), participants who were older than 74 years of age produced narrative descriptions with more morphological errors, leading to fewer complete sentences than in younger groups of individuals aged from 20 to 60 years.

These lexical difficulties that affect grammatical processing may be at least partly related to the decline in both attention and phonological working memory, which is frequently observed in the elderly. For example, in Kemper et al. (2004), a group of participants aged 70 to 80 years produced sentences that were less complex than those generated by younger participants aged 18 to 28 years in a sentence-generation task. In this task, they were asked to produce, as fast as possible, sentences using previously memorized sentence fragments formed by three words. Interestingly, the performance of younger adults was affected by the complexity of the syntactic manipulation, whereas that of the older ones was not. This suggests that processing limitations (e.g., reduced phonological working memory skills) also might hamper the ability of older adults to retain all necessary information for further syntactic processing.

Conclusions and Future Directions

This chapter focused on the alterations induced by healthy aging on discourse production skills, also considering the effects of cognitive decline. Overall, the available evidence suggests that aging affects production in different ways. Some skills tend to be preserved, whereas others, especially if related to cognitive abilities that suffer from the aging process, are weakened by aging. The mental lexicon keeps growing with age. Therefore, lexical knowledge is incremental and older individuals tend to know more words than younger people do. Nonetheless, older people often experience word-finding difficulties that may be associated with difficulties in a range of cognitive skills involved in the process of lexical selection and/or access such as phonological working memory, inhibitory control, and attention. The available evidence also

suggests that grammatical production may be affected by aging but apparently relies more on cognitively induced lexical (e.g., morphosyntactic and morphologic) difficulties than on purely grammatical skills (e.g., on procedural processes such as those involved in Merge).

Accumulating evidence suggests that aging significantly affects the ability to correctly organize a narrative discourse in terms of local and global coherence. Narrative production in older adults appears to be not simply due to a linguistic weakening but also to a more general cognitive weakening affecting sustained and selective attention, executive functions, and working memory. Such difficulties determine a reduced ability to adequately plan a discourse, monitor what has been already said and what still needs to be communicated, and inhibit the introduction of irrelevant pieces of information. Therefore, the different stages of discourse production in older persons are constantly influenced by a general cognitive decline.

As a final remark, it is important to highlight the clinical usefulness of procedures of discourse analysis in the assessment of language production in healthy individuals as well as in patients with brain lesions (e.g., Barker et al., 2017; Bryant et al., 2016) and/or neurodegenerative diseases (e.g., Carlomagno et al., 2005). Accumulating evidence suggests that the analysis of connected speech allows both clinicians and scholars to retrieve relevant information about actual linguistic abilities at both macro- (i.e., discourse planning and organization) and microlinguistic (i.e., lexical and grammatical) levels of processing. Among other things, this analysis shows the potential relations between these two levels of linguistic processing and the effects of other cognitive skills. For example, Marini et al. (2008) showed that, in a group of participants with schizophrenia, the difficulty observed in the ability to generate coherent samples of narrative discourse was affected by their executive impairments, which triggered the production of semantic and morphological errors. This finding supports the hypothesis of a significant interrelation between these levels of language processing. The clinical usefulness of procedures for the analysis of connected speech has been further confirmed in a recent investigation by Mazzon et al. (2019). In their study, measures of micro- and macrolinguistic processing derived from a multilevel procedure for discourse analysis discriminated older participants with a diagnosis of mild cognitive impairment who were developing Alzheimer's disease from those who did not have dementia.

In conclusion, the available evidence supports the idea that discourse production is the result of a complex interplay between linguistic and cognitive skills whose integrity is, for the most part, affected by aging. A critical issue concerns the notable interindividual variability that characterizes the deterioration of discourse production skills. Such variability likely depends on both genetic and environmental factors such as the level of formal education and/or socioeconomic status of the individual (e.g., Juncos-Rabadán, 1996). Further investigations are needed to deepen our understanding of the cognitive and neural underpinnings of interindividual differences in discourse production in the elderly.

References

Albert, M. L., Spiro, A., Sayers, K. J., Cohen, J. A., Brady, C. B., Goral, M., & Obler, L. K. (2009). Effects of health status on word finding in aging. *Journal of the American Geriatrics Society, 57*(12), 2300–2305. https://doi.org/10.1111/j.1532-5415.2009.02559.x

Arbuckle, T. Y., & Gold, D. P. (1993). Aging, inhibition, and verbosity. *Journal of Gerontology, 48*(5), 225–232. https://doi.org/10.1093/geronj/48.5.p225

Au, R., Joung, P., Nicholas, M., Obler, L. K., Kass, R., & Albert, M. L. (1995). Naming ability across the adult life span. *Aging, Neuropsychology, and Cognition, 2*(4), 300–311. https://doi.org/10.1080/13825589508256605

Baghel, M. S., Singh, P., Srivas, S., & Thakur, M. K. (2017). Cognitive changes with aging. *The Proceedings of the National Academy of Sciences, India, Section B: Biological Sciences, 89*(3), 1–9. https://doi.org/10.1007/s40011-017-0906-4

Barker, M. S., Young, B., & Robinson, G. A. (2017). Cohesive and coherent connected speech deficits in mild stroke. *Brain and Language, 168*, 23–36. https://doi.org.10.1016/j.bandl.2017.01.004

Berg, E. A. (1948). A simple objective technique for measuring flexibility in thinking. *Journal of General Psychology, 39*(1), 15–22. https://doi.org/10.1080/00221309.1948.9918159

Bryant, L., Ferguson, A., & Spencer, E. (2016). Linguistic analysis of discourse in aphasia: A review of the literature. *Clinical Linguistics and Phonetics, 30*(7), 489–518. https://doi.org/10.3109/02699206.2016.1145740

Buckner, R. L., & Carroll, D. C. (2007). Self-projection and the brain. *Trends in Cognitive Sciences, 11*(2), 49–57. https://doi.org/10.1016/j.tics.2006.11.004

Burke, D. M., & Shafto, M. A. (2004). Aging and language production. *Current Directions in Psychological Science, 13*(1), 21–24. https://doi.org/10.1111/j.0963-7214.2004.01301006.x

Carlomagno, S., Santoro, A., Menditti, A., Pandolfi, M., & Marini, A. (2005). Referential communication in Alzheimer's type dementia. *Cortex, 41*(4), 520–534. https://doi.org/10.1016/s0010-9452(08)70192-8

Carriere, J. S., Cheyne, J. A., Solman, G. J., & Smilek, D. (2010). Age trends for failures of sustained attention. *Psychology and Aging, 25*(3), 569–574. https://doi.org/10.1037/a0019363

Chomsky, N. (1995). *The minimalist program.* MIT Press.

Cohen, R., Masiske, M. M., & Smith, G. E. (2019). Neuropsychology of aging. In S. T. DeKosky & S. Asthana (Eds.), *Handbook of Clinical Neurology–Geriatric Neurology* (pp. 149–180). Elsevier.

Connor, L. T., Spiro, A., Obler, L. K., & Albert, M. L. (2004). Change in object naming ability during adulthood. *The Journals of Gerontology, Series B: Psychological Sciences, 59*(5), 203–209. https://doi.org/10.1093/geronb/59.5.p203

Drag, L. L., & Bieliauskas, L. A. (2010). Contemporary review 2009: Cognitive aging. *Journal of Geriatric Psychiatry and Neurology, 23*(2), 75–93. https://doi.org/10.1177/0891988709358590

Ellis, C., Henderson, A., Wright, H. H., & Rogalski, Y. (2016). Global coherence during discourse production in adults: A review of the literature. *International Journal of Language and Communication Disorders, 51*(4), 359–367. https://doi.org/10.1111/1460-6984.12213

Frau, F., Hilviu, D., Parola, A., Gabbatore, I., Bosco, F. M., & Marini, A. (2021, July 8–9). *Stability and decline of narrative abilities in healthy ageing* [Paper presentation]. 4th Experimental Pragmatics in Italy Conference–XPRAG.it 2020(21) [Virtual meeting]. https://doi.org/10.17605/OSF.IO/B4RFZ

Friederici, A., Chomsky, N., Berwick, R. C., Moro, A., & Bolhuis, J. J. (2017). Language, mind and brain. *Nature Human Behaviour, 1*(10), 713–722. https://doi.org/10.1038/s41562-017-0184-4

Gazzaley, A. (2012). Top-down modulation deficit in the aging brain: An emerging theory of cognitive aging. In D. T. Stuss & R. T. Knight (Eds.), *Principles of frontal lobe function* (pp. 593–608). Oxford University Press.

Gernsbacher, M. A. (1990). *Language comprehension as structure building.* Erlbaum.

Glisky, E. L. (2007). Changes in cognitive function in human brain aging models, methods, mechanisms. In D. R. Riddle (Ed.), *Brain aging: Models, methods, and mechanisms* (pp. 1–19). CRC Press.

Glosser, G., & Deser, T. (1992). A comparison of changes in macrolinguistic and microlinguistic aspects of discourse production in normal aging. *Journal of Gerontology, 47*(4), 266–272. https://doi.org/10.1093/geronj/47.4.p266

Gold, D. P., & Arbuckle, T. Y. (1995). A longitudinal study of off-target verbosity. *Journal of Gerontology: Psychological Sciences B, 50*(6), 307–315. https://doi.org/10.1093/geronb/50b.6.p307

Goulet, P., Ska, B., & Kahn, H. J. (1994). Is there a decline in picture naming with advancing age? *Journal of Speech and Hearing Research, 37*(3), 629–644. https://doi.org/10.1044/jshr.3703.629

Haberlandt, K., Berian, C., & Sandson, J. (1980). The episodic schema in story processing. *Journal of Verbal Learning and Verbal Behavior, 19*(6), 635–650. https://doi.org/10.1016/S0022-5371(80)90331-X

Harada, C. N., Love, M. C. N., & Triebel, K. L. (2013). Normal cognitive aging. *Clinics in Geriatric Medicine, 29*(4), 737–752. https://doi.org/10.1016/j.cger.2013.07.002

Hardy, S. M., Segaert, K., & Wheeldon, L. (2020). Healthy aging and sentence production: Disrupted lexical access in the context of intact syntactic planning. *Frontiers in Psychology, 11,* 257. https://doi.org/10.3389/fpsyg.2020.00257

Hasher, L., & Zacks, R. T. (1988). Working memory, comprehension, and aging: A review and a new view. *Psychology of Learning and Motivation, 22,* 193–225. https://doi.org/10.1016/S0079-7421(08)60041-9

Hasher L., Zacks, R. T., & May, C. P. (1999). Inhibitory control, circadian arousal and age. In D. Gopher & A. Koriat (Eds.), *Attention and performance. Cognitive regulation of performance: Interaction of theory and application* (pp. 653–675). MIT Press.

Heller, R. B., & Dobbs, A. R. (1993). Age differences in word finding in discourse and non-discourse situations. *Psychology and Aging, 8*(3), 443–450. https://doi.org/10.1037/0882-7974.8.3.443

Indefrey, P., & Levelt, W. J. M. (2000). The neural correlates of language production. In M. S.

Gazzaniga (Ed.), *The new cognitive neurosciences* (pp. 845–865). MIT Press.

James, L. E. (2004). Meeting Mr. Farmer versus meeting a farmer: Specific effects of aging on learning proper names. *Psychology and Aging, 19*(3), 515–522. https://doi.org/10.1037/0882-7974.19.3.515

James, L. E., Burke, D. M., Austin, A., & Hulme, E. (1998). Production and perception of "verbosity" in younger and older adults. *Psychology and Aging, 13*(3), 355–367. https://doi.org/10.1037//0882-7974.13.3.355

Johnson-Laird, P. N. (1983). *Mental models.* Cambridge University Press.

Juncos-Rabadán, O. (1996). Narrative speech in the elderly: Effects of age and education on telling stories. *International Journal of Behavioral Development, 19*(3), 669–685. https://doi.org/10.1080/016502596385758

Kavé, G., & Goral, M. (2017). Do age-related word retrieval difficulties appear (or disappear) in connected speech? *Neuropsychology, Development, and Cognition. Section B, Aging, Neuropsychology and Cognition, 24*(5), 508–527. https://doi.org/10.1080/13825585.2016.1226249

Kemper, S. (1990). Adults' diaries: Changes made to written narratives across the life span. *Discourse Processes, 13*(2), 207–223. https://doi.org/10.1080/01638539009544754

Kemper, S., Herman, R. E., & Liu, C.-J. (2004). Sentence production by young and older adults in controlled contexts. *The Journals of Gerontology Series B: Psychological Sciences and Social Sciences, 59*(5), 220–224. https://doi.org/10.1093/geronb/59.5.P220

Kemper, S., Rash, S., Kynette, D., & Norman, S. (1990). Telling stories: The structure of adults' narratives. *European Journal of Cognitive Psychology, 2*(3), 205–228. https://doi.org/10.1080/09541449008406205

Kemper, S., & Sumner, A. (2001). The structure of verbal abilities in young and older adults. *Psychology and Aging, 16*(2), 312–322. https://doi.org/10.1037/0882-7974.16.2.312

Kintsch, W., & van Dijk, T. (1978). Toward a model of text comprehension and production. *Psychological Review, 85*(5), 363–394. https://doi.org/10.1037/0033-295X.85.5.363

Le, K., Coelho, C. A., Mozeiko, J., Krueger, F., & Grafman, J. (2012). Predicting story goodness performance from cognitive measures following traumatic brain injury. *American Journal of Speech-Language Pathology, 21*(2), S115–S125. https://doi.org/10.1044/1058-0360(2012/11-0114)

Levelt, W. J. M. (1989). *Speaking: From intention to articulation.* MIT Press.

Levelt, W. J. M. (2001). Spoken word production: A theory of lexical access. *Proceedings of the National Academy of Sciences, 98*(23), 13464–13471. https://doi.org/10.1073/pnas.231459498

Lezak, M. D., Howieson, D. B., Bigler, E. D., & Tranel, D. (2012). *Neuropsychological assessment* (5th ed.). Oxford University Press.

Lindenberger, U., & Baltes, P. B. (1997). Intellectual functioning in old and very old age: Cross-sectional results from the Berlin Aging Study. *Psychology and Aging, 12*(3), 410–432. https://doi.org/10.1037//0882-7974.12.3.410

MacKay, A., Connor, L. T., Albert, M. L., & Obler, L. K. (2002). Noun and verb retrieval in healthy aging. *Journal of the International Neuropsychological Society, 8*(1), 764–770. https://doi.org/10.1017/s1355617702860040

Mani, T. M., Bedwell, J. S., & Miller, L. S. (2005). Age-related decrements in performance on a brief continuous performance test. *Archives of Clinical Neuropsychology, 2*(5), 575–586. https://doi.org/10.1016/j.acn.2004.12.008

Marini, A., & Andreetta, S. (2016). Age-related effects on language production: A combined psycholinguistic and neurolinguistic perspective. In H. H. Wright (Ed.), *Cognition, language and aging* (pp. 55–79). John Benjamins Publishing Company.

Marini, A., Andreetta, S., del Tin, S., & Carlomagno, S. (2011). A multilevel approach to the analysis of narrative language in aphasia. *Aphasiology, 25*(11), 1372–1392. https://doi.org/10.1080/02687038.2011.584690

Marini, A., Boewe, A., Caltagirone, C., & Carlomagno, S. (2005). Age-related differences in the production of textual descriptions. *Journal of Psycholinguistic Research, 34*(5), 439–

463. https://doi.org/10.1007/s10936-005-6203-z

Marini, A., Ferretti, F., Chiera, A., Magni, R., Adornetti, I., Nicchiarelli, S., . . . Valeri, G. (2019). Episodic future thinking and narrative discourse generation in children with autism spectrum disorders. *Journal of Neurolinguistics*, *49*, 178–188. https://doi.org/10.1016/j.jneuroling.2018.07.003

Marini, A., Spoletini, I., Rubino, I. A., Ciuffa, M., Banfi, G., Siracusano, A., . . . Spalletta, G. (2008). The language of schizophrenia: An analysis of micro- and macrolinguistic abilities and their neuropsychological correlates. *Schizophrenia Research*, *105*(1–3), 144–155. https://doi.org/10.1016/j.schres.2008.07.011

Mattay, V. S., Fera, F., Tessitore, A., Hariri, A. R., Berman, K. F., Das, S., . . . Weinberger, D. R. (2006). Neurophysiological correlates of age-related changes in working memory capacity. *Neuroscience Letters*, *39*(1–2), 32–37. https://doi.org/10.1016/j.neulet.2005.09.025

Mazzon, G., Ajčević, M., Cattaruzza, T., Menichelli, A., Guerriero, M., Capitanio, S., . . . Marini, A. (2019). Connected speech deficit as an early hallmark of CSF-defined Alzheimer's disease and correlation with cerebral hypoperfusion pattern. *Current Alzheimer Research*, *16*(6), 1–12. https://doi.org/10.2174/1567205016666190506141733

Mozeiko, J., Le, K., Coelho, C., Krueger, F., & Grafman, J. (2011). The relationship of story grammar and executive function following TBI. *Aphasiology*, *25*, 826–835. https://doi.org/10.1080/02687038.2010.543983

Nippold, M. A., Cramon, P. M., & Hayward-Mayhew, C. (2014). Spoken language production in adults: Examining age-related differences in syntactic complexity. *Clinical Linguistics and Phonetics*, *28*(3), 195–207. https://doi.org/10.3109/02699206.2013.841292

Obler, L. K., Au, R., Kugler, J., Melvold, J., Tocco, M., & Albert, M. L. (1994). Intersubject variability in adult normal discourse. In R. L. Bloom, L. K. Obler, S. D. Santi, & J. S. Ehrlich (Eds.), *Discourse analysis and applications. Studies in adult clinical population* (pp. 15–27). Lawrence Erlbaum Associates.

Pistono, A., Pariente, J., Bézy, C., Pastor, J., Tran, T. M., Renard, A., . . . Jucla, M. (2017). Inter-individual variability in discourse informativeness in elderly populations. *Clinical Linguistics and Phonetics*, *31*(5), 391–408. https://doi.org/10.1080/02699206.2016.1277390

Rabaglia, C. D., & Salthouse, T. A. (2011). Natural and constrained language production as a function of age and cognitive abilities. *Language and Cognitive Processes*, *26*(10), 1505–1531. https://doi.org/10.1080/01690965.2010.507489

Reitan, R. M. (1992). *Trail making test*. Reitan Neuropsychology Laboratory.

Roelofs, A. (1992). A spreading activation theory of lemma retrieval in speaking. *Cognition*, *42*(1–3), 107–142. https://doi.org/10.1016/0010-0277(92)90041-F

Rönnlund, M., Nyberg, L., Bäckman, L., & Nilsson, L. G. (2005). Stability, growth, and decline in adult life span development of declarative memory: Cross-sectional and longitudinal data from a population-based study. *Psychology and Aging*, *20*(1), 3–18. https://doi.org/10.1037/0882-7974.20.1.3

Ruitenberg, M. F. L., Santens, P., & Notebaert, W. (2020). Cognitive and affective theory of mind in healthy aging. *Experimental Aging Research*, *46*(5), 382–395. https://doi.org/10.1080/0361073X.2020.1802980

Salthouse, T. A. (1996). The processing-speed theory of adult age differences in cognition. *Psychological Review*, *103*(3), 403–428. https://doi.org/10.1037/0033-295x.103.3.403

Sander, M. C., Werkle-Bergner, M., & Lindenberger, U. (2012). Amplitude modulations and intertrial phase stability of alpha-oscillations differentially reflect working memory constraints across the life span. *Neuroimage*, *59*(1), 646–654. https://doi.org/10.1016/j.neuroimage.2011.06.092

Schank, R. C., & Abelson, R. P. (1977). *Scripts, plans, goals and understanding: An inquiry into human knowledge structures*. Lawrence Erlbaum Associates.

Segaert, K., Lucas, S. J. E., Burley, C. V., Segaert, P., Milner, A. E., Ryan, M., & Wheeldon, L. (2018). Higher physical fitness levels are associated with less language decline in healthy ageing. *Scientific Reports, 8,* 6715. https://doi.org/10.1038/s41598-018-24972-1

Shadden, B. (1997). Discourse behaviors in older adults. *Seminar in Speech and Language, 18*(2), 156–147. https://doi.org/10.1055/s-2008-1064069

Thomson, D. R., & Hasher, L. (2017). On the preservation of vigilant attention to semantic information in healthy aging. *Experimental Brain Research, 235*(7), 2287–2300. https://doi.org/10.1007/s00221-017-4969-5

Thornton, R., & Light, L. L. (2006). Language comprehension and production in normal aging. In J. E. Birren & K. W. Schaie (Eds.), *Handbook of the psychology of aging* (pp. 261–287). Academic Press.

Thornton, R., Skovbroten, K., & Burke, D. M. (2004, November 18–21). *Grammatical agreement processes in young and older adults* [Paper presentation]. Psychonomic Society 45th Annual Meeting, Minneapolis, MN.

Trunk, D. L., & Abrams, L. (2009). Do younger and older adults' communicative goals influence off-topic speech in autobiographical narratives? *Psychology and Aging, 24*(2), 324–337. https://doi.org/10.1037/a0015259

Verhaegen, C., & Poncelet, M. (2012). Changes in naming and semantic abilities with aging from 50 to 90 years. *Journal of the International Neuropsychological Society, 19*(2), 119–126. https://doi.org/10.1017/S1355617712001178

Wills, C. L., Capilouto, G. J., & Wright, H. H. (2012). Attention and off-topic speech in the recounts of middle-age and elderly adults: A pilot investigation. *Contemporary Issues in Communication Sciences and Disorders, 39,* 105–112. PMCID: PMC3571724

Wright, H. H., Koutsoftas, A. D., Capilouto, G. J., & Fergadiotis, G. (2014). Global coherence in younger and older adults: Influence of cognitive processes and discourse type. *Aging, Neuropsychology, and Cognition: A Journal on Normal and Dysfunctional Development, 21*(2), 1–23. https://doi.org/10.1080/13825585.2013.794894

Zanto, T. P., & Gazzaley, A. (2019). Aging of the frontal lobe. In M. D'Esposito & J. H. Grafman (Eds.), *Handbook of clinical neurology-The frontal lobes* (p. 369–384). Elsevier.

3 Discourse Processing in Older Adults: Considering Discourse Elicitation Tasks

Stephen Kintz and Hana Kim

Introduction

Aging impacts communication. Healthy older adults often complain of difficulty in remembering names and words. These complaints illuminate one manifestation of how language changes as people age, yet there is substantial evidence for age-related changes to language abilities, particularly discourse (Wright, 2016). For example, older adults often produce discourse that is less coherent (Wright et al., 2014) but more lexically diverse (Fergadiotis et al., 2011). Discourse is of particular interest to aging and language researchers because (a) it more closely mimics real-life communication activities compared to other measures of language, and (b) it is the most comprehensive method for studying the different facets of language and how these facets interact with other cognitive systems.

Discourse is defined as any language produced beyond a single sentence or utterance with the purpose of communicating information (Gee & Hartford, 2012), and it is composed of many different forms of language, including conversations, descriptions, instructions, monologues/speeches,

and narratives. Successful discourse requires a complex interaction between a speaker's language abilities (e.g., phonology, semantics, syntax) and their other cognitive domains, such as attention and memory (see Chapter 2). One important consideration for discourse analysis is discourse genre or type. Different genres and types of discourse impose different cognitive, structural, and linguistic demands, which may influence the quality of language samples (Marini et al., 2005; McCabe & Bliss, 2006; Nicholas & Brookshire, 1993; Van Leer & Turkstra, 1999). For example, recounts require a speaker to recall past actions and events that unfold spatially and temporally (Capilouto et al., 2006). These tasks rely on access to long-term memories. Procedural discourse requires the speaker to describe steps or provide instructions on how to do some task (Ulatowska et al., 1983). For these tasks, speakers must retrieve, plan, and organize information, which may rely on executive systems of organization and planning (Snow et al., 1997). Discourse analysis is further complicated by the specific tasks employed by clinicians and researchers (Olness, 2006; Wright & Capilouto, 2009). For example, single-picture description tasks require speakers to describe a picture. Yet if speakers are not prompted to produce a narrative with a beginning, middle, and end, they often only list the actions and items in the picture (Olness, 2006).

Specific discourse tasks can affect the quality and quantity of a speaker's discourse sample. Discourse genres, types, and tasks are also affected by age. While age affects discourse abilities (Wright, 2016), the research is generally mixed on whether specific abilities decline, remain stable, or even increase with age. Much of this variance may be explained by the different cognitive and linguistic demands of different discourse tasks. It is critical to understand how discourse tasks impact language samples to distinguish whether a speaker's performance is due to age or disorder. Therefore, the purpose of this chapter is to highlight how different discourse tasks impact specific language abilities that change as a function of age.

The chapter will first consider the different genres and types of discourse used, along with the different tasks employed, in collecting language samples for aging research. Next, the chapter will investigate how lexical diversity, syntactic complexity, cohesion, and coherence change across the life span with a focus on the specific discourse tasks that generate variance.

Discourse Genre and Type

There are several different genres of discourse: conversation, expository, narrative, and procedural (Table 3–1). Conversational discourse is a dialogue where speakers and listeners exchange information in a cooperative manner. It requires a variety of skills, such as topic maintenance, turn taking, appropriate referencing, and sensitivity to the conversational partner's ability and knowledge (Coelho et al., 2003). Yet some

Table 3–1. Discourse Genres and Types

	Definitions
Conversation	Discourse between two or more speakers
Expository	Discourse used to describe events, facts, or opinions
Informative	Expository discourse used to describe facts or opinions
Persuasive	Expository discourse used to describe facts or opinion with the intent to persuade
Narrative	Monologue with spatial or temporal organization
Single Picture	Narratives using single pictures
Sequential Picture	Narratives using sequential pictures
Recounts	Narratives using past events
Storytelling	Narratives using prompts or pictures to elicit stories
Story Retelling	Narratives told and retold by the speaker

of the linguistic and cognitive demands may be supported or offloaded onto a speaker's conversational partner (Moscoso del Prado Martín, 2017). While conversational discourse may be the most often used form of discourse in the real world, it is the least studied discourse genre in the aging literature, and it will only be briefly considered in this chapter (see Chapter 4 for more information on aging and conversation).

Expository Discourse

Expository discourse is when a speaker conveys factual or interpretative information about a topic (Bliss, 2002). Examples of expository task probes are provided in Box 3–1.

BOX 3–1. Examples of Expository Task Probes

Tell us about your work.

Tell us about your family.

Do you agree or disagree with homeschool?

Should healthcare be a right or privilege?

Who was the greatest president?

What do you like most about living here?

What was the most significant invention of the 20th century?

Expository discourse is often composed of concepts, explanations, and comments on cause and effect (Longacre, 1996). Due to the factual and opinionated structure of expository discourse, it may require more complex linguistic structures and a specific lexicon to successfully execute compared to the other forms of discourse (Nippold et al., 2014). Expository discourse can be further subdivided into two specific discourse types: informative and persuasive. Informative discourse simply requires describing facts or opinions. Persuasive discourse requires describing facts and opinions, but it has the added difficulty of requiring the speaker to consider the opinions and mindset of the listener to persuade. Expository discourse research is not used very often with typical older adults.

Narrative Discourse

Narrative discourse is a monologue where the speaker conveys actions and events that unfold spatially and temporally (Capilouto et al., 2006; see Chapter 2). Narratives are the most utilized discourse genre in aging research. Narrative discourse can be further subdivided into single-picture descriptions, sequential-picture descriptions, recounts, storytelling, and story retelling. The most common single pictures include "Picnic Scene" from the *Western Aphasia Battery* (Kertesz, 1982) and "Cookie Theft" from the *Boston Diagnostic Aphasia Examination* (Goodglass et al., 2001). Sequential pictures may include comic strips or wordless picture books, such as *Cinderella* (Grimes, 1993) or *Good Dog Carl* (Day, 1986). Sequential pictures may support the temporal and spatial sequencing of events more so than the static single picture (Babaei et al., 2019). Recounts require speakers to recall past events from their life (see probes in Box 3–2). Storytelling requires speakers to tell a story. This may be in the form of a parable, such as "The Boy Who Cried Wolf." Story retelling requires speakers to hear and then retell a story.

BOX 3–2. Examples of Recount Task Probes

What was your favorite vacation?

What was your favorite holiday?

What did you do last weekend?

Tell us about a past injury.

Procedural Discourse

Procedural discourse requires a speaker to describe or provide instructions on how to complete a task (see Box 3–3 for examples of procedural task probes). It is hierarchically organized into the different steps, substeps, target steps, optional steps, and alternative steps (Ulatowska et al., 1983). Procedural discourse requires speakers to retrieve, plan, and sequentially organize information. This may be particularly difficult if the procedure is complex or unknown (Snow et al., 1997).

BOX 3–3. Examples of Procedural Task Probes

How do you mail a letter?

How do you make a peanut butter and jelly sandwich?

How do you plant a flower?

How do you shop for groceries/clothing?

Discourse Measures and Analyses

Lexical Diversity

Lexical diversity (LD) is defined as the range of vocabulary items used by a speaker within a specific context (Fergadiotis et al., 2011). It reflects a speaker's crystalized lexical knowledge (i.e., vocabulary) and the semantic/executive retrieval processes used to access words. There are a variety of methods for estimating LD, but many of the most common estimates, such as the number of different words (NDW) and type-token ratio (TTR), are influenced by not only discourse type but also sample length. More robust measures exist, including the measure D, which accounts for samples of different lengths, moving-average type-token ratio (MATTR), and measures of textual lexical diversity (MTLD; Fergadiotis et al., 2013; Kintz et al., 2016; Table 3–2).

For healthy aging, there is general agreement that LD remains stable or increases across the life span (Boucher et al., 2019; Capilouto et al., 2016; Cooper, 1990; Dennis & Hess, 2016; Fergadiotis et al., 2011; Glosser & Deser, 1992; James et al., 1998; Juncos-Rabadán et al., 2005; Kavé et al., 2009; Kemper et al., 2010; Kynette & Kemper, 1986; Ostrand & Gunstad, 2020; Rabaglia & Salthouse, 2011; Wright & Capilouto, 2009). Similarly, single-item vocabulary tests show an expanding vocabulary until an individual is in their 60s or 70s (Albert et al., 1988; Feyereisen, 1997). The majority of these studies investigating LD and aging have utilized narrative tasks (Capilouto et al., 2016; Cooper, 1990; Dennis & Hess, 2016; Fergadiotis et al., 2011; James et al., 1998; Juncos-Rabadán et al., 2005; Kavé et al., 2009; Kynette & Kemper, 1986; Rabaglia

Measure	Calculation
Table 3–2. Different Measures of Lexical Diversity	
NDW[1]	The number of different words (types)
TTR[2]	The number of different words (types) divided by total number of words (tokens)
VocD[3]	Program takes 100 random samples of 35 tokens and calculates TTR. This is repeated for a 36-token sample to 50-token sample. The program uses this to produce a TTR curve. The D coefficient is then used to produce a theoretical curve that fits the empirical data. This procedure is done three times, and the Ds are averaged together.
MATTR[4]	Program calculates TTR for successive nonoverlapping segments of predetermined size. So the program takes a TTR for words 1 to 10, 2 to 11, 3 to 12, etc. This continues until the end of the sample. These TTRs are averaged together.
MTLD[5]	Program calculates TTR for increasingly longer token samples until TTR drops below a threshold, a factor count is increased by 1, and the TTR evaluations are reset. The program resumes from where it stopped. This is repeated until all tokens are part of a TTR estimate. Next, the total words (tokens) are divided by the factor count. This is done forwards and backwards. Both these numbers are averaged together.

Notes: [1]Number of Different Words; [2]Type–Token Ratio; [3] Vocabulary Diversity; [4]Moving Average Type–Token Ratio; [5]Measure of Textual Lexical Diversity (Note: D refers to analyses that address issues of samples of unequal lengths [Wright, 2003]). See also Chapter 5, Box 5–1.

& Salthouse, 2011; Wright & Capilouto, 2009), though there are a handful of studies examining procedural (Fergadiotis et al., 2011) and expository tasks as well (Glosser & Deser, 1992; Kemper et al., 2010; Ostrand & Gunstad, 2020). When examining the LD scores of the most commonly used discourse tasks across all age groups, procedural tasks have the least diverse vocabulary, whereas conversations have the most diverse vocabulary (Table 3–3). It is theorized that the supportive role of the conversational partners may ease processing loads, which in turn could free up resources to access a wider range of vocabulary items (Moscoso del Prado Martín, 2017).

Whether LD is stable or increases as a function of age depends on whether the discourse task utilizes pictorial or nonpictorial stimuli. Boucher et al. (2019) used the "Picnic Scene" and "Cookie Theft" pictures to elicit discourse from younger and older adults. They did not find a significant difference between younger and older adults in TTR or D. They did find that older adults produced words with lower frequencies and interpreted this as evidence of older adults possessing a larger vocabulary that was not fully utilized in the picture description task. Their results agree with other researchers who used single-picture line drawings (Cooper, 1990; Fergadiotis et al., 2011; James et al., 1998; Kavé et al., 2009) or historical paintings (James et al., 1998).

Fergadiotis et al. (2011) investigated the influence of different elicitation tasks on

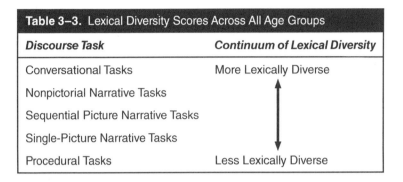

Table 3–3. Lexical Diversity Scores Across All Age Groups

Discourse Task	Continuum of Lexical Diversity
Conversational Tasks	More Lexically Diverse
Nonpictorial Narrative Tasks	
Sequential Picture Narrative Tasks	
Single-Picture Narrative Tasks	
Procedural Tasks	Less Lexically Diverse

LD in 43 younger and 43 older adults using *D* as an estimate of LD. Language samples were collected using four discourse tasks: single-picture descriptions, sequential-picture descriptions from wordless picture books, recounts, and procedural discourse. The researchers found that older adults produced higher LD only for the recounts and procedural discourse. There was no difference between the groups for single or sequential pictures. These results are consistent with other studies (Capilouto et al., 2016; James et al., 1998).

Taken together, findings indicate that pictorial stimuli may result in similar LD scores between age groups, though not all studies agree (Kynette & Kemper, 1986). It is possible that the stimuli provide a common pool of lexical items between the younger and older adults. Nonpictorial stimuli do not provide a common pool of lexical items and may allow older adults to use a more archaic but familiar vocabulary. Wright et al. (2014) argued that older adults' ability to suppress irrelevant information declines with age, with older adults tending to produce more off-topic comments. The lack of pictorial stimuli may prompt more off-topic comments, which may inflate LD scores. However, James et al. (1998) still found that narratives of older adults were longer even after controlling for off-topic content.

The researchers argued that the reason for the differential findings is that when older adults talk about their personal life, which encompasses mostly nonpictorial narratives or expository opinions, it is considered a more interesting and important topic compared to unfamiliar pictorial tasks.

Elicitation modality also matters. Rabaglia and Salthouse (2011) elicited written discourse samples from 85 younger adults, 169 middle-aged adults, and 145 older adults on two discourse tasks: a single-picture description and an expository discourse task asking people, "Who do you admire most?" The researchers found that older adults use a more diverse vocabulary on both tasks as measured by TTR. Since they analyzed written samples, they argued their results may be a better estimate of vocabulary size. During the written discourse tasks, people had more time to generate a response and consider their words, which may have eased the demands placed on word retrieval, which is known to decline with age (Kavé & Goral, 2017).

In conclusion, LD generally remains stable or increases across the life span. The variance of results may be explained by whether or not the discourse uses pictorial stimuli, since single and sequential description tasks do not show a difference between younger and older adults. Yet LD scores do show a difference between younger and older adults for nonpictorial description tasks, procedural tasks, and some expository tasks (Table 3–4). When selecting discourse tasks, clinicians should remember that more complex discourse tasks require more cognitive resources that are not available for word retrieval and may lead to decline in LD. Easier discourse tasks raise LD scores because cognitive resources are freed up for word retrieval. This demonstrates the importance of considering the type of discourse task and elicitation methods when determining whether LD scores are due to age or disorder.

Syntactic Complexity

Grammatical processing is often assessed by measuring the syntactic complexity of a speaker's utterance. There are numerous ways to estimate syntactic complexity, but they can be divided into (a) the quantity or quality of syntactic elements produced by the speaker, and (b) the number of morphological and syntactic errors. The quantity or quality of syntactic elements is measured through utterance length or clausal density; the number of adverbials, nominal, or relative clauses; the number of embeddings; or the percentage of grammatical utterances. Syntactic complexity is also measured to

determine the errors produced. These errors include the number of bound morpheme errors, syntactic omissions, or verbal paraphasias (Table 3–5).

There is a general consensus that syntactic complexity declines with age (see Marini & Andreetta, 2016, for review), though women may maintain grammatical processing abilities longer than men (Moscoso del Prado Martín, 2017). Older adults often produce shorter, less complex utterances (Shadden, 1997), more morphological errors (Marini et al., 2005), and referential errors (Heller & Dobbs, 1993). These declines are seen in single-picture description tasks (Bates et al., 1995; Capilouto et al., 2016; Gamm, 2014; Liu & Wang, 2019; Marini et al., 2005; Rabaglia & Salthouse, 2011), sequential-picture description tasks (Capilouto et al., 2016; Gamm, 2014; Marini et al., 2005), and nonpictorial narrative tasks such as recounts and interviews (Capilouto et al., 2016; Gamm, 2014; Kynette & Kemper, 1986; see trends in Table 3–6).

Marini et al. (2005) conducted single-picture and sequential-picture narrative tasks for healthy adults divided into five age groups. They measured syntactic complexity and grammatical errors. Syntactic complexity was the ratio of complex utterances compared to all utterances, and errors were a ratio of grammatical errors, such as bound morphemes and missing/incorrect

Table 3–4. Trends for Lexical Diversity Changes Across the Life Span	
Discourse Tasks	*Trends Across the Life Span*
Pictorial Description Tasks	Stable
Nonpictorial Description Tasks	Increases
Expository Tasks	Mixed
Procedural Tasks	Increases

Table 3–5. Measures of Syntactic Complexity

	Definitions
Utterance Length	The number of words or morphemes in a single utterance, or the average number of words or morphemes in all utterances
Clausal Density	The total number of clauses (nominal, adverbial, relative, etc.) divided by the number of utterances
Percentage of Grammatical Utterances	The number of utterances without grammatical errors divided by the total number of clauses
Percentage of Complex Utterances	The number of utterances with an independent and dependent clause divided by total utterances
Number of Adverbial Clauses	The number of adverbial clauses, which are dependent clauses that function as adverbs by modifying a verb, adjective, or another adverb (e.g., **Even if I run to the next gate**, I will not make my flight)
Number of Nominal Clauses	The number of nominal clauses, which are dependent clauses that contain a noun and a conjugated verb that acts as a noun (e.g., The reason for the positive book review is that **it covered my favorite topic**)
Number of Relative Clauses	The number of relative clauses, which are clauses that modify nouns or noun phrases (e.g., The cat went to the vet, **who gave her a shot**)
Bound Morpheme Errors	The number of missing or incorrect bound morphemes. These include tense and agreement (e.g., She **hate** the cold. Hate needs an –s suffix for agreement).
Syntactic Omissions	The number of open and closed class words missing
Verbal Paraphasia	The number of word substitutions (e.g., If the speaker said **cat** but meant **dog**)

Table 3–6. Trends for Syntactic Complexity Across the Life Span

Discourse Tasks	Trends Across the Life Span
Single-Picture Narrative Tasks	Declines
Sequential Picture Narrative Tasks	Declines
Nonpictorial Narrative Tasks	Declines
Procedural Tasks	Declines
Expository Tasks	Mixed
Conversational Tasks	Mixed

function words, divided by all words. They found that syntactic complexity had a linear decline with a sharp decrease in performance of participants over the age of 75 and a linear increase in the number of errors across the different age groups. These results agreed with others who have found a decline in syntactic complexity starting around the seventh decade of life (Capilouto et al., 2016; Kemper & Anagnopoulos, 1989; Kemper & Sumner, 2001; Nippold et al., 2014) where older adults produce fewer complex utterances in English (Kemper & Anagnopoulos, 1989) and Chinese (Liu & Wang, 2019), as well as for written samples (Rabaglia & Salthouse, 2011).

In contrast, Glosser and Deser (1992) tested middle-aged adults (43–61 years) and healthy older adults (67–88 years). Participants were asked to describe family or work experiences from their past. To measure syntactic complexity, the researchers measured complete/incomplete utterances, syntactic omissions, and the weighted index of subordination that followed the guidelines from Loban (1976). They did not find any difference between the research topic (family or work), nor did they find a significant difference between the groups with respect to syntactic complexity. Unfortunately, the low number of participants may have influenced the researchers' ability to find a significant difference.

In conclusion, syntactic complexity often declines as a function of age, except for expository and conversational discourse tasks, where the research is mixed. Nippold et al. (2014) argued that expository discourse tasks require more complex language to communicate a speaker's ideas and intentions compared to narrative or procedural tasks. If true, older adults may be capable of producing complicated syntax when necessary but rely on simpler syntactic forms

for ease of processing. Moscoso del Prado Martín (2017) provided further evidence of spared syntactic complexity by demonstrating a linear increase in the variety of syntactic forms used during a conversational task until speakers were in their early 60s. Conversational discourse may be the result of partner support or perhaps navigating the complexities of turn taking and other pragmatics issues requiring more complex language than simply narrating a monologued story.

Cohesion

Cohesion in discourse refers to the linkage of meaning across sentences or utterance by means of cohesion devices (Halliday & Hasan, 1976). These devices are linguistic elements that serve to form structural or semantic relationships between elements of a text and contribute to the continuity and coherence of the discourse. Inappropriate use or absence of cohesion devices appears to cause discontinuity in discourse (Ripich & Terrell, 1988). Cohesion has been primarily investigated by using the five cohesive categories suggested by Halliday and Hasan (Table 3–7) and the number of errors produced when one of these cohesive categories is wrong.

There is general agreement that cohesion declines as a function of age. This may present as a reduction of the number of cohesive ties per utterance (Babaei et al., 2019), an increase in the number of referential errors, including ambiguous nouns and pronouns (Juncos-Rabadán et al., 2005; Kemper et al., 1990; Pratt et al., 1989; Ulatowska et al., 1986), and a reduced ability to repair cohesive errors through repetition (Saling et al., 2012). Yet, some researchers have found no difference in the use of appropriate or

Table 3–7. Halliday and Hasan's Cohesive Categories

Cohesive Tie	Example
Reference	Definition: A word or phrase that references a previous word or phrase. Example: **Sarah** went to the store. **She** needed to buy milk. **She** references **Sarah**.
Substitution	Definition: A word or phrase replaced by another word to avoid repetition. Example: The old **truck** wouldn't start. He should get a new **one**. **One** replaces **truck** to avoid wordiness.
Ellipsis	Definition: An omission of a word or phrase. Example: Jessica **cooked** the turkey. Amanda … the mashed potatoes. The "…" reflects the omission of the word **cooked**.
Conjunction	Definition: A word or phrase that provides grammatical connections, such as coordinating conjunctions (for, and, nor, but, or, yet, so) or adverbial/prepositional expressions (furthermore, actually, as a result of). Example: Alice jumped down the hole, **and** she started to fall very slowly. **And** is a coordination conjunction.
Lexicalization	Definition: Cohesion expressed through the selection of vocabulary. Example: That **cat** is pretty. I think it is a **calico**. **Calico** is a more specific form of the word **cat**.

incomplete cohesive ties (Glosser & Deser, 1992) or in subjective ratings of cohesion (Leon et al., 2019). Again, some of these differences may be the result of the discourse type and elicitation techniques used.

Babaei et al. (2019) showed that older adults produce fewer cohesive ties in discourse compared to younger adults in a story retelling task utilizing single and sequential pictures. The researchers found that older adults produced significantly fewer cohesive ties per utterance compared to younger adults within the story retelling task but not a persuasive task. Consistent with this finding, Marini et al. (2005) systematically examined cohesion utilizing single- and sequential-picture storytelling tasks and found a sharp decline in the appropriate use of cohesive ties within the oldest group.

The inappropriate use of cohesive ties was found to gradually increase with age, starting around 50 years old.

Glosser and Deser (1992) investigated referential and lexical cohesive ties in middle-aged and older adults. Cohesiveness was estimated by counting the number of ambiguous prenominal and nominal referents in the preceding verbalization. Cohesion errors were estimated by counting the absence of lexical and anaphoric referents in the preceding verbalization. They found no differences between the two groups. More recently, Leon et al. (2019) reported no age-related differences in cohesion based on the subjective ratings of a panel of judges in a storytelling task. Unfortunately, the limited scope of the cohesive ties and errors analyzed in Glosser and Deser, as well as the subjective and very different nature of Leon's measure, may have influenced the results, making interpretation difficult.

If the above results are taken at face value, life span changes in cohesion do not seem to follow the same trajectory as lexical diversity (LD.) LD scores are stable across the life span for pictorial description tasks and increase for older adults when nonpictorial and procedural tasks are used. In contrast, for cohesion, most commonly studied with pictorial description tasks, there is a general decline across the life span (e.g., fewer cohesive ties and more cohesive errors). No significant differences between younger and older adults are found using nonpictorial narrative, expository and procedural discourse tasks, which are less frequently studied (see Table 3–8 for life span cohesion trends).

In general, pictorial tasks, whether single or sequential, may provide visual support of the logical sequence of events, making it easier to use cohesive ties. Unfortunately, older adults may receive less support from these visual cues (Babaei et al., 2019), causing Sherratt and Bryan (2019) to conclude that pictorial tasks are ideal to elicit cohesive ties within language samples and analyze age-related changes in cohesion. However, more research is needed to understand why older adults cannot seem to utilize the support offered by pictorial tasks.

Coherence

Coherence is often defined as the ability of a speaker to maintain a topic (Glosser & Deser, 1992), maintain a specific theme (Agar & Hobbs, 1982), or the ability of the listener to derive meaning from the speaker (Ripich & Terrell, 1988) within a specific context. In general, coherence is divided into two types: local coherence and global coherence (Glosser & Deser, 1992. Local coherence refers to how adjacent utterances within discourse are linked meaningfully; it is the ability of a speaker to incorporate information from one utterance into the next utterance. Global coherence is the ability to organize the discourse around a central theme or topic (Ellis et al., 2016). Researchers and clinicians have developed a variety of methods for estimating coherence. These measures may include subjective Likert-based rating systems (Glosser & Deser, 1992; Wright et al., 2014), main concept/proposition analysis (Capilouto et al., 2005), coherence error analysis (Marini et al., 2005), and schema/structural analysis (Saling et al., 2012). Table 3–9 describes each measure further.

In general, coherence declines as a function of age (Duong, 2001; Whitworth et al., 2015; Wright et al., 2014). Within narrative tasks, older adults produce fewer main ideas/events (Capilouto et al., 2005; Duong, 2001) compared to younger adults. Marini

Table 3–8. Trends of Cohesiveness Across the Life Span	
Discourse Tasks	**Trends Across the Life Span**
Pictorial Narrative Tasks	Declines
Nonpictorial Narrative Tasks	Stable
Expository Tasks	Stable
Procedural Tasks	Stable

Table 3–9. Measures of Coherence	
	Definition
Rating Scales	Subjective rating scales on a Likert-based scale. They can be used to analyze local or global coherence. This method was used by Glosser and Deser (1992) and Wright et al. (2014).
Main Concept Analysis	Counts or ratios of the number of main ideas or propositions that are necessary for successful discourse. These methods are often unique to the specific discourse.
Errors Analysis	Counts or ratios of errors produced. For local coherence, these errors include ambiguous referents or semantic shifts. For global coherence, these errors often include tangential utterances or conceptually incongruent utterances.
Schema Analysis	Coding utterances or sections of discourse as belonging to a macrostructure or superstructure (story grammar)

et al. (2005) found an increase in coherence errors. Older adults produced a larger number of ambiguous referents and semantic shifts compared to younger adults. Other researchers have found an increase in the number of global coherence errors, such as off-topic or tangential utterances (Hoffman, Loginova, et al., 2018; James et al., 1998).

Yet there appears to be a slight divide between pictorial and nonpictorial narrative tasks. Older adults did not produce fewer main events for single-picture description tasks (Wright et al., 2011), but they did score lower on subjective, Likert-based rating scales for recount tasks (Wright et al., 2014). While cohesion scores showed the greatest difference between younger and older adults utilizing pictorial stimuli, coherence scores show the greatest difference between the age groups when utilizing nonpictorial narrative tasks. It is interesting to note that cohesion is partly a linguistic/ grammatical process, whereas coherence is typically thought to be an executive system process. Though pictorial stimuli do not support or cue cohesive abilities, pictorial stimuli do appear to support and cue the logical organization and sequencing of discourse elements.

Procedural discourse differed in the number of steps provided with younger adults providing more steps (Whitworth et al., 2015). North et al. (1986) found mixed results with older adults producing significantly fewer steps for one type of procedural discourse (i.e., how to shop) but not others (i.e., mail a letter and polish shoes), and Wright et al. (2014) found there was no difference between age groups for procedural discourse when estimating coherence with a 4-point rating scale. North et al. (1986) suggested that the difficulty of a procedural discourse may play an important role in whether there are differences between younger and older adults since "how to shop" is more difficult than "make a peanut butter and jelly sandwich," "plant a flower," "mail a letter," or "polish shoes." However, there is evidence that older adults are more tangential and egocentric with procedural discourse (Barnett & Coldiron, 2021).

Expository tasks have clearer results. There appears to be a decline in coherence for older adults (Babaei et al., 2019; Glosser

& Deser, 1992; Hoffman, McClelland, et al., 2018; Kemper et al., 2010; Whitworth et al., 2015). Hoffman, Loginova, et al. (2018) investigated global coherence in younger adults and older adults by eliciting language samples by asking about general knowledge. Latent Semantic Analysis (LSA; Landauer et al., 1998) was used to measure coherence. LSA is a computational method in natural language processing used to derive contextual meaning of words. The method assumes words that appear in similar context must have similar meanings. This analysis can be used with other monologic discourse genres.

Hoffman, Loginova, et al. (2018) found that older adults produced less coherent samples compared to younger adults, which was mainly explained by measures of semantic memory and executive function. In an unpublished study, Kim and Wright also found that coherence was correlated with executive function. Expository discourse is similar to narrative recounts in having little stimulus support and requiring more organizational structure compared to descriptive tasks. This may make it an excellent task for studying the coherence abilities of healthy older adults.

Taken together, coherence does appear to decline as a function of age. Since the different types of discourse require different skills, it is not surprising that older adults' coherence performance varied as a function of discourse type. Life span coherence performance trends are shown in Table 3–10.

Conclusions

A wide range of acquired neurogenic disorders are associated with changes in communication, often evident in discourse behaviors. This chapter has provided an overview of the complexity of factors that influence discourse performance, including specific genres and tasks, elicitation stimuli and methods, and targeted outcomes. Understanding this complexity is particularly critical when considering the ways in which aging is associated with changes in discourse abilities. As can be seen in Table 3–11, there is no one trend that characterizes these abilities across the life span.

For example, lexical diversity, general knowledge, and other forms of crystalized knowledge appear to increase in healthy adults until much later in life. This increase in lexical diversity is most evident when utilizing nonpictorial discourse tasks that do not constrain the speaker to specific concepts and topics. In contrast, syntactic complexity is reduced as working memory declines, with older adults producing shorter utterances with fewer complex clauses and embeddings but increased grammatical errors. Once again, the discourse task matters; most age-associated syntactic decline is observed with descriptive and narrative genres.

Cohesion and coherence are also influenced by task. Cohesion declines with age are associated with fewer ties between

Table 3–10. Trends in Coherence Across the Life Span

Discourse Tasks	Trends Across the Life Span
Pictorial Narrative Tasks	Mixed (but general decline)
Nonpictorial Narrative Tasks	Declines
Expository Tasks	Declines
Procedural Tasks	Mixed

Table 3–11. General Trends Across the Life Span for Discourse Genre

	Lexical Diversity	Syntactic Complexity	Cohesion	Coherence
Conversation Genre	Increases	Mixed	No Data	Decreases
Expository Genre	Mixed	Mixed	Stable	Decreases
Narrative Genre	Increases	Decreases	Mixed	Mixed
Procedural Genre	Increases	Decreases	Stable	Mixed

utterances and more referential errors. This pattern is seen with pictorial stimuli in either descriptive or narrative tasks. However, narrative recounts produce more cohesive ties, possibly because speakers can focus on previously learned relationships. There are also declines in coherence with aging, with changes most pronounced for narrative and expository discourse. Unlike cohesion, nonpictorial tasks elicit the most differences in coherence between younger and older adults. The lack of pictorial support may free the speaker to produce tangential/off-topic information.

Hopefully, clinicians and researchers will be increasingly aware that choices of tasks, stimuli, and measures can and will influence discourse performance and can be systematically manipulated to learn more about and better serve clients with acquired neurogenic communication disorders. In addition, since many of these clients are older, understanding the contribution of the healthy or typical aspects of an aging person's discourse behaviors can help define what is normative and guide assessment choices and treatment design.

References

Agar, M., & Hobbs, J. (1982). Interpreting discourse: Coherence and the analysis of ethnographic enterviews. *Discourse Processes*, 5(1), 1–32. https://doi.org/10.1080/0163853 8209544529

Albert, M. S., Heller, H. S., & Milberg, W. (1988). Changes in naming ability with age. *Psychology and Aging*, 3(2), 173–178. https://doi.org/10.1037/0882-7974.3.2.173

Babaei, Z., Ghayoumi-Anaraki, Z., & Mahmoodi-Bakhtiari, B. (2019). Discourse in aging: Narrative and persuasive. *Dementia and Neuropsychologia*, 13(4), 444–449. https://doi.org/10.1590/1980-57642018dn13-040012

Barnett, M., & Coldiron, A. (2021). Off-topic verbosity: Relationships between verbal abilities and speech characteristics among young and older adults. *Applied Neuropsychology: Adult*, 1–7. https://doi.org/10.1080/2327909 5.2021.1878461

Bates, E., Harris, C., Marchman, V., Wulfeck, B., & Kritchevsky, M. (1995). Production of complex syntax in normal ageing and Alzheimer's disease. *Language and Cognitive Processes*, 10(5), 487–539. https://doi.org/10 .1080/01690969508407113

Bliss, L. S. (2002). *Discourse impairments: Assessment and intervention applications*. Allyn & Bacon. https://www.pearson.com/us/higher-education/program/Bliss-Discourse-Impair ments-Assessment-and-Intervention-Appli cations/PGM231549.html

Boucher, J., Slegers, A., & Brambati, S. M. (2019). Cross-sectional analysis of picture descriptions of healthy young and older adults. *Neuropsychologie Clinique et Appliquée*, 3(Fall 2019), 132–145. https://doi.org/10.46278/j .ncacn.20190714

Capilouto, G. J., Wright, H. H., & Maddy, K. M. (2016). Microlinguistic processes that contribute to the ability to relay main events: Influence of age. *Aging, Neuropsychology, and Cognition, 23*(4), 445–463. https://doi.org/10.1080/13825585.2015.1118006

Capilouto, G. J., Wright, H. H., & Wagovich, S. A. (2005). CIU and main event analyses of the structured discourse of older and younger adults. *Journal of Communication Disorders, 38*(6), 431–444. https://doi.org/10.1016/j.jcomdis.2005.03.005

Capilouto, G. J., Wright, H. H., & Wagovich, S. A. (2006). Reliability of main event measurement in the discourse of individuals with aphasia. *Aphasiology, 20*(2–4), 205–216. https://doi.org/10.1080/02687030500473122

Coelho, C., Youse, K., Le, K., & Feinn, R. (2003). Narrative and conversational discourse of adults with closed head injuries and non-brain-injured adults: A discriminant analysis. *Aphasiology, 17*(5), 499–510. https://doi.org/10.1080/02687030344000111

Cooper, P. V. (1990). Discourse production and normal aging: Performance on oral picture description tasks. *Journal of Gerontology, 45*(5), P210–P214. https://doi.org/10.1093/geronj/45.5.P210

Day, A. (1986). *Good dog Carl.* Simon & Schuster.

Dennis, P. A., & Hess, T. M. (2016). Aging-related gains and losses associated with word production in connected speech. *Aging, Neuropsychology, and Cognition, 23*(6), 638–660. https://doi.org/10.1080/13825585.2016.1158233

Duong, A. (2001). Production of narratives: Picture sequence facilitates organizational but not conceptual processing in less educated subjects. *Brain and Cognition, 46*(1–2), 121–124. https://doi.org/10.1016/S0278-2626(01)80047-6

Ellis, C., Henderson, A., Wright, H. H., & Rogalski, Y. (2016). Global coherence during discourse production in adults: A review of the literature. *International Journal of Language and Communication Disorders, 51*(4), 359–367. https://doi.org/10.1111/1460-6984.12213

Fergadiotis, G., Wright, H. H., & Capilouto, G. J. (2011). Productive vocabulary across discourse types. *Aphasiology, 25*(10), 1261–1278. https://doi.org/10.1080/02687038.2011.606974

Fergadiotis, G., Wright, H. H., & West, T. M. (2013). Measuring lexical diversity in narrative discourse of people with aphasia. *American Journal of Speech-Language Pathology, 22*(2), S397. https://doi.org/10.1044/1058-0360(2013/12-0083)

Feyereisen, P. (1997). A meta-analytic procedure shows an age-related decline in picture naming: Comments on Goulet, Ska, and Kahn (1994). *Journal of Speech, Language, and Hearing Research, 40*(6), 1328–1333. https://doi.org/10.1044/jslhr.4006.1328

Gamm, K. N. (2014). The influence of task type and working memory on the syntactic complexity of narrative discourse production in healthy aging adults. *Theses and Dissertations–Communication Sciences and Disorder, 3.*

Gee, J. P., & Hartford, M. (Eds.). (2012). *The Routledge handbook of discourse anaylsis.* Routledge.

Glosser, G., & Deser, T. (1992). A comparison of changes in macrolinguistic and microlinguistic aspects of discourse production in normal aging. *Journal of Gerontology, 47*(4), P266–P272. https://doi.org/10.1093/geronj/47.4.P266

Goodglass, H., Kaplan, E., & Barresi, B. (2001). *The Boston Diagnostic Aphasia Examination.* Lippincott Williams & Wilkins.

Grimes, N. (1993). *Cinderella.* Random House Books.

Halliday, M. A. K., & Hasan, R. (1976). *Cohesion in English.* Longman.

Heller, R. B., & Dobbs, A. R. (1993). Age differences in word finding in discourse and non-discourse situations. *Psychology and Aging, 8*(3), 443–450. https://doi.org/10.1037/0882-7974.8.3.443

Hoffman, P., Loginova, E., & Russell, A. (2018). Poor coherence in older people's speech is explained by impaired semantic and executive processes. *ELife, 7,* 1–29. https://doi.org/10.7554/eLife.38907

Hoffman, P., McClelland, J. L., & Lambon Ralph, M. A. (2018). Concepts, control, and context: A connectionist account of normal and disordered semantic cognition. *Psychological Review, 125*(3), 293–328. https://doi.org/10.1037/rev0000094

James, L. E., Burke, D. M., Austin, A., & Hulme, E. (1998). Production and perception of "verbosity" in younger and older adults. *Psychology and Aging, 13*(3), 355–367. https://doi.org/10.1037/0882-7974.13.3.355

Juncos-Rabadán, O., Pereiro, A. X., & Rodríguez, M. S. (2005). Narrative speech in aging: Quantity, information content, and cohesion. *Brain and Language, 95*(3), 423–434. https://doi.org/10.1016/j.bandl.2005.04.001

Kavé, G., & Goral, M. (2017). Do age-related word retrieval difficulties appear (or disappear) in connected speech? *Neuropsychology, Development, and Cognition. Section B, Aging, Neuropsychology and Cognition, 24*(5), 508–527. https://doi.org/10.1080/13825585.2016.1226249

Kavé, G., Samuel-Enoch, K., & Adiv, S. (2009). The association between age and the frequency of nouns selected for production. *Psychology and Aging, 24*(1), 17–27. https://doi.org/10.1037/a0014579

Kemper, S., & Anagnopoulos, C. (1989). Language and aging. *Annual Review of Applied Linguistics, 10*, 37–50. https://doi.org/10.1017/s0267190500001203

Kemper, S., Rash, S., Kynette, D., & Norman, S. (1990). Telling stories: The structure of adults' narratives. *European Journal of Cognitive Psychology, 2*(3), 205–228. https://doi.org/10.1080/09541449008406205

Kemper, S., Schmalzried, R., Hoffman, L., & Herman, R. (2010). Aging and the vulnerability of speech to dual task demands. *Psychology and Aging, 25*(4), 949–962. https://doi.org/10.1037/a0020000

Kemper, S., & Sumner, A. (2001). The structure of verbal abilities in young and older adults. *Psychology and Aging, 16*(2), 312–322. https://doi.org/10.1037/0882-7974.16.2.312

Kertesz, A. (1982). *The Western Aphasia Battery.* Grune & Stratton.

Kintz, S., Fergadiotis, G., & Wright, H. H. (2016). Aging effects on discourse production. In H. H. Wright (Ed.), *Cognition, language and aging* (pp. 81–106). John Benjamins Publishing. https://doi.org/10.1075/z.200.04kin

Kynette, D., & Kemper, S. (1986). Aging and the loss of linguistic complexity [Data set]. In

Language and Communication, 6(1/2), 65–72. https://doi.org/10.1037/e665402011-291

Landauer, T. K., Foltz, P. W., & Laham, D. (1998). An introduction to latent semantic analysis. *Discourse Processes, 25*(2–3), 259–284. https://doi.org/10.1080/01638539809545028

Leon, S. A., Altmann, L. J. P., Abrams, L., Gonzalez Rothi, L. J., & Heilman, K. M. (2019). Novel associative processing and aging: Effect on creative production. *Aging, Neuropsychology, and Cognition, 26*(6), 807–822. https://doi.org/10.1080/13825585.2018.1532067

Liu, X., & Wang, H. (2019). A study of syntactic complexity in language production by Chinese-speaking older adults. *Studies in Linguistics and Literature, 3*(1), 79. https://doi.org/10.22158/sll.v3n1p79

Loban, W. (1976). *Language development: Kindergarten through grade 12.* National Council of Teachers of English.

Longacre, R. E. (1996). *The grammar of discourse.* Plenum Press.

Marini, A., & Andreetta, S. (2016). Age-related effects on language production. In H. H. Wright (Ed.), *Cognition, language and aging* (pp. 55–80). John Benjamins Publishing.

Marini, A., Boewe, A., Caltagirone, C., & Carlomagno, S. (2005). Age-related differences in the production of textual descriptions. *Journal of Psycholinguistic Research, 34*(5), 439–463. https://doi.org/10.1007/s10936-005-6203-z

McCabe, A., & Bliss, L. S. (2006). Struggling to make sense: Patterns of impairment in adult narrative discourse. *Imagination, Cognition, and Personality, 25*(4), 321–336. https://doi.org/10.2190/P60L-40M2-7354-8U2V

Moscoso del Prado Martín, F. (2017). Vocabulary, grammar, sex, and aging. *Cognitive Science, 41*(4), 950–975. https://doi.org/10.1111/cogs.12367

Nicholas, L. E., & Brookshire, R. H. (1993). A system for quantifying the informativeness and efficiency of the connected speech of adults with aphasia. *Journal of Speech, Language, and Hearing Research, 36*(2), 338–350. https://doi.org/10.1044/jshr.3602.338

Nippold, M. A., Cramond, P. M., & Hayward-Mayhew, C. (2014). Spoken language production in adults: Examining age-related differences in syntactic complexity. *Clinical Linguistics and Phonetics*, *28*(3), 195–207. https://doi.org/10.3109/02699206.2013.841292

North, A. J., Ulatowska, H. K., Macaluso-Haynes, S., & Bell, H. (1986). Discourse performance in older adults. *The International Journal of Aging and Human Development*, *23*(4), 267–283. https://doi.org/10.2190/BPF0-2BWD-BGNQ-HWCW

Olness, G. S. (2006). Genre, verb, and coherence in picture-elicited discourse of adults with aphasia. *Aphasiology*, *20*(2–4), 175–187. https://doi.org/10.1080/02687030500472710

Ostrand, R., & Gunstad, J. (2020). Using automatic assessment of speech production to predict current and future cognitive function in older adults. *Journal of Geriatric Psychiatry and Neurology*, *34*(5), 357–369. https://doi.org/10.1177/0891988720933358

Pratt, M. W., Boyes, C., & Robins, S. (1989). Telling tales: Aging, working memory, and the narrative cohesion of story retellings. *Developmental Psychology*, *25*(4), 628–635. https://doi.org/10.1037/0012-1649.25.4.628

Rabaglia, C. D., & Salthouse, T. A. (2011). Natural and constrained language production as a function of age and cognitive abilities. *Language and Cognitive Processes*, *26*(10), 1505–1531. https://doi.org/10.1080/01690965.2010.507489

Ripich, D. N., & Terrell, B. Y. (1988). Patterns of discourse cohesion and coherence in Alzheimer's disease. *Journal of Speech and Hearing Disorders*, *53*(1), 8–15. https://doi.org/10.1044/jshd.5301.08

Saling, L. L., Laroo, N., & Saling, M. M. (2012). When more is less: Failure to compress discourse with retelling in normal ageing. *Acta Psychologica*, *139*(1), 220–224. https://doi.org/10.1016/j.actpsy.2011.10.005

Shadden, B. B. (1997). Discourse behaviors in older adults. *Seminars in Speech and Language*, *18*(2), 143–157. https://doi.org/10.1055/s-2008-1064069

Sherratt, S., & Bryan, K. (2019). Textual cohesion in oral narrative and procedural discourse: The effects of ageing and cognitive skills. *International Journal of Language and Communication Disorders*, *54*(1), 95–109. https://doi.org/10.1111/1460-6984.12434

Snow, P. C., Douglas, J. M., & Ponsfordoe, J. L. (1997). Conversational assessment following traumatic brain injury: A comparison across two control groups. *Brain Injury*, *11*(6), 409–429. https://doi.org/10.1080/026990597123403

Ulatowska, H. K., Doyel, A. W., Stern, R. F., Haynes, S. M., & North, A. J. (1983). Production of procedural discourse in aphasia. *Brain and Language*, *18*(2), 315–341. https://doi.org/10.1016/0093-934X(83)90023-8

Ulatowska, H. K., Hayashi, M. M., Cannito, P., & Fleming, S. G. (1986). Disruption of reference in aging. *Brain and Language*, *28*(1), 24–41. https://doi.org/10.1016/0093-934x(86)90088-x

Van Leer, E., & Turkstra, L. (1999). The effect of elicitation task on discourse coherence and cohesion in adolescents with brain injury. *Journal of Communication Disorders*, *32*(5), 327–349. https://doi.org/10.1016/S0021-9924(99)00008-8

Whitworth, A., Claessen, M., Leitão, S., & Webster, J. (2015). Beyond narrative: Is there an implicit structure to the way in which adults organise their discourse? *Clinical Linguistics and Phonetics*, *29*(6), 455–481. https://doi.org/10.3109/02699206.2015.1020450

Wright, H. H. (2016). *Cognition, language, and aging*. John Benjamins Publishing.

Wright, H. H., & Capilouto, G. J. (2009). Manipulating task instructions to change narrative discourse performance. *Aphasiology*, *23*(10), 1295–1308. https://doi.org/10.1080/02687030902826844

Wright, H. H., Capilouto, G. J., Srinivasan, C., & Fergadiotis, G. (2011). Story processing ability in cognitively healthy younger and older adults. *Journal of Speech, Language, and Hearing Research*, *54*(3), 900–917. https://doi.org/10.1044/1092-4388(2010/09-0253)

Wright, H. H., Koutsoftas, A. D., Capilouto, G. J., & Fergadiotis, G. (2014). Global coherence in younger and older adults: Influence of cognitive processes and discourse type. *Aging, Neuropsychology, and Cognition*, *21*(2), 174–196. https://doi.org/10.1080/13825585.2013.794894

4 Conversation and Typical Aging

Marion Leaman and Aviva Lerman

Introduction

Conversation is at the core of everyday interaction. People converse with one another to accomplish many interpersonal goals, including sharing and exchanging information, building and negotiating relationships, reminiscing about the past, and planning for the future. Conversation is the communication activity that adults engage in most often (Davidson et al., 2003), and it is a critical component for developing and maintaining social relationships (Azios et al., 2022; Davidson et al., 2008; Palmer et al., 2019). During the aging process, regular stimulating social interactions are key to cognitive health (Kelly et al., 2017). Further, an important developmental stage for older adults is reflection and integration of life events to develop an understanding of self (Erikson, 1959; Erikson & Erikson, 1997), which is accomplished at least in part through conversation with others. In this chapter we consider changes in conversation that may occur during the aging process to support clinicians and researchers in differentiating between features of conversation that may be related to typical aging from those that are likely related to acquired neurological conditions.

Interpreting Conversational Research

Conversation is a commonplace and routine daily activity that often feels simple and effortless. People may converse with little overt awareness of how their interactional and language behaviors and choices are influenced by the conversational context (Gumperz, 1992). For instance, contextual factors that must be kept in mind when interpreting the literature on conversation and aging include the conversation partner, the relationship between the partners, the location and purpose of the conversation, and the interpersonal and cultural expectations for what should occur during that kind of interaction (Goodwin & Duranti, 1992; Goffman, 1974).

For instance, clinical conversations between patients and medical personnel (including speech-language pathologists) are characterized by an interview format in which the healthcare provider is expected to ask questions while the patient is expected to respond (e.g., Frankel, 1990). A power imbalance revolving around the clinician's expertise often exists, and the interaction often restricts features of conversation such as the topic and level of formality (Drew & Heritage, 1992; Maynard, 1991). Thus, a conversation that is an interview is very different, for example, from a casual conversation between two close friends.

Although research regarding aging and conversation has been ongoing for nearly 40 years, the result is a limited number of studies across a broad spectrum of conversation and partner types and partner instructions. For example, studies vary from highly structured conversational tasks in which partners must describe pictures to one another in a conversational interaction (e.g., Hupet et al., 1993), to unstructured spontaneous conversation (e.g., Mackenzie, 2000). Partners are sometimes restricted to making minimal responses, such as saying "yes" or requesting more information without adding information (e.g., Horton et al., 2010). In other studies, the conversation partners are unrestricted and are asked to carry out open-ended conversations (e.g., Boden & Bielby, 1983, 1986).

In addition, studies investigate and compare a variety of age cohorts, making an "older group" in one study perhaps the "younger group" in another study. For example, the "older group" in a study by Nippold et al. (2014) was aged 60 to 69 in comparison to the "younger group" of 61 to 73 years of age in another study by Horton et al. (2010). Researchers have also used a broad number of measures, many of them without interrater reliability or test-retest stability, to evaluate the resulting samples. For instance, measures vary from interactional behaviors such as turn taking and topic initiation, to linguistic production of lexical items and syntactic structures, to productivity measures such as speaking rate and number of words or utterances produced.

Figure 4–1 illustrates these methodological choices made by researchers regarding conversational subtype, partners, measures, and elicitation procedures that introduce sample variability between studies. These differences make comparing findings across studies challenging because seemingly contradictory findings may be related to methodological differences. Thus, the literature regarding how conversation is impacted by typical aging is currently in an early phase and findings are not yet conclusive.

Lastly, we note that conversation often includes other discourse genres (Günthner, 2014). For instance, during conversation, people tell stories (narrative discourse), give instructions (procedural discourse), and explain ideas (expository discourse). None of the studies reviewed specified the extent to which other discourse genres occurred within the samples. However, when other discourse genres are embedded in conversation, they are integrated into the ongoing interaction and, as such, are implicitly included within conversational research.

In this chapter, we provide foundational information about sensory function, cognition, and bilingualism that contributes to conversational interactions in older populations. We then explore the current literature regarding typical aging and conversation and discuss clinical applications. In selecting studies for review, we used the definition of conversation provided by Levinson (1983), who described it as "that familiar predominant kind of talk in which two or more participants freely alternate in speaking, which generally occurs outside specific institutional settings like religious services, law courts, classrooms and the like" (p. 284). Further, our review includes only conversations be-

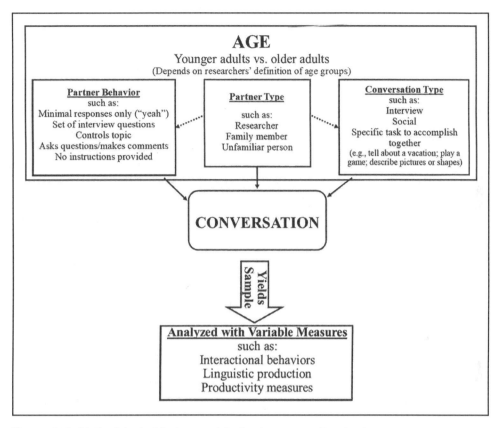

Figure 4–1. Methodological factors contributing to conversational outcomes.

tween two people (rather than groups) and focuses on expressive aspects of conversation.

Despite the challenges of methodological differences across studies, our intention is to summarize current knowledge regarding this important topic to support clinical decision making and to encourage future systematic research endeavors. While Figure 4–1 provides a visual schematic of relevant variables, the chapter's companion website provides a detailed table that includes methodological and contextual details about individual studies of conversational interaction. The reader is also referred to Chapters 7 and 10 for more information about conversational interactions.

Factors Contributing to Conversational Interactions

Hearing and Vision

Almost one fifth of U.S. citizens over the age of 70 report blindness in one or both eyes, and over one third report hearing loss (Crews & Campbell, 2004). By age 85, hearing and visual impairment occurs in about double the number of people compared to age 70 (Jacobs et al., 2012). The negative effects of vision and hearing loss on conversational skills in this population are both direct and indirect. For example, poor hearing limits participation in conversations taking place in noisy backgrounds, with many contributors, or if part or all of a conversation is whispered (Crews & Campbell, 2004). Furthermore, the ability to understand the pragmatic and emotional subtleties of language and communication are directly dependent on our vision and hearing. If one or both of these sensory channels are impaired, conversational skills will be affected (Charness, 2001) because successful conversation relies greatly on comprehending pragmatic features such as facial expressions, gestures, intonation, and figurative language. Add this to already declining pragmatic skills due to right cerebral hemisphere aging (Messer, 2015), and older adults with decreased hearing or vision acuity are at an evident disadvantage during conversation.

Dual sensory loss (i.e., both decreased vision and hearing) occurs in 8.6% of U.S. citizens over the age of 70 and becomes increasingly more common in the very old (Crews & Campbell, 2004; Yorkston et al., 2010). Consequences include salient and frequent difficulties conducting conversations, which can cause misunderstanding and misplaced negative reactions (Yorkston et al., 2010). It is also recognized that uncorrected declining vision or hearing acuity can result in cognitive decline in older adults, such as declining working memory (e.g., Jacobs & Stessman, 2020; Keller et al., 1999; Lin et al., 2013; Rogers & Langa, 2010), thus indirectly affecting conversational skills.

Cognition

Cognitive changes in aging are well documented (see Chapter 2). While there is consensus that general cognitive slowing in old age is due to decreased processing speed (e.g., Madden et al., 2017; Salthouse, 1996),

not all cognitive processes decline equally across the life span, if at all (e.g., Burke & MacKay, 1997; Hartshorne & Germine, 2015).

In conversation, declining working memory—directly, as a result of aging (Hartshorne & Germine, 2015) or indirectly, as a result of sensory loss (e.g., Jacobs & Stessman, 2020; Keller et al., 1999; Lin et al., 2013; Rodgers & Langa, 2010)—might make it harder for older people to remember what has already been said or what they were about to say. Conversely, better-spared vocabulary, comprehension, and general knowledge (the latter sometimes continuing to improve up to age 70; Hartshorne & Germine, 2015) might result in richer conversations and thus compensate for working memory decline.

Moreover, a decline in word retrieval ability with increasing age is well documented, both for common nouns (e.g., Brady et al., 2005; Burke & MacKay, 1997; Goral et al., 2007) and proper nouns (Seidenberg et al., 2009). It has been attributed to cognitive decline such as decreased executive functioning, decreased processing speed, limited resource capacity, or episodic memory decline (e.g., Craik & Salthouse, 2000; Goral et al., 2007; Seidenberg et al., 2009). Difficulties with word retrieval can lead to dysfluency, a breakdown in the message being conveyed, or losing one's turn during a conversation. However, good vocabulary knowledge persisting into old age should allow for the retrieval of a variety of words and thus more lexical flexibility, which could compensate for specific retrieval difficulties during conversation. Additionally, the ability to inhibit interfering stimuli and irrelevant thoughts declines with age (e.g., Arbuckle & Gold, 1993; Troyer et al., 2006). Difficulty inhibiting interference, together with decreased processing speed, might also affect the ability to follow a conversation among many people, especially if the conversation is fast moving and switches between conversation partners frequently. This difficulty will be exacerbated further if vision or hearing decline is also an issue.

The interaction of lifetime experience, together with differential changes across different cognitive abilities, indicates that older adults are a particularly heterogeneous group when it comes to their language skills (Hartshorne & Germine, 2015; Ylikoski et al., 1999). The number of languages spoken further adds to the heterogeneity of this population.

Bilingualism

The impact of being bilingual on conversation in old age is important to consider. Bilingualism can influence language selection and maintenance and can result in better-spared cognitive skills in bilingual adults relative to monolingual older adults. Attrition of one or more languages due to sociolinguistic changes is also possible in older age. While conversational skills in older bilingual adults compared to monolingual adults have not been the focus of conversation research to date, bilingualism adds to the heterogeneous nature of the older adult population. We summarize some of the main issues relating to bilingualism, aging, and conversation in older adults in Box 4–1. These topics are important to explore in future research.

Changes in Conversation Related to Aging

Tip-of-Tongue Phenomenon and Vocabulary

Despite the frequent complaint of tip-of-tongue experiences by older adults, and a robust literature investigating this phenomenon in word-level tasks, there are few

---

BOX 4–1: Bilingualism, Aging, and Conversation Facts

■ Bilingual speakers must choose which language(s) to use for any given conversation based on the conversational partner.

■ In typically aging adults, maintaining one language and switching between languages during conversation is not expected to deteriorate with age due to a lifetime of practice switching languages (Bialystok et al., 2004, 2006; Green & Abutalebi, 2013; Salvatierra & Rosselli, 2011),

■ Suppression of the nontarget language is known to deteriorate with age (Ardila & Ramos, 2008; Kohnert, 2013; Mendez et al., 1999), but this difficulty is less salient in conversation than in structured tasks (Gollan & Ferreira, 2009; Gollan et al., 2011; Kavé et al, 2008; Kohnert, 2013).

■ In old age, there is a tendency to withdraw into single-language use, often the first-acquired language (L1) (Lerman & Obler, 2017):

  ■ Due to environmental changes around retirement age;
  ■ Potentially resulting in progressive loss (i.e., attrition) in the less-used language (Ardila & Ramos, 2008; Goral et al., 2008);
  ■ With associated challenges to maintaining the less-used language during conversation.

studies investigating this concern in either structured or unstructured conversations. This may be due in part to speakers' ability to quickly change vocabulary words or effectively use circumlocution to avoid tip-of-tongue occurrences in conversation (Brown, 1991). Further, although tip-of-tongue experiences are often frustrating (Schwartz & Metcalfe, 2011), they are relatively rare and thus the ability to capture spontaneous instances during conversation for the purpose of research is not predictable (Brown, 1991). Diary studies in which participants were asked to record spontaneously occurring tip-of-tongue experiences note that the phenomenon occurs approximately once a day for older adults in contrast to once a week for younger adults (Schwartz & Metcalfe, 2011). Despite this greater challenge of lexical retrieval, adults are reported to use a more diverse vocabulary as they age, and use words with similar frequency in English as younger adults (Horton et al., 2010).

Syntax

Older adults may produce longer utterances (Horton et al., 2010), yet the opposite has been reported as well, with no difference in the mean length of utterance between age groups (Nippold et al., 2014). Further, researchers have reported more words per clause in older adults (Gould & Dixon, 1993), while there are no differences in clausal density across age groups (Horten et al., 2010; Nippold et al., 2014). Nippold and colleagues (2014) also reported no differences between age groups for complex low-frequency syntactic structures, such as "rather than swimming in the ocean, her dog prefers to roll in the sand" (a complex left-branching structure).

Productivity Measures

Measures evaluating aspects of verbal production during conversation suggest that aging is associated with greater dysfluency (Bortfeld et al., 2001), more fillers (e.g., *uh* and *um*), more silent pauses (Horton et al., 2010), and a slower rate of speech (Bortfeld et al., 2001). Likewise, Gould and Dixon (1993) reported that a collaborative storytelling conversation took longer among older married couples than younger married couples, although there were no significant differences in words per second, total number of words, or mean clauses per topic between the two groups. Similarly, in another study, Nippold et al. (2014) reported no significant differences in the number of utterances used in a structured conversational task on familiar topics (e.g., family, pets, hobbies) between age groups.

Topic Initiation and Maintenance

A measure of conversational initiation, which evaluated the skills needed to maintain the flow of conversation (e.g., topic initiation), suggested no significant difference between a group of old-old adults (aged 75–88) and a combined group of middle-aged and old adults (aged 40–74) in 10-minute open-ended conversations (Mackenzie, 2000). However, differences between men and women were observed in a study by Gould and Dixon (1993), who evaluated the extent to which one partner monopolized topic-initiating turns in a joint conversational storytelling task in 20 male/female married couples. The females in the older group produced significantly more topics without participation from their partners than in the younger group, while there was no difference on this parameter among the males in each group. Conversely, in the younger group, the males produced all of the topics without contribution from the partner to a significantly greater extent than among the older couples.

Topic maintenance has been investigated in the extent and frequency of off-topic language, defined as abundant output with reduced focus (Gold et al., 1988; Pushkar, 2000). Off-topic language (often referred to as verbosity, talkativeness, or rambling language) is a common stereotype of older adults. The literature suggests that off-topic verbosity is not directly related to aging, but rather occurs secondary to cognitive changes (Gold et al., 1988), such as difficulty suppressing irrelevant information (Arbuckle & Gold, 1993) or reduced inhibitory control (Arbuckle et al., 2000; Pushkar et al., 2000), as discussed earlier.

Unlike other researchers, Mackenzie (2000) differentiated poor topic maintenance from verbosity. She defined topic maintenance as the extent to which a contribution is relevant to the ongoing topic, as opposed to verbosity, which she defined as "an inefficiency of conveying information due to inclusion of unnecessary or peripheral detail and repetition" (p. 273). She evaluated both topic maintenance and verbosity as parts of a measure comprised of five interactional components, each measured on a 5-point scale. For the topic maintenance measure, she found a significant interaction for age, such that the elderly group (aged 75–88) was less skilled in topic maintenance than the younger group (aged 40–74). Conversely, for verbosity, Mackenzie (2000) observed that the elderly group was "inclined to verbosity" (p. 279) in comparison to the younger group in an unstructured conversational format. However, in contrast, she reported no significant difference between the number of words, clauses, or utterances during conversation in association with aging. This finding is consistent with the above-reported productivity data (Gould & Dixon, 1993; Nippold et al., 2014).

Topic maintenance differences and off-topic verbosity in older adults have also been associated with being socially active, extroverted, not being concerned with others' impressions, and/or experiencing stress (Gold et al., 1988). Alternatively, Burke (1997) hypothesized that older adults demonstrate off-topic verbosity because they have different communication goals than younger adults. Burke posited that older adults with reduced social interaction opportunities may highly value verbal encounters, leading to increased talking and off-topic verbosity.

Topic Content

Several studies have considered differences in the content of the topics discussed across different age groups. Boden and Bielby (1983, 1986) reported that speakers over age 62 spoke more about the past than younger speakers (i.e., "students"). In another study, older adults were reported to speak significantly less about their personal futures than younger adults (Brianza & Demiray, 2019). The same group of researchers also reported that both older and younger adults talked significantly more about the past than the future, and that the two groups both talked most often about the present (Demiray et al., 2018). Further, during future talk that is specifically centered around oneself, older adults included talk about their friends significantly less frequently than the younger adults (Brianza & Demiray, 2019).

As a part of Gould and Dixon's (1993) study, content produced during a joint conversational storytelling task about a recent vacation was compared across the older and younger married couples. The authors found that while both groups of participants discussed the task itself and vacation itinerary topics to the same extent, the older couples described significantly more people and places, elaborated much more about the events, and provided far fewer descriptions of itineraries than the younger couples. In addition, older adults were rated as producing significantly more subjective content in their conversations, although, in apparent contradiction to this finding, no difference in topics that were categorized as subjective reactions and discussion about the task were reported.

Interactional Behaviors

In addition to the microlinguistic and macrolinguistic aspects of conversation discussed above, interactional aspects of conversation may vary with aging. Several studies investigating interactional behaviors across age groups have focused on frequency of requests for clarification, backchanneling (e.g., saying "mhm" to indicate interest), turn-taking skills, and the ability to tailor one's turn specific to the partner's background and knowledge and to the specific situation (referred to as *audience design*; Clark, 1996). Although these data are limited, they suggest that older adults request clarification more often than younger adults in structured conversational tasks (Hupet et al., 1993). Gould and Dixon (1993) also demonstrated significantly less frequent use of back-channeling in older married couples than younger married couples in their collaborative storytelling task. Mackenzie (2000) noted increased difficulty with turn taking in the very oldest of three groups (aged 75–88).

Audience design is often investigated in a task during which two participants engage in a conversation in which they need to provide detailed instructions or descriptions to one another about a novel picture or geometric figure while separated by a barrier so neither can see the item being described. As speakers become accustomed to one another and to the task items, they will tend to use shorter, abbreviated terms to refer to the pictures, a process referred to as collaborative referencing (Clark, 1996). This occurs because as they interact with one another, they collaboratively develop ways to refer to each item that become progressively more efficient.

Results of three studies using collaborative referencing to investigate audience design suggest that older adults are less efficient in the development of novel referencing terms for pictured items. For instance, they use significantly more words (Hupet et al., 1993) and turns (Hupet et al., 1993; Lysander & Horton, 2012) to arrive at the joint referent. Consistent with these findings, older adults take significantly more time to produce their turns (Hupet et al., 1993). Throughout the interaction, they use fewer overlapping lexical items with their partner (Horton & Spieler, 2007), more unique or idiosyncratic terms, and fewer definite references (i.e., they continue to say "a dog" even when a specific dog has already been established as a referent between the pair) (Hupet et al., 1993). Older adults also explicitly negotiate the specific term the dyad will use to refer to each referent over more turns than younger adults (Lysander & Horton, 2012). Once a reference term has been collaboratively developed between the pair, older adults use the term less often (Hupet et al., 1993), although the length of the referencing term and the extent of tailoring to the partner's knowledge level do not differ between age cohorts (Yoon & Stine-Morrow, 2019).

Clinical Applications and Future Research

Clinical application of this literature can be guided by the summary of the research findings in Box 4–2. Overall, the literature suggests that during conversation, aging may be associated with an increase in the tip-of-tongue experiences (i.e., lexical retrieval difficulty). In addition, and aligned with this finding, there is evidence that older adults converse at a slower rate, produce more dysfluencies, and experience more filled and silent pauses than younger adults (Bortfeld et al., 2001; Gould & Dixon, 1993). Older adults have also been reported to demonstrate reduced efficiency when compared to younger adults in the number of turns and length of time needed to establish a joint referent to describe a novel picture (Hupet et al., 1993; Lysander & Horton, 2012). Thus, when working with clinical populations, it is important to keep in mind that findings in these areas may be reflective of typical aging and not necessarily the communication disorder being evaluated.

Currently clinicians and researchers must use clinical judgement in evaluating tip-of-tongue behavior and joint referencing abilities because no measures with psychometric or normative data are available. However, since tip-of-tongue experiences reflect lexical retrieval difficulty, clinicians may evaluate this phenomenon with several other recent measures of lexical

---

BOX 4–2. *Conversation and Aging: A Summary of the Findings to Date*

- Lexical retrieval and vocabulary
  - Older adults: more diverse vocabulary and more lexical retrieval difficulty than younger adults
- Syntax
  - Mixed findings/conflicting evidence
- Productivity measures
  - Older adults: more dysfluencies, slower rate of speech than younger adults
  - No difference in numbers of words, utterances, and similar language units
- Topic initiation
  - No differences overall
    - Possible interaction of gender and age
- Topic maintenance
  - Older adults maintain topic less than younger adults
- Verbosity
  - Conflicting evidence
  - Related to cognitive skills, rather than aging *per se*
- Topic content
  - Differences between older and younger adults
    - Older adults: more focus on past than future
    - Older adults: more focus on setting than events
- Interactional behaviors
  - Older adults:
    - Request more clarifications
    - Use back channeling less frequently
    - Experience more difficulty with turn taking
    - Are less efficient in development of novel referencing than younger adults

retrieval in conversation. Examples include Correct Information Unit in Conversation (CIUconv; Leaman & Edmonds, 2019b, 2021a), or the Complete Utterance, which includes a measure of relevancy with which the words are produced (CU; Leaman & Edmonds, 2019a, 2021a). These measures have been shown to be reliable and stable, and have normative data available. Another set of measures for conversational language is the Profile of Word Errors and Retrieval in Speech (POWERS; Herbert et al., 2012), which includes seven reliable measures of noun and content word production. Most of these measures show adequate stability, although normative data are not available.

In measuring the extent of dysfluencies during conversation, one measure, LEXbeh, evaluates pauses, false starts, and repetitions in people with mild to severe aphasia. LEXbeh may be useful for measuring productivity efficiency in conversations of older adults (Leaman & Edmonds, 2019a). While this measure demonstrates adequate reliability, it has not yet undergone further psychometric evaluation (e.g., for test-retest stability), nor does it have normative data available. There is a need for future research assessing the use of LEXbeh in both neurotypical older adults and those with communication disorders.

In addition to considering which language skills may decline in association with aging, evaluation can be informed by changes in language skills not expected to decline in aging. For instance, a decline that is observed where none is expected in an older adult may be an indication that neurological changes are occurring that warrant further investigation. For example, productivity measures such as number of words, clauses, and utterances should not change in typical aging (Gould & Dixon, 1993; Mackenzie, 2000; Nippold et al., 2014). Similarly, assuming that cognitive skills are within normal limits relative to age, the extent of off-topic language, or verbos-

ity (e.g., meta-talk, subjective utterances, and/or commentary utterances) has been observed to be comparable between older and younger adults (Carlson et al., 2020; Gould & Dixon, 1993; Hummert et al., 1998; Mackenzie, 2000; Richeson & Shelton, 2008). Consequently, declining topic maintenance or increasing verbosity may be suggestive that neurological changes are occurring, indicating consideration for medical follow up and communication assessment. One measure that may be helpful in evaluating topic maintenance is the Global Coherence Scale in Conversation (Leaman & Edmonds, 2021b) adapted from Wright and Capilouto's monologue-level Global Coherence Scale (2012). These measures use a 4-point scale to evaluate the coherence of each utterance to the topic. The companion website provides a scored example.

Finally, it is clear from the conversation and aging literature to date that there is a need for a methodology for collecting conversation samples, because highly variable procedures across research groups contribute to challenges in interpreting findings. Recent advances in assessing conversation in clinical populations provide several relevant practical tools for conversation sampling and measurement that clinicians and researchers can apply to typically aging individuals to increase standardization of collection procedures for unstructured social conversations (e.g., RHDBank Discourse Protocol, Minga et al., 2021; Kennedy et al., 1994; Mediated Discourse Elicitation Procedure, Hengst & Duff, 2007; Social Conversation Collection Protocol, Leaman & Edmonds, 2019a, 2021a), social conversations with a predetermined initial topic (e.g., Dyad Conversastion Protocol, King et al., 2007) or problem-focused topical conversations (e.g., Conversation Sample Procedures; Iwashita & Sohlberg, 2019).

Improved interpretability of research findings will support a more precise ability to differentiate older adults with mild language impairment from typically aging adults. Such differentiation is important clinically for diagnosis of progressive diseases affecting language (see Chapters 13 to 16) and for recognition of mild language impairments in people with sudden onset conditions such as aphasia following stroke. Further, differentiation of these two groups will support clinicians in substantiating a need for intervention, in developing relevant treatment plans, and in measuring outcomes and/or changes over time.

In closing, while additional focused research is clearly needed to more fully understand conversational changes associated with typical aging, clinicians can inform their practice with the research findings, protocols, and measures we have discussed. As the population continues to age, speech-language pathologists have a critical role in discerning subtle communication changes contributing to comprehensive identification, assessment, and diagnosis of communication disorders. This is essential, because even mild difficulty with conversational discourse can impact social networks, maintenance of friendships, and psychosocial well-being, all of which contribute to overall cognitive health.

Acknowledgments. We would like to express thanks to research assistants Iman Aly and Zoey Devney who contributed to this work by completing the preliminary review of many, many abstracts relevant to the discourse and aging literature.

References

Arbuckle, T. Y., & Gold, D. P. (1993). Aging, inhibition, and verbosity. *Journal of Gerontology: Psychological Sciences, 48*(5), 225–232. https://doi.org/10.1037/0882-7974.15.1.65

Arbuckle, T. Y., Nohara-LeClair, M., & Pushkar, D. (2000). Effect of off-topic verbosity on communication efficiency in a referential communication task. *Psychology and Aging, 15*(1), 65–77. https://doi.org/10.1037/0882-7974.15.1.65

Ardila, A., & Ramos, E. (2008). Normal and abnormal aging in bilinguals. *Dementia and Neuropsychologia, 2*(4), 242–247. https://doi.org/10.1590%2FS1980-57642009DN20400002

Azios, J. H., Strong, K. A., Archer, B., Douglas, N. F., Simmons-Mackie, N. N., & Worrall, L. (2022). Friendship matters: A research agenda for aphasia. *Aphasiology, 36*(3) 317–336. https://doi.org/10.1080/02687038.2021.1873908

Bialystok, E., Craik, F. I. M., Klein, R., & Viswanathan, M. (2004). Bilingualism, aging, and cognitive control: Evidence from the Simon task. *Psychology and Aging, 19*(2), 290–303. https://doi.org/10.1037/0882-7974.19.2.290

Bialystok, E., Craik, F. I. M., & Ryan, J. (2006). Executive control in a modified antisaccade task: Effects of aging and bilingualism. *Journal of Experimental Psychology: Learning, Memory, and Cognition, 32*(6), 1341–1354. https://doi.org/10.1037/0278-7393.32.6.1341

Boden, D., & Bielby, D. D. (1983). The past as a resource: A conversational analysis of elderly talk. *Human Development, 26*(6), 308–319. https://doi.org/10.1159/000272892

Boden, D., & Bielby, D. D. (1986). The way it was: Topical organization in elderly conversation. *Language and Communication, 6*(1/2), 73–89. https://doi.org/10.1037/0278-7393.32.6.1341

Bortfeld, H., Leon, S. D., Bloom, J. E., Schober, M. F., & Brennan, S. E. (2001). Disfluency rates in conversation: Effects of age, relationship, topic, role, and gender. *Language and Speech, 44*(2), 123–147. https://doi.org/10.1177/00238309010440020101

Brady, C. B., Spiro, A., III, & Gaziano, J. M. (2005). Effects of age and hypertension status on cognition: The Veterans Affairs Normative Aging Study. *Neuropsychology, 19*(6), 770. https://doi.org/10.1037/0894-4105.19.6.770

Brianza, E., & Demiray, B. (2019). Future time perspective and real-life utterances about the future in young and older adults. *GeroPsych,*

32(4), 161–173. https://doi.org/10.1024/1662-9647/a000216

Brown, A. S. (1991). A review of the tip-of-the-tongue experience. *Psychological Bulletin*, *109*(2), 204–223. https://doi.org/10.1037/0033-2909.109.2.204

Burke, D. (1997). Language, aging, and inhibitory deficits: Evaluation of a theory. *Journal of Gerontology: Psychological Sciences, 52B*(6), 254–264. https://doi.org/10.1093/geronb/52B.6.P254

Burke, D. M., & MacKay, D. G. (1997). Memory, language, and ageing. *Philosophical Transactions of the Royal Society of London. Series B: Biological Sciences, 352*(1363), 1845–1856. https://dx.doi.org/10.1098%2Frstb.1997.0170

Carlson, K. J., Black, D. R., Holley, L. M., & Coster, D. C. (2020). Stereotypes of older adults: Development and evaluation of an updated stereotype content and strength survey. *The Gerontologist, 60*(5), e347–e356. https://doi.org/10.1093/geront/gnz061

Charness, N. (2001). Aging and communication: Human factors issues. In N. Charness, D. C. Park, & B. A. Sabel (Eds.), *Communication, technology and aging: Opportunities and challenges for the future* (pp. 1–29). Springer.

Clark, H. H. (1996). *Using language.* Cambridge University Press.

Craik, F. I. M., & Salthouse, T. A. (Eds.) (2000). *The handbook of aging and cognition* (2nd ed). Lawrence Erlbaum Associates. https://doi.org/10.4324/9780203837665

Crews, J. E., & Campbell, V. A. (2004). Vision impairment and hearing loss among community-dwelling older Americans: Implications for health and functioning. *American Journal of Public Health, 94*(5), 823–829. https://doi.org/10.2105%2Fajph.94.5.823

Davidson, B., Howe, T., Worrall, L., Hickson, L., & Togher, L. (2008). Social participation for older people with aphasia: The impact of communication disability on friendships. *Topics in Stroke Rehabilitation, 15*(4), 325–340. https://doi.org/10.1310/tsr1504-325

Davidson, B., Worrall, L., & Hickson, L. (2003). Identifying the communication activities of older people with aphasia: Evidence from

naturalistic observation. *Aphasiology, 17*(3), 243–264. https://doi.org/10.1080/729255457

Demiray, B., Mehl, M. R., & Martin, M. (2018). Conversational time travel: Evidence of a retrospective bias in real life conversations. *Frontiers in Psychology, 9*(2160). https://doi.org/10.3389/fpsyg.2018.02160

Drew, P., & Heritage, J. (1992). Analysing talk at work: An introduction. In P. Drew & J. Heritage (Eds.), *Talk at work: Interaction in institutional settings* (pp. 3–65). Cambridge.

Erikson, E. H. (1959). *Identity and the life cycle.* International Universities.

Erikson, E. H., & Erikson, J. M. (1998). *The life cycle completed: Extended version.* W. W. Norton.

Frankel, R. (1990). Talking in interviews: A dispreference for patient-initiated questions in physician-patient encounters. In G. Psathas (Ed.), *Interaction competence* (pp. 231–262). University Press of America.

Goffman, E. (1974). *Frame analysis: An essay on the organization of experience.* Harper & Row.

Gold, D., Andres, D., Arbuckle, T., & Schwartzman, A. (1988). Measurement and correlates of verbosity in elderly people. *Journal of Gerontology: Psychological Sciences, 43*(2), 27–33. https://doi.org/10.1093/geronj/43.2.P27

Gollan, T. H., & Ferreira, V. S. (2009). Should I stay or should I switch? A cost–benefit analysis of voluntary language switching in young and aging bilinguals. *Journal of Experimental Psychology: Learning, Memory, and Cognition, 35*(3), 640–665. https://doi.org/10.1037/a0014981

Gollan, T. H., Sandoval, T., & Salmon, D. P. (2011). Cross-language intrusion errors in aging bilinguals reveal the link between executive control and language selection. *Psychological Science, 22*(9), 1155–1164. https://doi.org/10.1177/0956797611417002

Goodwin, C., & Duranti, A. (1992). Rethinking context: An introduction. In A. Duranti & C. Goodwin (Eds.), *Rethinking context* (pp. 1–42). Athenæum Press.

Goral, M., Libben, G., Obler, L. K., Jarema, G., & Ohayon, K. (2008). Lexical attrition in younger and older bilingual adults. *Clinical*

Linguistics and Phonetics, 22(7), 509–522. https://doi.org/10.1080/02699200801912237

Goral, M., Spiro, A., Albert, M. L., Obler, L. K., & Connor, L. (2007). Change in lexical retrieval ability during adulthood. *The Mental Lexicon, 2*(2), 215–238. http://doi.org/10.1075/ml.2.2.05gor

Gould, O. N., & Dixon, R. A. (1993). How we spent our vacation: Collaborative storytelling by young and old adults. *Psychology and Aging, 8*(1), 10–17. https://doi.org/10.1037/0882-7974.8.1.10

Green, D. W., & Abutalebi, J. (2013) Language control in bilinguals: The adaptive control hypothesis. *Journal of Cognitive Psychology, 25*(5), 515–530. https://doi.org/10.1080/20445911.2013.796377

Gumperz, J. J. (1992). Contextualization and understanding. In A. Duranti & C. Goodwin (Eds.), *Rethinking context: Language as an interactive phenomenon* (pp. 229–252). Cambridge.

Günthner, S. (2014). Discourse genres in linguistics: The concept of "communicative genres." In M. Fludernik & D. Jacob (Eds.), *Linguistics and literary studies* (pp. 307–331). De Gruyter.

Hartshorne, J. K., & Germine, L. T. (2015). When does cognitive functioning peak? The asynchronous rise and fall of different cognitive abilities across the life span. *Psychological Science, 26*(4), 433–443. https://doi.org/10.1177/0956797614567339

Hengst, J. A., & Duff, J. A. (2007). Clinicians as communication partners: Developing a mediated discourse elicitation protocol. *Topics in Language Disorders, 27*(1), 37–49. https://doi.org/10.1097/00011363-200701000-00005

Herbert, R., Best, W., Hickin, J., Howard, D., & Osborne, F. (2012). *POWERS: Profile of Word Errors and Retrieval in Speech.* J & R Press Ltd. https://www.jr-press.co.uk/word-errors-retrieval-speech.html

Horton, W. S., & Spieler, D. H. (2007). Age-related differences in communication and audience design. *Psychology and Aging, 22*(2), 281–290. https://doi.org/10.1037/0882-7974.22.2.281

Horton, W. S., Spieler, D. H., & Shriberg, E. (2010). A corpus analysis of patterns of age-related change in conversational speech. *Psychology and Aging, 25*(3), 708–713. https://doi.org/10.1037/a0019424

Hummert, M. L., Shaner, J. L., Garstka, T. A., & Henry, C. (1998). Communication with older adults: The influence of age stereotypes, context, and communicator age. *Human Communication Research, 25*(1), 124–151. https://doi.org/10.1111/j.1468-2958.1998.tb00439.x

Hupet, M., Chantraine, Y., & Nef, F. (1993). References in conversation between young and old normal adults. *Psychology and Aging, 8*(3), 339–346. https://doi.org/10.1037/0882-7974.8.3.339

Iwashita, H., & Sohlberg, M. M. (2019). Measuring conversations after acquired brain injury in 30 minutes or less: A comparison of two pragmatic rating scales. *Brain Injury, 33*(9), 1219–1233. https://doi.org/10.1080/02699052.2019.1631487

Jacobs, J. M., Maaravi, Y., Cohen, A., Bursztyn, M., Ein-Mor, E., & Stessman, J. (2012). Changing profile of health and function from age 70 to 85 years. *Gerontology, 58*(4), 313–321. https://doi.org/10.1159/000335238

Jacobs, J., & Stessman, J. (2020). Visual impairment at age 85 predicts subsequent cognitive decline at age 90. *Innovation in Aging, 4*(Suppl. 1), 216. https://doi.org/10.1093/geroni/igaa057.699

Kavé, G., Eyal, N., Shorek, A., & Cohen-Mansfield, J. (2008). Multilingualism and cognitive state in the oldest old. *Psychology and Aging, 23*(1), 70–78. https://doi.org/10.1037/0882-7974.23.1.70

Keller, B. K., Morton, J. L., Thomas, V. S., & Potter, J. F. (1999). The effect of visual and hearing impairments on functional status. *Journal of the American Geriatrics Society, 47*(11), 1319–1325. https://doi.org/10.1111/j.1532-5415.1999.tb07432.x

Kelly, M. E., Duff, H., Kelly, S., Power, J. E. M., Brennan, S., Lawlor, B. A., & Loughrey, D. G. (2017). The impact of social activities, social networks, social support and social relationships on the cognitive functioning of healthy older adults: A systematic review. *Systematic Reviews, 6*(259), 1–18. https://doi.org/10.1186/s13643-017-0632-2

Kennedy, M. R., Strand, E. A., Burton, W., & Peterson, C. (1994). Analysis of first-encounter conversation of right hemisphere-damaged adults. *Clinical Aphasiology, 22,* 67–80. http://aphasiology.pitt.edu/id/eprint/159

King, J. M., Alarcon, N., & Rogers, M. A. (2007). Primary progressive aphasia. In D. R. Beukelman, K. L. Garrett, & K. M. Yorkston (Eds.), *Augmentative communication strategies for adults with acute and chronic medical condition* (pp. 243–266). Paul H. Brookes.

Kohnert, K. (2013). *Language disorders in bilingual children and adults* (2nd ed.). Plural Publishing.

Leaman, M. C., & Edmonds, L. A. (2019a). Conversation in aphasia across communication partners: Exploring stability of microlinguistic measures and communicative success. *American Journal of Speech-Language Pathology, 28*(1S), 359–372. https://doi.org/10.1044/2018_AJSLP-17-0148

Leaman, M. C., & Edmonds, L. A. (2019b). Revisiting the correct information unit: Measuring informativeness in unstructured conversations of people with aphasia. *American Journal of Speech-Language Pathology, 28*(3), 1099–1114. https://doi.org/10.1044/2019_AJSLP-18-0268

Leaman, M. C., & Edmonds, L. A. (2021a). Assessing language in unstructured conversation in people with aphasia: Methods, psychometric integrity, normative data, and comparison to a structured narrative task. *Journal of Speech, Language, and Hearing Research, 64*(11), 4344–4365. https://doi.org/10.1044/2021_JSLHR-20-00641

Leaman, M. C., & Edmonds, L. A. (2021b). Measuring global coherence of people with aphasia during unstructured conversation. *American Journal of Speech-Language Pathology, 30*(S1), 359–375. https://doi.org/10.1044/2020_AJSLP-19-00104

Lerman, A., & Obler, L. (2017). Aging in bilinguals: Normal and abnormal. In A. Ardila, A. B. Cieslicka, R. R. Heredia, & M. Rosselli (Eds.), *Psychology of bilingualism: The cognitive world of bilinguals.* Springer.

Levinson, S. C. (1983). *Pragmatics.* Cambridge University Press.

Lin, F. R., Yaffe, K., Xia, J., Xue, Q. L., Harris, T. B., Purchase-Helzner, E., . . . Group, F. T. (2013). Hearing loss and cognitive decline in older adults. *JAMA Internal Medicine, 173*(4), 293–299. https://doi.org/10.1001/jamainternmed.2013.1868

Lysander, K., & Horton, W. S. (2012). Conversational grounding in younger and older adults: The effect of partner visibility and referent abstractness in task-oriented dialogue. *Discourse Processes, 49*(1), 29–60. https://doi.org/10.1080/0163853X.2011.625547

Mackenzie, C. (2000). Adult spoken discourse: The influences of age and education. *International Journal of Language and Communication Disorders, 35*(2), 269–285. https://pubmed.ncbi.nlm.nih.gov/10912255/

Madden, D. J., Parks, E. L., Tallman, C. W., Boylan, M. A., Hoagey, D. A., Cocjin, S. B., . . . Diaz, M. T. (2017). Sources of disconnection in neurocognitive aging: Cerebral white-matter integrity, resting-state functional connectivity, and white-matter hyperintensity volume. *Neurobiology of Aging, 54,* 199–213. https://doi.org/10.1016/j.neurobiolaging.2017.01.027

Maynard, D. W. (1991). Interaction and asymmetry in clinical discourse. *The American Journal of Sociology, 97*(2), 448–495. https://www.jstor.org/stable/2781383

Mendez, M. F., Perryman, K. M., Pontón, M. O., & Cummings, J. L. (1999). Bilingualism and dementia. *Journal of Neuropsychiatry and Clinical Neuroscience, 11*(3), 411–412. https://doi.org/10.1176/jnp.11.3.411

Messer, R. H. (2015). Pragmatic language changes during normal aging: Implications for health care. *Healthy Aging and Clinical Care in the Elderly, 7*(1), 1–7. https://doi.org/10.4137/HaCCe.S22981

Minga, J., Johnson, M., Blake, M. L., Fromm, D., & MacWhinney, B. (2021). Making sense of right hemisphere discourse using RHDBank. *Topics in Language Disorders, 41*(1), 99–122.

https://doi.org/10.1097/TLD.00000000000 00244

Nippold, M. A., Cramond, P. M., & Hayward-Mayhew, C. (2014). Spoken language production in adults: Examining age-related differences in syntactic complexity. *Clinical Linguistics and Phonetics*, *28*(3), 195–207. https://doi .org/10.1044/2016_JSLHR-L-16-0124

Palmer, A. D., Carder, P. C., White, D. L., Sanders, G., Woo, H., Graville, D. J., & Newsom, J. T. (2019). The impact of communication impairments on the social relationships of older adults: Pathways to psychological well-being. *Journal of Speech, Language, and Hearing Research*, *62*(1), 1–21. https://doi.org/10 .1044/2018_JSLHR-S-17-0495

Pushkar, D., Basevitz, P., Arbuckle, T., Nohara-LeClair, M., Lapidus, S., & Peled, M. (2000). Social behavior and off-target verbosity in elderly people. *Psychology and Aging*, *15*(2), 361–374. https://doi.org/10.1037/0882-7974 .15.2.361

Richeson, J. A., & Shelton, J. N. (2008). A social psychological perspective on the stigmatization of older adults. In L. L. Carstensen & C. R. Hartel (Eds.), *When I'm 64* (pp. 179–208). National Academies.

Rogers, M.A., & Langa, K.M. (2010). Untreated poor vision: A contributing factor to late-life dementia. *American Journal of Epidemiology*, *171*(6), 728–735. https://doi.org/10.1093/aje/ kwp453

Salthouse, T. A. (1996). The processing-speed theory of adult age differences in cognition. *Psychological Review*, *103*(3), 403–428. https://doi.org/10.1037/0033-295X.103.3.403

Salvatierra, J., & Rosselli, M. (2011). The effect of bilingualism and age on inhibitory control. *International Journal of Bilingualism*, *15*(1), 26–37. https://doi.org/10.1177/13670069103 71021

Schwartz, B. L., & Metcalfe, J. (2011). Tip-of-the-tongue (TOT) states: Retrieval, behavior, and experience. *Memory and Cognition*, *39*(5), 737–749. https://doi.org/10.3758/s13421-010-0066-8

Seidenberg, M., Guidotti, L., Nielson, K. A., Woodard, J. L., Durgerian, S., Zhang, Q., . . . Rao, S. M. (2009). Semantic knowledge for famous names in mild cognitive impairment. *Journal of the International Neuropsychological Society*, *15*(1), 9–18. https://doi.org/10.10 17/S1355617708090103

Troyer, A. K., Leach, L., & Strauss, E. (2006). Aging and response inhibition: Normative data for the Victoria Stroop Test. *Aging, Neuropsychology, and Cognition*, *13*(1), 20–35. https://doi.org/10.1080/138255890968187

Wright, H. H., & Capilouto, G. J. (2012). Considering a multilevel approach to understanding maintenance of global coherence in adults with aphasia. *Aphasiology*, *26*(5), 656–672. https://doi.org/10.1080/02687038.2012.676 855

Ylikoski, R., Ylikoski, A., Keskivaara, P., Tilvis, R., Sulkava, R., & Erkinjuntti, T. (1999). Heterogeneity of cognitive profiles in aging: Successful aging, normal aging, and individuals at risks for cognitive decline. *European Journal of Neurology*, *6*(6), 645–652. https://doi .org/10.1046/j.1468-1331.1999.660645.x

Yoon, S. O., & Stine-Morrow, E. A. L. (2019). Evidence of preserved audience design with aging in interactive conversation. *Psychology and Aging*, *34*(4), 613–623. https://doi .org/10.1037/pag0000341

Yorkston, K. M., Bourgeois, M. S., & Baylor, C. R. (2010). Communication and aging. *Physical Medicine and Rehabilitation Clinics*, *21*(2), 309–319. https://doi.org/10.1016/j .pmr.2009.12.011

SECTION II
Discourse in Aphasia

Mary Boyle, Topic Chair

Aphasia's Effects on Discourse

The linguistic impairments caused by aphasia are well known, and we have made progress in understanding how they affect discourse production. Speakers with aphasia convey less information and convey it less efficiently than speakers without aphasia (Nicholas & Brookshire, 1993). Word-retrieval difficulty, whether it results in paraphasias, neologisms, or frank retrieval failures, interferes with the ability to communicate a message and to link ideas clearly to each other (cohesion) and to the topic of discussion (global coherence) (Andreetta et al., 2012; Andreetta & Marini, 2015). Omissions and other syntactic errors make it difficult to produce accurate or complete sentences. Omitting verbs and predicate arguments, a common problem in nonfluent aphasia, makes it difficult for people with aphasia to convey complex ideas. Beeke et al. (2003) reported that this syntactic difficulty can result in people with aphasia creating their own grammar in conversations to compensate for their sentence production difficulties. In fluent aphasia, the paragrammatic substitution of grammatic morphemes can interfere with the cohesion and coherence of a discourse,

making it difficult for a listener to follow. All of these aphasic impairments can lead to conversational breakdowns that can be challenging for the person with aphasia to repair, prompting collaboration from conversational partners. Sometimes this collaborative repair is successful, but sometimes the repair process causes further disruption to the conversation.

Given the centrality of discourse in the everyday communication of adults, these discourse impairments create serious participation barriers for people with aphasia. Although assessing and treating discourse impairments is currently an active area of clinical research and practice, this focus on discourse is relatively recent.

The Evolution of Discourse Analysis in Aphasia

Before 1980, publications that focused on discourse in aphasia were primarily concerned with developing criteria for distinguishing fluent from nonfluent aphasia (Berko Gleason et al., 1980). In the 1980s, attention shifted to differentiating the discourse of people with aphasia from that of neurotypical adults or of people with other neurogenic communication disorders.

Researchers approached discourse assessment from a variety of different theoretical perspectives, focused on different aspects and genres of discourse, and employed a wide variety of methods to elicit and analyze the discourse sample (Armstrong, 2000). While this resulted in a surge in our knowledge about aphasic discourse, the theoretical and methodological differences made it difficult to see connections across studies or to fully appreciate the way that language impairments affected everyday communication. The disparate approaches also resulted in a proliferation of outcome measures that have left clinicians and researchers confused about which to use, but reluctant to agree on a common set of measures (Bryant et al., 2016, 2017; Dietz & Boyle, 2018; Pritchard et al., 2017).

At the same time, the revision of the World Health Organization's (WHO, 2001) model of functioning and disability expanded clinical focus from the traditional impairment level to include the levels of activity and participation, often considered to be more functional than impairment-level measures. This, in turn, caused third-party payers and research funders to expect activity- and participation-level outcomes to be reported. Because the everyday communication activities of most adults take the form of discourse, the expanded focus on functional outcomes emphasized the need for capturing change in discourse. It also highlighted the need to enhance our understanding of whether improving performance in one part of the WHO model affects performance at levels other than the level that is targeted in treatment. For example, if an individual improves at the impairment level, are changes in communication activities and participation apparent? If a person with aphasia participates in conversational dyads or groups, does that have a positive outcome at the language impairment level? These questions are among those being investigated currently.

Another factor increasing interest in discourse assessment in aphasia was the Life Participation Approach to Aphasia (LPAA; LPAA Project Group, 2000). This approach emphasizes meaningful real-life outcomes that enhance quality of life. Its ultimate goal is reengagement into everyday social life. Because the social life of adults involves discourse-level communication, the need for discourse-level assessment is apparent. The LPAA was influential in broadening assessment and treatment to include communication partners of people with aphasia. It also reminds us that communication involves more than language, so that assessing behaviors that accompany or replace language, such as facial expressions, drawings, or gestures, is important to consider. While earlier studies of discourse in aphasia concentrated on monologues and structured tasks, the increased attention to the social role of communication has expanded discourse assessment to include conversation. Often, studies of conversational discourse in aphasia examine natural conversations with the usual communication partners rather than conversations about topics chosen by and discussed with investigators or clinicians.

Cultural differences influence communication on many levels. Multicultural caseloads are increasing (Centeno et al., 2020), and speech-language pathologists are increasingly likely to find themselves assessing clients from a culture other than their own. Studies of multilingual speakers with aphasia typically focus on how aphasia differentially impacts the languages at the word level or on how the languages recover differentially in the context of aphasia (Centeno et al., 2022). The importance of cultural differences in interactional behaviors is acknowledged, but few, if any, studies focus on how discourse is affected in multilingual individuals. This is an area that requires much more attention.

Sufficient studies of discourse assessment and treatment in aphasia have been published that meta-analyses and systematic reviews have begun to appear (see for example Bryant et al., 2016; Dipper et al., 2021; Pritchard et al., 2017). This has led to a consensus that the large number of discourse assessments is creating barriers to their use (Bryant et al., 2017; Dietz & Boyle, 2018). Another area of consensus is that more attention needs to be paid to the psychometric properties of the measures, especially if they are to be used to assess treatment-related change (Dietz & Boyle, 2018). The growing consensus around these issues has resulted in the formation of a working group of clinical researchers focused on standardizing assessment of spoken discourse in aphasia (Stark et al., 2021).

The Chapters in This Section

The chapters in this section reflect the broad range of approaches that currently characterize discourse assessment in aphasia. They discuss choosing tasks to elicit discourses and assessments to measure them, along with the rationale for the choices. They provide examples of various assessment methods and discuss how the results might be used to inform treatment.

Chapter 5 by Lucy Bryant focuses on linguistic analysis of discourse. It discusses what we know about linguistic impairment of discourse production in aphasia. Bryant explains the microstructural and macrostructural levels of discourse and provides suggestions of different analysis methods targeted at each level. Examples throughout the chapter highlight the dif-

ferent information gained from these varied assessment methods and different discourse genres, illustrating how each can enhance our insight into the challenges and strengths of a particular person with aphasia. Bryant addresses the differing needs and constraints of front-line clinicians versus clinical researchers, and she provides suggestions about which assessments might be better suited to each group. The chapter also reports the outcomes of a study designed to train student clinicians in linguistic discourse analysis. The study showed that such training increased knowledge and confidence about discourse analysis and improved awareness of how linguistic impairments affected discourse production, even when the analyses themselves could not be applied in intense acute-care environments.

In Chapter 6, Lucy Dipper and Madeline Cruice also address the differing needs of clinicians and researchers by sharing their experience of co-designing a clinically feasible discourse assessment and treatment package with front-line clinicians. This chapter focuses on narrative discourse, specifically a personal story generated by a person with aphasia. It provides a multi-level (microstructure, macrostructure, and superstructure) assessment approach, giving clear explanations of what each measure tells us. Although it might seem that this chapter would overlap extensively with the Bryant chapter, that is not the case. Different assessments are addressed in each of the chapters. Dipper and Cruice include a discussion about the differing perspectives that clinicians and researchers have regarding discourse assessment and the choice of measures. Reading this interesting discussion can enlighten members of each group about why the other group does things as they do. Such understanding might lead to treatment studies that are more easily transferable to the clinic, and might lessen the frustration felt by clinicians when they read about methods that are too time consuming to apply in their workplace. The chapter includes a very helpful theoretical model that integrates the discourse levels with the communication skills needed for them. The co-designers ultimately decided to choose two assessment protocols: one for clinicians and another for researchers. The measures for each protocol are explained, with examples of how to perform the assessments and use the results to guide treatment decisions.

Chapter 7 by Jamie Azios and Nina Simmons-Mackie addresses clinical applications of conversation analysis. It gives a clear, thorough, easily understandable explanation of the many aspects of conversation and its analysis. For those who have not received training in this approach to discourse analysis, this chapter provides a comfortable and accessible way to learn about the process. Examples of how each aspect of the method applies to people with aphasia appear throughout the chapter. Azios and Simmons-Mackie address sampling, transcribing, and analyzing a conversational sample from a speaker with aphasia, and they include "clinical hacks" to make the process practical for a front-line clinician. They discuss how this approach differs from impairment-based analyses in that it searches for behaviors that help or hinder the flow of conversation in each conversational participant rather than focusing on linguistic errors produced by the person with aphasia. These behaviors can serve as treatment targets, and a conversational participant can be guided to increase a helpful behavior, reduce a problematic behavior, or replace a hindering behavior with one that is more helpful to reduce or repair communication breakdowns. Examples of commonly targeted behaviors and strategies to modify them are included.

In Chapter 8, Elizabeth Armstrong and colleagues, though focused on the indigenous population of Australia, provide valuable information and insights for any clinician or researcher who is evaluating someone from a different culture. For example, their discussion about how Grice's principles of conversation have been altered to reflect differences in Aboriginal versus majority-Australian culture alerts us that familiar "principles" that we accept unquestioningly may not apply to someone from a culture other than our own. The authors specifically note that behaviors that speech-language pathologists from a mainstream Western culture would identify as communication problems are not considered to be problems in some non-Western cultures. Similarly, usual communication partners might include a much wider circle than clinicians generally consider, and some of these less typical partners might actually be more appropriate choices than the spouse or child who would usually be nominated for that role by a clinician.

Conclusion

The chapters in this section of the book provide clinicians and clinical researchers who are interested in discourse analysis with a variety of assessment approaches that are covered in an accessible way and that include relevant examples of their application. The Companion Website materials that accompany each chapter, including worked clinical examples, will provide further demonstrations of each method's usefulness. We hope that these chapters can make the sometimes overwhelming topic of discourse assessment in aphasia one that readers can approach with better understanding and greater confidence.

References

Andreetta, S., Cantagallo, A., & Marini, A. (2012). Narrative discourse in anomic aphasia. *Neuropsychologia, 50*(8), 1787–1793. https://doi.org/10.1016/j.neuropsychologia.2012.04.003

Andreetta, S., & Marini, A. (2015). The effect of lexical deficits on narrative disturbances in fluent aphasia. *Aphasiology, 29*(6), 705–723. https://doi.org/10.1080/02687038.2014.979394

Armstrong, E. (2000). Aphasic discourse analysis: The story so far. *Aphasiology, 14(9)*, 875–892. https://doi.org/10.1080/02687030050127685

Beeke, S., Maxim, J., & Wilkinson, R. (2003). Exploring aphasic grammar 1: A single case analysis of conversation. *Clinical Linguistics and Phonetics, 17*(2), 81–107. https://doi.org/10.1080/0269920031000061795

Berko Gleason, J., Goodglass, H., Obler, L., Green, E., Hyde, M. R., & Weintraub, S. (1980). Narrative strategies of aphasic and normal-speaking subjects. *Journal of Speech and Hearing Research, 23*(2), 370–382. https://doi.org/10.1044/jshr.2302.370

Bryant, L., Ferguson, A., & Spencer, E. (2016). Linguistic analysis of discourse in aphasia: A review of the literature. *Clinical Linguistics and Phonetics, 30*(7), 489–518. https://doi.org/10.3109/02699206.2016.1145740

Bryant, L., Spencer, E., & Ferguson, A. (2017). Clinical use of linguistic discourse analysis for the assessment of language in aphasia. *Aphasiology, 31*(10), 1105–1126. https://doi.org/10.1080/02687038.2016.1239013

Centeno, J., Kiran, S., & Armstrong, E. (2020). Editorial: Aphasia management in growing multiethnic populations. *Aphasiology, 34*(11), 1314–1318. https://doi.org/10.1080/02687038.2020.1781420

Centeno, J. G., Ghazi-Aaidi, L., & Ansaldo, A. I. (2022). Aphasia management in ethnoracially diverse multilingual populations. In I. Papathansiou & P. Coppens (Eds.), *Aphasia and related neurogenic communication disorders* (3rd ed., pp. 379–401). Jones & Bartlett Learning.

Dietz, A., & Boyle, M. (2018). Discourse measurement in aphasia: Consensus and caveats. *Aphasiology, 32*(4), 487–492. https://doi.org/10.1080/02687038.2017.1398814

Dipper, L., Marshall, J., Boyle, M., Botting, N., Hersh, D., Pritchard, M., & Cruice, M. (2021). Treatment for improving discourse in aphasia: A systematic review and synthesis of the evidence base. *Aphasiology, 35*(9), 1125–1167. https://doi.org/10.1080/02687038.2020.1765305

LPAA Project Group (in alphabetical order): Chapey, R., Duchan, J. F., Elman, R. J., Garcia, L. J., Kagan, A., Lyon, J. G., & Simmons-Mackie, N. (2000). Life participation approach to aphasia: A statement of values for the future. *ASHA Leader, 5*(3), 4–6. https://doi.org/10.1044/leader.FTR.05032000.4

Nicholas, L. E., & Brookshire, R. H. (1993). A system for quantifying the informativeness and efficiency of the connected speech of adults with aphasia. *Journal of Speech, Language, and Hearing Research, 36*(2), 338–350. https://doi.org/10.1044/jshr.3602.338

Pritchard, M., Hilari, K., Cocks, N., & Dipper, L. (2017). Reviewing the quality of discourse information measures in aphasia. *International Journal of Language and Communication Disorders, 52*(6), 689–732. https://doi.org/10.1111/1460-6984.12318

Stark, B. C., Dutta, M., Murray, L. L., Bryant, L., Fromm, D., MacWhinney, B., . . . Sharma, S. (2021). Standardizing assessment of spoken discourse in aphasia: A working group with deliverables. *American Journal of Speech-Language Pathology, 30*(1S), 491–502. https://doi.org/10.1044/2020_ajslp-19-00093

World Health Organization. (2001). *International Classification of Functioning, Disability and Health (ICF)*. https://www.who.int/classifications/international-classification-of-functioning-disability-and-health

5 Analyzing Linguistic Features of Discourse in People With Aphasia

Lucy Bryant

Introduction

Linguistic analysis is a prominent approach to discourse used in the aphasia literature and has grown in popularity over the past several decades. With more than 500 different linguistic measures used in research to analyze the language of people with aphasia (Bryant et al., 2016), the opportunities to understand the linguistic competence and difficulties of people with aphasia are numerous. However, applications of linguistic discourse analysis within clinical settings are often limited despite a growing evidence base and efforts to encourage translation of research to practice (Bryant et al., 2017; Stark et al., 2021). The approach to linguistic analysis discussed in this chapter draws on the implementation approach used in an educational program for speech-language pathologists (Bryant, 2018; Bryant et al., 2019) and is available online as an appendix to Bryant's doctoral thesis (Bryant, 2018; http://hdl.handle.net/1959.13/1388301).

Viewed through a linguistic lens, discourse is the *process* of communication. It includes the expression of words and sentences that convey meaning, the person producing that meaning, their environ-ment, and the social and cultural content that influences meaning and its interpre-tation (Sutherland, 2016). Drawing from these definitions, analysis of the linguistic features of discourse places the focus on the expression of words and sentences, forming the foundation of discourse as a communi-cative *transaction*. When we communicate, we engage in communicative transaction by exchanging information through the forma-tion of words and sentences to construct and express "factual or propositional infor-mation" (Brown & Yule, 1983, p. 2). The effectiveness of the transaction is influenced by a number of external factors, including social relationships and personal attitudes, forming the *interactional* elements of dis-course (see Chapter 7). However, commu-nicative success is built on the foundation of the linguistic structure of meaning.

For people with aphasia, impairments at a linguistic, transactional level can limit communicative success and their ability to convey meaning in an effective way. Dif-ficulty with the accurate use of words and grammar can have a pervasive effect on the ability to convey meaning in discourse. At a word level, differing patterns of noun and verb retrieval across aphasia types can limit the word classes to which the person with aphasia has access (Gordon, 2008), and therefore, result in impaired sentence structure. People with aphasia also show marked decreases in their ability to use inflections such as tense, aspect, and agreement, which can further limit their ability to communicate meaning, particularly in relation to time and when an event occurred (Bastiaanse et al., 2011). Through analyzing these linguistic features in discourse, researchers and clinicians can better understand the underlying mechanisms that may affect overall communicative competence at a discourse level.

There are a number of tools at the disposal of researchers and clinicians who wish to understand the linguistic structures and functions used by a person with aphasia as they affect discourse and meaning. Standardized tests draw on naming, verbal fluency, and sentence completion and formulation tasks to address vocabulary and grammar in isolation. These discrete tasks examine one linguistic feature at a time. For example, a task requiring a person to name an action may examine their vocabulary and word retrieval, or it may assess their knowledge of morphology (e.g., past tense *clapped* versus the progressive *clapping*). However, discrete assessment tasks rarely consider the cognitive demands required to combine linguistic structures simultaneously as needed in everyday communication. Grammatical morphemes, rules of syntax, and lexemes are not used as separate entities but are instead combined as we speak to express complex ideas and meaning. By analyzing linguistic features of language in the context of discourse, we gain a true picture of how language is used in everyday living. This analysis may reveal areas of proficiency or new deficits that are not otherwise apparent as a person draws on linguistic strengths to compensate for weaknesses.

The examples used throughout this chapter serve to illustrate how linguistic analysis can highlight strengths and deficits in the discourse of a woman with aphasia that were not evident in standardized testing. This 76-year-old woman, E. C., was diagnosed with mild anomic aphasia (AQ = 89) using the Western Aphasia Battery–Revised (Kertesz, 2006), though she reported considerable difficulty communicating. A more thorough analysis of her standardized test scores and the results of a linguistic discourse analysis can be found on the companion website to this text.

Levels of Linguistic Analysis

The theoretical perspective underlying the linguistic analysis of discourse transaction draws from structural/cognitivist approaches to discourse (also called *formalist*; Schiffrin, 1994). Within this view, discourse is seen as the sum of its parts: words, phrases, sentences, and the rules that govern how these are combined to form meaning. To break this down further, an analysis of linguistic transaction considers: morphology—the structure and form of words; lexicology—vocabulary and the use of words; syntax—the use of rules governing the combination of words into sentences; and semantics—how all of these elements work together to create meaning (Crystal, 2008).

In examining each of these linguistic features, a thorough linguistic analysis requires the completion of three tasks, informed by the linguistic conceptualization of Ulatowska et al. (1981). The first task examines the microlinguistic features of language, lexical units, and the rules that govern how they are combined; that is, words and sentences. The second task looks more specifically at cohesion and how ideas are combined within and between structures (sentences) to create a meaningful whole. The third and final task requires examination of the macrolinguistic level of language—how ideas are structured to meet different purposes.

These three linguistic tasks identified by Ulatowska et al. (1981) correspond with three levels of linguistic analysis. The first level, the microlinguistic level, is the surface-level representation of language in discourse, the words and phrases used to communicate meaning, and the grammar used to create words and sentences. Shadden (1998) called this the sentential/surface-level analysis. The second level of analysis looks at the continuity of meaning and grammar between sentences, used to create a meaningful whole. Cohesion analysis (Liles & Coelho, 1998) examines linguistic units that rely on other units for meaning and the consistency with which grammatical rules are upheld within and between sentences. The third and final level, the macrolinguistic level, is the overarching level of analysis. Macrolinguistic analysis looks at how ideas are structured to create meaning and achieve different goals in the use of language. Within this level, analysis of information content examines how linguistic devices are used to create and structure meaning to establish the gist, theme, or main ideas of discourse. Analyses at each level provide insight into linguistic competence and communication in aphasia.

Microlinguistic Word- and Sentence-Level Analysis

Analysis of discourse at the microlinguistic level examines the natural units of language output that are encoded immediately prior to speech. The focus is on the utterance or sentence level and on words and how they are organized to create meaning; that is, lexemes, lexicosemantics, morphemes, and syntax.

Lexical Content and Diversity

Lexical analysis primarily focuses on vocabulary diversity and productivity measures that are particularly useful as they provide direct insight into the central anomic impairment experienced by many people with aphasia. Analyses examining vocabulary quantify the use of different words in a sample, providing insight into access to the foundational units used to construct meaning and achieve the communicative purpose of the discourse. Variations on vocabulary measures may examine specific lexical word classes, such as nouns or verbs, to understand further nuances in lexical ability. Bryant and colleagues (2013) analyzed interview samples of 50 people with aphasia using the most basic measure of lexical diversity, a count of the number of different words, to examine vocabulary. Statistical analysis showed that increased aphasia severity was significantly correlated with decreases in the number of different words used, supporting the notion that aphasia limits access to vocabulary.

Other measures of lexical diversity include analysis of different words (*types*) as a proportion of total words (*tokens*; type-token ratio [TTR]), and statistical variations of that measurement. For example, moving average type-token ratio (MATTR) measures sequential parts of the sample and averages TTR across those parts (Box 5–1). Fergadiotis et al. (2013) compared several versions of TTR measurement and identified MATTR as the best measure for

---

BOX 5–1. Methods for Evaluating MATTR

Manual Analysis of MATTR

1. Follow methods described by Shadden (1998) for calculating type-token ratio (TTR). See companion website.
2. Complete TTR analysis for words 1–50.
3. Repeat TTR calculation for words 2–51, 3–52, 4–53 . . . until the end of the sample.
4. Average the TTR scores across each calculation.

Automated Analysis of MATTR

The following tools compute MATTR automatically from an appropriately formatted transcript:

1. Computerized Language Analysis (MacWhinney, 2000)
2. Systematic Analysis of Language Transcripts (Miller et al., 2020)
3. MATTR (Covington & McFall, 2010)

---

capturing lexical diversity of people with aphasia because it is free from confounding influences such as text length that affect other versions of the measure.

The degree of linguistic and statistical knowledge, and the time and attention required to calculate TTR and its variations, can be tedious. As such, clinicians, and researchers in the 21st century often rely on computer programs and software to complete descriptive linguistic analyses (see Box 5–1). Linguistic analysis software uses part-of-speech tagging and recognition of words, codes, and punctuation to quantify linguistic content and structures. Commercially available software platforms that perform suites of analysis (for example Computerized Language Analysis [CLAN; MacWhinney, 2000; see also Chapter 17] or Systematic Analysis of Language Transcripts [SALT; Miller et al., 2020]) are reported frequently in aphasia research literature (Bryant et al., 2016) and by clinicians (Bryant et al., 2017).

As an alternative to often labor-intensive and time-consuming descriptive analysis of lexical content, clinicians and researchers can use comparative methods to analyze vocabulary, whereby a discourse sample is analyzed with reference to an expert model or data set to identify if target words have been included. These methods may be more clinically viable and preferred by clinicians who frequently reported using transcriptionless analysis to qualitatively evaluate the linguistic content and structures used in discourse as it was spoken (Bryant et al., 2017).

Core lexicon (also called CoreLex) has recently emerged as a means to assess lexical retrieval and vocabulary in the discourse of people with aphasia. The core lexicon approach suggests that when producing structured discourse samples (like a picture description or standard narrative retell), neurologically healthy speakers draw on an essential vocabulary—the core lexicon. By compiling that essential vocabulary into a list, the researcher or clinician can easily compare an elicited discourse sample to the master list to identify what core lexemes are evident in the discourse of a person with aphasia, and which are omitted (Box 5–2). Research has suggested that this type of comparative analysis correlates with over-

> **BOX 5–2. Core Lexicon Analysis of an Excerpt From E. C.'s Cinderella Story**
>
> The Core Lexicon used for comparison was drawn from the 10 most frequent nouns and 10 most frequent verbs used by nonaphasic speakers in the *Cinderella* story retell (MacWhinney et al., 2010).
>
> *And she looks up and here's this little old lady.*
>
> *She <u>said</u>, "<u>I'm</u> your **fairy godmother**."*
>
> *She said, "<u>I've</u> got a magic wand and you can <u>go</u> to the **ball**."*
>
> *She said, "and when you're ready I've <u>got</u> something special for you."*
>
> *She waved a wand and (ah) **Cinderella** was belle of the ball.*
>
> *She handed her a pair of glass **slippers**.*
>
> *They would have been the most uncomfortable thing you ever put on your feet ever.*
>
> *(she just put the, sh) she wore them to the ball.*
>
> Excerpt contains five of 10 nouns (in **bold**: *fairy, godmother, Cinderella, ball, slippers*) and five nouns not mentioned (*prince, mother/stepmother, dress, daughter/stepdaughter, sister/stepsister*)
>
> Excerpt contains five of 10 verbs (<u>underlined</u>: *said, have, go, be, get*) and five verbs not mentioned (*come, do, try, marry, know*)

all semantic content in the main concepts or ideas present in the discourse (Dalton & Richardson, 2015). Similarly, an analysis of spoken discourse of Italian speakers with and without aphasia showed that difficulties with the microlinguistic level of lexical content correlated with difficulties in establishing coherence in a narrative sample (Andreetta et al., 2012). With this in mind, comparative measures can provide more in-depth information about linguistic content and structure beyond the content explicitly assessed.

Because the discourse sample being assessed—the one produced by the person with aphasia—must be comparable to the reference set, comparative analysis methods can be applied only to certain discourse samples that contain similar content between speakers. For example, a picture description, narrative retell (e.g., the *Cinderella* story), or familiar procedure (e.g., making a peanut butter and jelly sandwich) contain the same general semantic content regardless of who produces the sample. Individualized samples such as personal narratives will not contain comparative content between individuals, so are not suitable for comparative analysis. Similarly, comparative analysis typically relates to semantic content, and the linguistic representation of meaning using words and phrases as content is more consistent and comparable between individuals. Morphosyntactic structure (i.e., analysis of word and sentence grammar) is much more variable within and between speakers, and cannot typically be analyzed using comparative methods. These linguistic structures can be better understood using descriptive analysis. (See Chapter 6 for additional methods of analyzing discourse at the word level.)

Morphosyntactic Structure

Microlinguistic analysis of morphology and syntax provides a detailed assessment of the use of linguistic structures, grammatical rules, and encoding. Disruptions to the use of these structures can lead to breakdowns in the semantic relationships between words and interrupt the natural flow of language. Syntactic analysis requires close examination of sentences and sentence structure in discourse. However, sentence boundaries are not always clear in spoken discourse, and the discourse is often broken down into smaller units based on linguistic units of meaning. There is no single agreed method by which clinicians and researchers segment the discourse into smaller linguistic units for analysis. Utterances, C-units, and T-units all appear in the discourse literature (Bryant et al., 2016), and each defines an individual unit differently (see Table 5–1 for definitions). The method used for segmentation is at the discretion of the person performing the analysis, though methods that are more clearly defined for the purposes of segmenting spoken discourse (that is, C-units or utterances) are recommended when analyzing spoken discourse. Therefore, an analysis might examine the number or proportion of complete and grammatical C-units rather than sentences.

One common measure of morphosyntactic complexity used in discourse studies across the life span is the mean length of utterance (MLU) in morphemes. This measure averages the number of morphemes, including bound grammatical morphemes of derivation and inflection and free morphemes (i.e., root words) per utterance in a discourse sample. A higher number indicates greater length and com-

Table 5–1. Definitions of Units for Segmenting Spoken Discourse

Segmented Unit	Reference	Definition	Additional Units
T-unit	Hunt (1965)	A main clause and all of its subordinating clauses	None Does not include partial sentences
C-unit	Loban (1976)	A main clause and its predicates	Sentence fragments Elliptical responses Yes/no responses Affirmations
Utterance	Owens (2013)	A spoken unit defined by changes in intonation, pauses, and breaks for inhalation	Compound sentences Complex sentences Commands

plexity of individual utterances. As would be expected, such morphosyntactic measures show significant linear correlation with aphasia severity, with MLU declining as aphasia becomes more severe (Bryant et al., 2013; Grande et al., 2008). MLU is also lower, indicating reduced syntactic complexity, for adults with nonfluent aphasia (Grande et al., 2008), which is unsurprising given the central agrammatic impairment of many nonfluent aphasias. While MLU is a more common measure in the language of children, its use to assess adult discourse clearly differentiated adults with aphasia from those with right-hemisphere brain damage, left-hemisphere damage without aphasia, and non-brain-injured controls (Bates et al., 2001).

Because sentences themselves can be difficult to analyze, syntactic analysis of the spoken discourse of people with aphasia may focus on verbs as the central component of a sentence (Halliday & Matthiessen, 2004). A complete and grammatical sentence may be defined as one containing a main verb and all required verb arguments in the correct place and order and including the correct verb morphology. This is also consistent with the aforementioned definitions of a C-unit as consisting of a main clause and its predicates. Analysis of discourse changes in three Italian speakers with aphasia following therapy suggested that an increase in the number of verbs directly correlated with increases in the proportion of grammatically complete sentences (Marini et al., 2007). This focus on verbs informs many popular aphasia treatments such as Verb Network Strengthening Treatment (VNeST; Edmonds & Babb, 2011) or Treatment of Underlying Forms (TUF; Thompson & Shapiro, 2005) that aim to improve production and retrieval of verbs and their arguments to improve the

verbal expression of people with aphasia. In such cases, analysis of verbs and verb arguments in discourse is likely to be the most appropriate measure of generalization of treatment effects beyond the sentence level.

Thompson and colleagues (2013) utilized analysis of verbs and verb argument structures (a method proposed by Thompson et al. [1995]) to measure the outcomes of a treatment that trained verb and verb argument production in people with aphasia. Using this method, verbs are categorized as intransitive, transitive, or ditransitive (that is, requiring one, two, or three arguments). Verbs were analyzed based on whether obligatory and optional arguments were used including agents (the person performing the action) and themes (the object acted upon). Using this analysis, the identification of verbs with three arguments (either optional or obligatory) and the addition of complements (i.e., arguments that are clauses on their own) would indicate longer and more complex syntactic structures in discourse. These were seen less frequently in the discourse of people with aphasia when compared to controls (Thompson et al., 1995). An example is shown in Box 5–3. A simplified means of conducting a similar analysis involves quantifying the ratio of the number of nouns to the number of verbs in a discourse sample. As each argument, typically representing a subject, direct object, or indirect object of the verb, would necessarily contain a noun, a larger ratio could indicate greater syntactic complexity with more arguments for each verb. While the simplified analysis permits automated analysis using computational software, it does not allow for the examination of the appropriateness of argument use and whether obligatory arguments are used as required. (See Chapter 6 for another method of analyzing predicate argument structures.)

BOX 5–3. Verb and Verb Argument Structure Analysis of E. C.'s Cinderella Story Excerpt

[She]_{AGENT} **_looks_** [up]_{ADJUNCT}.

And [here]_{ADVERB} **_is_** [this little old lady]_{AGENT}.

[She]_{AGENT} **_said_** ["I'm your fairy godmother"]_{SENTENTIAL COMPLEMENT}.

[She]_{AGENT} **_said_** ["I've got a magic wand and you can go to the ball"]_{SENTENTIAL COMPLEMENT}.

[She]_{AGENT} **_said_** ["and when you're ready, I've got something special for you"] _{SENTENTIAL COMPLEMENT}.

[She]_{AGENT} **_waved_** [a wand]_{THEME}.

And [Cinderella]_{AGENT} was [belle of the ball]_{PREDICATE NP}.

[She]_{AGENT} **_handed_** [her]_{THEME} [a pair of glass slippers]_{GOAL}.

[They]_{AGENT} **_would have been_** [the most uncomfortable thing]_{THEME} [you ever put on your feet] _{SENTENTIAL COMPLEMENT} ever.

[She]_{AGENT} **_wore_** [them]_{THEME} [to the ball]_{GOAL}.

In excerpt:	In main clauses (excluding sentential complements):
Total verbs = 20	Intransitive verbs = 2
Total nouns (including pronouns) = 34	Transitive verbs = 2
Noun:verb ratio = 1.7	Ditransitive verbs = 1
Mean length of C-unit (in words) = 7.9	Optional transitive verbs = 0
	Optional ditransitive verbs = 2
	Complement verbs = 3

Linguistic Analysis of Cohesion in Discourse

Linguistic devices and grammatical rules operate within discourse beyond the level of the sentence to link syntactic units and create a meaningful whole. This process of connecting units is known as *cohesion*. The analysis of cohesion is considered by some as a step that bridges the gap between the micro- and macrolinguistic elements of discourse (Peach & Coelho, 2016), while others consider cohesion within a microlinguistic analysis of discourse (Leaman & Edmonds, 2019). Regardless, prior research has largely agreed that the linguistic devices that create cohesion in discourse are significantly reduced in people with aphasia and vary depending on aphasia type (Zhang et al., 2021). Halliday and Hasan (1976) defined six different cohesive devices that may be observed in discourse, including reference, substitution, ellipsis, reiteration, collocation, and conjunctions (Table 5–2). Liles and Coelho (1998) provided a comprehen-

Table 5–2. Cohesive Devices Defined by Halliday and Hasan (1976) With Examples

Cohesive Device	Definition	Example
Grammatic Devices		
Reference	The use of words whose semantic value is drawn from elsewhere in the text and not from the lexeme itself	*She had a stepmother and two stepsisters, and they were cruel. They used her as a servant.*
Substitution	The interchange of one lexeme item with another, where both refer to the same semantic unit	*When the stepmother got an invitation, she got a new dress. The father was very weak, he should have stood up to the old woman.*
Ellipsis	A form of substitution where the lexeme is substituted with an omission and its meaning is implied	*She was running down the stairs (of the palace)OMITTED. She got out of the palace.*
Conjunction	The use of this specific word class that, by design, links pieces of information. They create relationships of coordination or subordination.	*When the stepmother got an invitation, she got a new dress, and the stepsisters got a new dress and Cinderella didn't get anything.*
Lexical Devices		
Reiteration	The repetition of a lexeme or a synonym, near-synonym, or subordinate of that lexeme with the same referent	*She left it on the stair. She was coming down the stairs, running down the stairs. She got out of the palace.*
Collocation	The use of lexical items that generally appear in similar contexts or are closely associated (e.g., antonyms) to connect adjacent syntactic units	*Her mother passed away and her father remarried.*

sive tutorial to guide the analysis of these cohesive devices in discourse.

From a linguistic perspective, consistency of grammar including tense morphemes and the agreement between nouns and verbs, nouns and articles, nouns and pronouns, and pronouns and the gender of the person they represent create cohesion between sentences. While the linguistic devices that contribute to discourse can be analyzed at the microlinguistic level, their contribution to meaning extends beyond individual words and sentences. For example, in examining *reference* as a measure of cohesion, we may look at the use of pronouns and demonstratives. An analysis of pronouns (*he/she/they/it*) can be used to assess perspective, and analysis of demonstratives (*this/that*) may be used to assess grammatical completeness at the microlinguistic level. However, the semantic content of these words is determined by other lexical items, called antecedents, that appear in adjacent clauses or sentences. In examining reference as an element of narrative competence in aphasia, Ulatowska and colleagues (2013) found that most people with aphasia made errors in failing to provide adequate reference or providing a referent that did not agree with its antecedent (e.g., using a masculine pronoun for a female antecedent). They did note that these reference errors had minimal qualitative impact on the overall *coherence* of the narrative; that is, on the listeners' ability to comprehend meaning.

The agreement between nouns and verbs (i.e., use of singular nouns with singular verbs, and plural nouns with plural verbs) and the consistent use of verb inflection throughout discourse also aid in the maintenance of cohesion at a grammatical level. Electrophysiological analysis of event-related potentials in adults with Broca's aphasia during sentence comprehension tasks illustrated that people with Broca's aphasia had markers of difficulty related to maintaining the information across clausal boundaries required to establish agreement between subjects and verbs (Wassenaar et al., 2004). Similarly, studies of verb tense inflection by people with agrammatic aphasia suggest that the use of past tense morphology in particular is impaired (Bastiaanse et al., 2011) and may be more prominent than difficulties with agreement (Clahsen & Ali, 2009). While switching between tenses may not affect the overall coherence of the discourse, the effects on cohesion are noticeable, as seen in Box 5–4.

BOX 5–4. Verb Tense Switching in an Excerpt From E. C.'s Cinderella Story

She [was weeping]PAST CONTINUOUS *near the stove, and she [heard]*PAST SIMPLE *a noise.*

And she [looks]PRESENT SIMPLE *up and* [here's]PRESENT SIMPLE *this little old lady.*

She [said]PAST SIMPLE, *"I'm your fairy godmother."*

Analyzing Macrolinguistic Structure and Meaning

The macrolinguistic level of discourse relates heavily to semantics and the structure and communication of meaning. Several analyses appear in the aphasia literature aimed at quantifying the linguistic representation of meaning and the gist, theme, or main ideas of discourse. Repeated studies of discourse in aphasia suggest that macrolinguistic structure and meaning are areas of relative strength for people with aphasia, who are often able to successfully convey meaning despite errors in microlinguistic content, structure, and cohesion (e.g., Altman et al., 2012; Ulatowska et al., 1983). Therefore, analysis of meaning is essential to understand relative communicative strengths.

One well known early example of macrolinguistic analysis of meaning is content unit analysis, applied to the Cookie Theft picture description by Yorkston and Beukelman (1980). Content units (CUs) were defined as semantic units composed of one or more words used at least once by a group of "normal speakers" in describing the Cookie Theft picture. The descriptive discourse of the person with aphasia could then be analyzed to determine semantic content based on the number of content units expressed and the efficiency with which semantic content was communicated based on content units expressed per minute (Box 5–5). This comparative analysis has also been updated for the 21st century and extended to differentiate between semantic information depicted in the left- or right-hand side of the picture to assess hemispheric neglect alongside the analysis of linguistic content (Berube et al., 2019).

While content units examine the quantity and efficiency of information content

---

BOX 5–5. *Content Unit Analysis of E. C.'s Cookie Theft Picture Description*

Units of analysis for comparison drawn from Yorkston and Beukelman (1980).

<u>A catastrophe</u>.

Something's blocking the sink.

She's very slow on the uptake.

*He knows <u>**mum**</u>'s in strife.*

*He's <u>**taking**</u> the goodies <u>**out of the jar**</u> while he can if he doesn't break his neck in the meantime.*

Examiner's prompt: What else can you see?

*The daughter <u>**laughing**</u>.*

See the trees and see the flowers out the window.

Examiner's prompt: Is there anything else?

Yeah there's, I'd say it's a vegetable garden to the left.

A garden of some sort, and there's a garden (round the) round the other side.

I thought at first there might have been chooks pecking round.

Total content units (of 57) = 5

E. C.'s description shows impoverished content compared to Yorkston and Beukelman's (1980) sample average: 14.7 CUs for healthy geriatric adults; 16.4 CUs for mild aphasia; 14.6 CUs for high-moderate aphasia; 10.5 CUs for low-moderate aphasia.

---

in discourse, they do not permit analysis of the quality and completeness of information content. Nicholas and Brookshire's (1995) main concepts add to the information analyses by also quantifying the accuracy and completeness of information in a discourse sample. Main concepts, defined linguistically as units containing a subject, main verb, object, and any subordinating clause, are predefined units that identify the gist or essential information in a discourse sample. Each unit is assessed for its presence or absence and completeness to provide analysis of the quantity and quality of the information included. Dalton and Richardson (2019) showed that main concept analysis was effective in measuring the information content of discourse in people with aphasia, showing significant reductions in information particularly for those with Broca's and Wernicke's aphasia.

As main concepts are compiled in a predefined list for the discourse elicitation material (e.g., retelling of the fairy tale

Cinderella; Richardson & Dalton, 2016), this analysis is also performed comparatively. However, information content can also be examined descriptively without the need for a comparison dataset. One of the most frequent measures used in the analysis of any aphasic discourse (Bryant et al., 2016) is the correct information unit (CIU) analysis initially reported by Nicholas and Brookshire (1993). CIUs are defined as words that are "accurate, relevant, and informative relative to the eliciting stimulus" (Nicholas & Brookshire, 1993, p. 340). The CIU analysis is popular due to its strongly established psychometric properties (Pritchard et al., 2017) and reliability in assessing discourse in aphasia (Boyle, 2014). Indeed, the reliability of the CIU measure has resulted in a clear indication that a change of 19 CIUs and 9 CIUs/minute between samples represents a reliable indication of change between testing periods, for example if comparing the information content of language pre- and post-treatment (Boyle, 2014).

Interpreting Meaning from Linguistic Discourse Analysis

To properly interpret linguistic discourse analysis, researchers and clinicians need to understand the linguistic function of the content and structures they analyze, and the specific linguistic targets of the measures used. Both descriptive and comparative measures provide a numeric representation of linguistic content or structure in discourse, and how the speaker uses the rules of language to construct meaning. Unfortunately, comparison to large norm-referenced data sets is not yet a possibility in discourse research, though calls to arms

to develop psychometric foundations for discourse measures (Stark et al., 2021) and a core outcome set for discourse measures (Dietz & Boyle, 2018) will no doubt lead to change in the future. Therefore, clinicians and researchers are left to find other methods of interpreting the numeric data associated with linguistic discourse measures.

When measuring the change over time, the natural variability in discourse can further complicate this interpretation. Boyle (2014) used minimally detectable change to identify the number that represented "real" change in discourse and not just natural variation. The caveat, however, was that this measure could only be used in analyses that were sufficiently stable to allow clinical decision making. Results identified four lexical measures that were suitably stable: two efficiency measures (words per minute and CIUs per minute), and two fluency measures (percent T-units with time fillers and percent T-units with delays); and numeric values that represented meaningful change in each measure. Of many hundreds of linguistic measures, these are a few with clear numeric data to support interpretation. For the many other measures with no clear interpretative data, further research is needed to establish valid and reliable interpretation.

Discourse Sampling and Linguistic Analysis

Discourse elicitation tasks are discussed in detail in Chapter 3, though elicitation tasks and the types of discourse they create (also referred to as *genres*) warrant further discussion here due to the differential impact that they have on linguistic form and content. Different genres, including descriptive, narrative, procedural, persuasive, expository, and conversational discourse, are defined as such by the purpose for which they are used. However, in achieving that purpose, speakers draw on unique grammatical structures and lexical patterns, meaning that each genre has inherent differences. The discourse samples in Boxes 5–6, 5–7, and 5–8 illustrate the use of pronouns and verb inflection across three discourse excerpts from a person with mild aphasia. While the focus here is on only two linguistic elements, other measures also vary across genres.

BOX 5–6. E. C.'s Narrative Discourse Sample: Cinderella Story Retell

She had to scuttle round and find a rat for (the) the coachman, and (ah) I think used a rabbit for the coach.

And (ah) she got (four mouse) four mice.

They were the horses.

And (ah) she waved her magic wand.

And there was the lovely coach (s) there with four horses and the coachman, all in his fancy gear.

Off they went to the ball.

In the narrative sample, E. C. is using a combination of simple and past perfect tenses to retell the narrative of *Cinderella*. This is evident in the use of past-tense morphology (*-ed*). The story is told using the third-person perspective, illustrated in the use of pronouns (*she/they*). Event sequence is created in the use of coordinating con-

junctions (*and*), and most utterances have relatively simple syntactic structure.

BOX 5–7. E. C.'s Procedural Discourse Sample: Making Scrambled Eggs

Get a flat pan and, (it) could be (a) a pan that's nonstick.

Or (if) if it's not a nonstick pan, smear it with butter.

Crack the (e e) eggs in a bowl (and a) and (ah) whisk.

Put a bit of pepper and salt in but not much salt.

And I have always found that (i) it's (ea) easiest to have a (w) wood spatula (t) to move it over.

(I adore) I always (like) mix up the eggs and cream.

(but ah) And if you want to take that eggy taste out, it doesn't hurt to have a (sc) scraping of nutmeg.

In comparison to the narrative, the same person with aphasia is using primarily simple present tense in the procedural discourse to provide instructions, so the verb morphology used in the narrative is not evident in this sample. The instructions are given in a second-person perspective, using the pronoun *you*, though some first-person commentary is also given. The steps are provided in sequence, though there is no explicit linking of events using conjunctions or temporal words. The syntax shows greater variation, with subordinating clauses used within steps to qualify if and when certain actions should occur.

> ### BOX 5–8. E. C.'s Descriptive Discourse Sample: Cookie Theft Picture Description (Goodglass et al., 2001)
>
> (Note: This is the same sample discourse shown in Box 5–5, though a different analysis is applied.)
>
> *Something's blocking the sink.*
>
> *She's very slow on the uptake.*
>
> *He knows mum's in strife (he, he, I).*
>
> *He's taking the goodies out of the jar while he can, if he doesn't break his neck in the meantime.*
>
> *The daughter laughing (ah).*
>
> *See the trees and see the flowers out the window.*
>
> *I'd say it's a vegetable garden to the left (and the), a garden of some sort, and there's a garden (round the) round the other side.*

The morphology again differs in the picture description discourse sample with verbs expressed in the present progressive tense (*is, -ing*). Like the narrative, the person with aphasia used the third-person perspective with pronouns (*he/she/they*). There is little to no connection between utterances, with each utterance referring to an element of the picture, and the presence of the picture providing the only cohesive connection between the speaker and listener during the discourse production. Utterances again have relatively simple syntactic structure of subject-verb-object.

While this is a simple illustration of the effects of discourse type on linguistic content, research also provides insight into the effects of genre on linguistic structure. In categorising different discourse genres by their level of complexity, studies suggest that picture descriptions often have the most complex grammar, followed by narratives and expositions (Li et al., 1996), while the grammar used to provide a procedural discourse varied depending on the speaker's familiarity with the topic (Williams et al., 1994). When examining the narrative, expository, and procedural discourse of people with aphasia, Stark (2019) identified significantly fewer verbs and a greater noun-to-verb ratio in procedural discourse, suggesting minimal grammatical complexity, greater propositional density, lower lexical diversity, and a slower rate of speech in narratives.

Acknowledging, then, that different discourse types will allow a person with aphasia to use different linguistic structures, researchers and clinicians must consider whether they want to elicit a single piece of discourse from one genre or multiple pieces of discourse of different types. This also means that researchers and clinicians should be careful in choosing a discourse task when assessing changes from an intervention. For example, a therapy that aims to increase the grammatical complexity of sentences may not show any treatment effect in procedural discourse types that typically have simple syntactic structures. The differences suggest that clinicians cannot assume performance in all discourse tasks based on the assessment of one task. Multiple different types of discourse should therefore be collected.

Discourse protocols such as Aphasia-Bank (see Chapter 17) provide a more comprehensive view of linguistic abilities by combining multiple discourse types; however, collapsing a number of discourse tasks to create a single sample may not allow the assessor to draw meaningful conclusions about language and discourse ability (Stark & Fukuyama, 2021). For example, when considering use of conjunctions as a measure of syntactic complexity, collapsing the procedural and discourse samples in Box 5–6, Box 5–7, and Box 5–8 results in a measure of 64% of C-units with conjunctions. This may hide the greater syntactic complexity shown in the procedural sample where 100% of C-units contain conjunctions, compared to the much simpler syntax used in the picture description. Multiple discourse samples of different types are therefore preferable, though these should be analyzed separately to examine linguistic content and structure within and between discourse tasks.

Clinical Implementation and Implications

Linguistic analysis of discourse is prevalent in the aphasia literature; however, surveys investigating the use of discourse analysis by clinicians show that applications in the clinical context are limited (Bryant et al., 2017; Stark et al., 2021). As a common theme, the time taken to thoroughly analyze linguistic features of morphology, lexicology, syntax, and semantics at the micro level, the level of cohesion, and macro-level structure often prohibits clinical application of these methods. Indeed, estimates in the research literature suggest that a thorough analysis of discourse may take up to 60 times as long as the time taken to elicit the sample itself in order to adequately transcribe, segment, code, and count all of the relevant linguistic features (Armstrong et al., 2007). In addition, clinicians appear to report low levels of knowledge and confidence that stand in the way of regular use of discourse analysis methods. Specialized linguistic knowledge

is needed not only to apply the analysis, but also to interpret the findings and understand the implications for everyday communication. Despite these barriers, researchers and clinicians seem to agree that linguistic analysis of discourse is a valuable tool to thoroughly understand communication ability and disability in people with aphasia. As such, it is important to identify strategies to enhance clinical implementation.

Bryant et al. (2019) used a training-based strategy to upskill student clinicians in linguistic discourse analysis and evaluated their ongoing use of learned skills over a 6-month period. While the training program did not bring about lasting change in the clinical use of linguistic analysis, trainees reported significant and lasting gains in confidence and knowledge. This illustrated that training alone is not sufficient to improve clinical use of linguistic discourse analysis. Other institutional barriers such as time and resource availability stood in the way of sustained use, particularly in high-demand acute clinical environments where barriers to implementation of evidence-based communication methods are well documented (see Foster et al., 2015; Simmons-Mackie et al., 2007).

Interestingly, the results of skills training showed that regardless of whether linguistic analysis was explicitly applied by clinicians to assess the language of people with aphasia, knowledge of those methods increased awareness of linguistic function. Following training, participants were better able to identify features of linguistic use and their impact on communication. They were also more likely to consider language use in their goal-setting and intervention planning than when evaluating the language of a person with aphasia using a standardized assessment alone (Bryant et al., 2019). This suggested that awareness of linguistic content and structure at a discourse level, even in absence of the actual analysis, reorients clinicians towards a more functional approach to assessment and intervention in aphasia.

References

Altman, C., Goral, M., & Levy, E. S. (2012). Integrated narrative analysis in multilingual aphasia: The relationship among narrative structure, gammaticality and fluency. *Aphasiology*, *26*(8), 1029–1052. https://doi.org/10.1080/02687038.2012.686103

Andreetta, S., Cantagallo, A., & Marini, A. (2012). Narrative discourse in anomic aphasia. *Neuropsychologia*, *50*(8), 1787–1793. https://doi.org/10.1016/j.neuropsychologia.2012.04.003

Armstrong, L., Brady, M., Mackenzie, C., & Norrie, J. (2007). Transcription-less analysis of aphasic discourse: A clinician's dream or a possibility? *Aphasiology*, *21*(3–4), 355–374. https://doi.org/10.1080/02687030600911310

Bastiaanse, R., Bamyaci, E., Hsu, C. J., Lee, J., Duman, T. Y., & Thompson, C. K. (2011). Time reference in agrammatic aphasia: A cross-linguistic study. *Journal of Neurolinguistics*, *24*(6), 652–673. https://doi.org/10.1016/j.jneuroling.2011.07.001

Bates, E., Reilly, J., Wulfeck, B., Dronkers, N., Opie, M., Fenson, J., . . . Herbst, K. (2001). Differential effects of unilateral lesions on language production in children and adults. *Brain and Language*, *79*(2), 223–265. https://doi.org/10.1006/brln.2001.2482

Berube, S., Nonnemacher, J., Demsky, C., Glenn, S., Saxena, S., Wright, A., . . . Hillis, A. E. (2019). Stealing cookies in the 21st century: Measures of spoken narrative in healthy versus speakers with aphasia. *American Journal of Speech-Language Pathology*, *28*(1s), 321–329. https://doi.org/10.1044/2018_ajslp-17-0131

Boyle, M. (2014). Test-retest stability of word retrieval in aphasic discourse. *Journal of Speech, Language and Hearing Research*, *57*(3), 966–978. https://doi.org/10.1044/2014_JSLHR-L-13-0171

Brown, G., & Yule, G. (1983). *Discourse analysis*. Cambridge University Press. https://doi.org/10.1017/CBO9780511805226

Bryant, L. (2018). *Investigating the implementation of linguistic discourse analysis for the assessment of aphasia in speech pathology practice*. University of Newcastle. http://hdl.handle.net/1959.13/1388301

Bryant, L., Ferguson, A., & Spencer, E. (2016). Linguistic analysis of discourse in aphasia: A review of the literature. *Clinical Linguistics and Phonetics*, *30*(7), 489–518. https://doi.org/10.3109/02699206.2016.1145740

Bryant, L., Ferguson, A., Valentine, M., & Spencer, E. (2019). Implementation of discourse analysis in aphasia: Investigating the feasibility of a knowledge-to-action intervention. *Aphasiology*, *33*(1), 31–57. https://doi.org/10.1080/02687038.2018.1454886

Bryant, L., Spencer, E., & Ferguson, A. (2017). Clinical use of linguistic discourse analysis for the assessment of language in aphasia. *Aphasiology*, *31*(10), 1105–1126. https://doi.org/10.1080/02687038.2016.1239013

Bryant, L., Spencer, E., Ferguson, A., Craig, H., Colyvas, K., & Worrall, L. (2013). Propositional idea density in aphasic discourse. *Aphasiology*, *27*(8), 992–1009. https://doi.org/10.1080/02687038.2013.803514

Clahsen, H., & Ali, M. (2009). Formal features in aphasia: Tense, agreement, and mood in English agrammatism. *Journal of Neurolinguistics*, *22*(5), 436–450. https://doi.org/10.1016/j.jneuroling.2009.02.003

Covington, M. A., & McFall, J. (2010). Cutting the Gordian Knot: The moving-average type–token ratio (MATTR). *Journal of Quantitative Linguistics*, *17*(2), 94–100. https://doi.org/10.1080/09296171003643098

Crystal, D. (2008). *A dictionary of linguistics and phonetics* (6th ed.). Blackwell Publishing. https://doi.org/10.1002/9781444302776

Dalton, S. G. H., & Richardson, J. D. (2015). Core-lexicon and main-concept production during picture-sequence description in adults without brain damage and adults with aphasia. *American Journal of Speech-Language Pathology*, *24*(4), S923–938. https://doi.org/10.1044/2015_ajslp-14-0161

Dalton, S. G. H., & Richardson, J. D. (2019). A large-scale comparison of main concept production between persons with aphasia and persons without brain injury. *American Journal of Speech-Language Pathology, 28*(1S), 293–320. https://doi.org/10.1044/2018_ajslp-17-0166

Dietz, A., & Boyle, M. (2018). Discourse measurement in aphasia research: Have we reached the tipping point? *Aphasiology, 32*(4), 459–464. https://doi.org/10.1080/02687038.2017.1398803

Edmonds, L. A., & Babb, M. (2011). Effect of verb network strengthening treatment in moderate to severe aphasia. *American Journal of Speech-Language Pathology, 20*(2), 131–145. https://doi.org/10.1044/1058-0360(2011/10-0036)

Fergadiotis, G., Wright, H. H., & West, T. M. (2013). Measuring lexical diversity in narrative discourse of people with aphasia. *American Journal of Speech-Language Pathology, 22*(2), S397–S408. https://doi.org/10.1044/1058-0360(2013/12-0083)

Foster, A. M., Worrall, L., Rose, M., & O'Halloran, R. (2015). "That doesn't translate": The role of evidence-based practice in disempowering speech pathologists in acute aphasia management. *International Journal of Language and Communication Disorders, 50*(4), 547–563. https://doi.org/10.1111/1460-6984.12155

Goodglass, H., Kaplan, E., & Barresi, B. (2001). *Boston Diagnostic Aphasia Examination* (3rd ed.). Lippincott Williams & Wilkins. https://doi.org/10.1007/978-0-387-79948-3_868

Gordon, J. K. (2008). Measuring the lexical semantics of picture description in aphasia. *Aphasiology, 22*(7–8), 839–852. https://doi.org/10.1080/02687030701820063

Grande, M., Hussmann, K., Bay, E., Christoph, S., Piefke, M., Willmes, K., & Huber, W. (2008). Basic parameters of spontaneous speech as a sensitive method for measuring change during the course of aphasia. *International Journal of Language and Communication Disorders, 43*(4), 408–426. https://doi.org/10.1080/13682820701685991

Halliday, M. A. K., & Hasan, R. (1976). *Cohesion in English.* Longman. https://doi.org/10.4324/9781315836010

Halliday, M. A. K., & Matthiessen, C. M. I. M. (2004). *An introduction to functional grammar* (3rd ed.). Routledge. https://doi.org/10.4324/9780203431269

Kertesz, A. (2006). *Western Aphasia Battery–Revised.* Pearson Assessments.

Leaman, M. C., & Edmonds, L. A. (2019). Conversation in aphasia across communication partners: Exploring stability of microlinguistic measures and communicative success. *American Journal of Speech-Language Pathology, 28*(15), 359–372. https://doi.org/10.1044/2018_AJSLP-17-0148

Li, E. C., Volpe, A. D., Ritterman, S., & Williams, S. E. (1996). Variations in grammatic complexity across three types of discourse. *Journal of Speech-Language Pathology and Audiology, 20*(3), 180–186. https://www.cjslpa.ca/download.php?file=/1996_JSLPA_Vol_20/No_03_169-217/Li_Ritterman_Volpe_JSLPA_1996.pdf

Liles, B. Z., & Coelho, C. A. (1998). Cohesion analysis. In L. R. Cherney, B. B. Shadden, & C. A. Coelho (Eds.), *Analyzing discourse in communicatively impaired adults* (pp. 65–84). Aspen.

MacWhinney, B. (2000). *The CHILDES Project: Tools for analyzing talk* (3rd ed.). Lawrence. https://doi.org/10.1177/026565909200800211

MacWhinney, B., Fromm, D., Holland, A., Forbes, M., & Wright, H. H. (2010). Automated analysis of the Cinderella story. *Aphasiology, 24*(6–8), 856–868. https://doi.org/10.1080/02687030903452632

Marini, A., Caltagirone, C., Pasqualetti, P., & Carlomagno, S. (2007). Patterns of language improvement in adults with nonchronic nonfluent aphasia after specific therapies. *Aphasiology, 21*(2), 164–186. https://doi.org/10.1080/02687030600633799

Miller, J., Gillon, G., & Westerveld, M. (2020). *Systematic Analysis of Language Transcripts (SALT).* In SALT Software, LLC (New Zealand/Australia Version 20).

Nicholas, L. E., & Brookshire, R. H. (1993). A system for quantifying the informativeness and efficiency of the connected speech of adults with aphasia. *Journal of Speech, Language and*

Hearing Research, 36(2), 338–350. https://doi.org/10.1044/jshr.3602.338

Nicholas, L. E., & Brookshire, R. H. (1995). Presence, completeness, and accuracy of main concepts in the connected speech of non-brain-damaged adults and adults with aphasia. *Journal of Speech, Language and Hearing Research, 38*(1), 145–156. https://doi.org/10.1044/jshr.3801.145

Peach, R. K., & Coelho, C. A. (2016). Linking inter- and intrasentential processes for narrative production following traumatic brain injury: Implications for a model of discourse processing. *Neuropsychologia, 80,* 157–164. https://doi.org/10.1016/j.neuropsychologia.2015.11.015

Pritchard, M., Hilari, K., Cocks, N., & Dipper, L. (2017). Reviewing the quality of discourse information measures in aphasia. *International Journal of Language and Communication Disorders, 52*(6), 689–732. https://doi.org/10.1111/1460-6984.12318

Richardson, J. D., & Dalton, S. G. (2016). Main concepts for three different discourse tasks in a large nonclinical sample. *Aphasiology, 30*(1), 45–73. https://doi.org/10.1080/02687038.2015.1057891

Schiffrin, D. (1994). *Approaches to discourse.* Blackwell.

Shadden, B. B. (1998). Sentential/surface-level analysis. In L. R. Cherney, B. B. Shadden, & C. A. Coelho (Eds.), *Analyzing discourse in communicatively impaired adults* (pp. 35–64). Aspen.

Simmons-Mackie, N., Kagan, A., O'Neill Christie, C., Huijbregts, M., McEwen, S., & Willems, J. (2007). Communicative access and decision making for people with aphasia: Implementing sustainable healthcare systems change. *Aphasiology, 21*(1), 39–66. https://doi.org/10.1080/02687030600798287

Stark, B. C. (2019). A comparison of three discourse elicitation methods in aphasia and age-matched adults: Implications for language assessment and outcome. *American Journal of Speech-Language Pathology, 28*(3), 1067–1083. https://doi.org/10.1044/2019_AJSLP-18-0265

Stark, B. C., Dutta, M., Murray, L. L., Fromm, D., Bryant, L., Harmon, T. G., . . . Roberts, A. C. (2021). Spoken discourse assessment and analysis in aphasia: An international survey of current practices. *Journal of Speech, Language and Hearing Research, 64*(11), 4366–4389. https://doi.org/10.1044/2021_JSLHR-20-00708

Stark, B. C., & Fukuyama, J. (2021). Leveraging big data to understand the interaction of task and language during monologic spoken discourse in speakers with and without aphasia. *Language, Cognition and Neuroscience, 36*(5), 562–585. https://doi.org/10.1080/23273798.2020.1862258

Sutherland, S. (2016). *A beginner's guide to discourse analysis.* Palgrave.

Thompson, C., & Shapiro, L. (2005). Treating agrammatic aphasia within a linguistic framework: Treatment of underlying forms. *Aphasiology, 19*(10–11), 1021–1036. https://doi.org/10.1080%2F02687030544000227

Thompson, C. K., Riley, E. A., den Ouden, D-B., Meltzer-Asscher, A., & Lukic, S. (2013). Training verb argument structure production in agrammatic aphasia: Behavioral and neural recovery patterns. *Cortex, 49*(9), 2358–2376. https://doi.org/10.1016/j.cortex.2013.02.003

Thompson, C. K., Shapiro, L. P., Li, L., & Schendel, L. (1995). Analysis of verbs and verb-argument structure: A method for quantification of aphasic language production. *Clinical Aphasiology, 23,* 121–140. http://aphasiology.pitt.edu/id/eprint/195

Ulatowska, H. K., Freedman-Stern, R., Doyel, A. W., Macaluso-Haynes, S., & North, A. J. (1983). Production of narrative discourse in aphasia. *Brain and Language, 19*(2), 317–334. https://doi.org/10.1016/0093-934x(83)90074-3

Ulatowska, H. K., North, A. J., & Macaluso-Haynes, S. (1981). Production of narrative and procedural discourse in aphasia. *Brain and Language, 13,* 345–371. https://doi.org/10.1016/0093-934X(81)90100-0

Ulatowska, H. K., Reyes, B., Santos, T. O., Garst, D., Vernon, J., & McArthur, J. (2013). Personal narratives in aphasia: Understanding narrative competence. *Topics in Stroke Reha-*

bilitation, 20(1), 36–43. https://doi.org/10.13 10/tsr2001-36

Wassenaar, M., Brown, C. M., & Hagoort, P. (2004). ERP effects of subject-verb agreement violations in patients with Broca's aphasia. *Journal of Cognitive Neuroscience, 16*(4), 553–576. https://doi.org/10.1162/0898929043230 57290

Williams, S. E., Li, E. C., Volpe, A. D., & Ritterman, S. (1994). The influence of topic and listener familiarity on aphasic discourse. *Journal of Communication Disorders, 27,* 207–222. https://doi.org/10.1016/0021-9924 (94)90001-9

Yorkston, K. M., & Beukelman, D. R. (1980). An analysis of connected speech samples of aphasic and normal speakers. *Journal of Speech and Hearing Disorders, 45*(1), 27–36. https://doi.org/10.1044/jshd.4501.27

Zhang, M., Geng, L., Yang, Y., & Ding, H. (2021). Cohesion in the discourse of people with post-stroke aphasia. *Clinical Linguistics and Phonetics, 35*(1), 2–18. https://doi.org/10.10 80/02699206.2020.1734864

6 Weaving Research Evidence and Clinical Expertise Together in Discourse Analysis of Spoken Personal Narratives in Aphasia

Lucy Dipper and Madeline Cruice

Introduction

In this chapter we propose a set of indicators for evaluating spoken discourse at different levels of language (word, sentence, and discourse superstructure). This proposal arises from a research project in which we created a new *assessment* and *treatment* package for discourse production in aphasia. This package is called Language Underpins Narrative in Aphasia (LUNA). LUNA was created specifically for evaluating and treating personal narratives, although the analyses described in this chapter can be used with any type of discourse. LUNA was developed through a systematic process in which we reviewed the evidence base, surveyed clinicians, and codesigned the content of the package itself with front line speech-language pathologists (SLPs) and people with aphasia.

The Importance of Personal Narratives in Living With Aphasia

In LUNA, discourse is addressed at word, sentence, and superstructure discourse levels, using a personal narrative told by the individual. Personal narratives are an appropriate assessment and treatment choice given their centrality in everyday communication, their multifunctional role (referential, evaluative, intra-, and interpersonal), and the opportunities they provide for personalization.

Personal narratives, and discourse more broadly, reflect communication activity in real-world settings, making discourse analysis an ideal primary outcome measure of functional communication. There is consensus among core stakeholders in aphasia rehabilitation that discourse is central in aphasia rehabilitation. People with aphasia identify improved discourse as a key priority (Wallace et al., 2017), and clinicians agree, indicating that treatment should support the person with aphasia to communicate more than their basic needs, such as memories and opinions (Wallace et al., 2017). Discourse treatment is highlighted in best practice guidelines; for example, it is recommended that treatment targets include communication in everyday environments (Power et al., 2015) to improve functional communication, including language therapy aimed at the production and comprehension of words, sentences, and superstructure discourse (Hebert et al., 2016).

Weaving Together Research Evidence and Clinical Expertise

LUNA was created to support evidence-based practice (EBP). The American Speech-Language-Hearing Association (ASHA) defines three pillars of EBP: the scientific literature, clinical expertise/expert opinion, and client/patient/caregiver perspectives (https://www.asha.org/research/ebp/). When these three knowledge bases are integrated, clinicians can make evidence-based decisions and provide services reflecting the values and choices of individuals with communication disorders (ASHA, 2021). This is an ambitious goal, and difficult to consistently achieve for all patients for two reasons. First, no clear, accessible tools exist that enable clinicians to do this integrated clinical reasoning on the front line. Second, EBP models have failed to consider the *clinical practice* knowledge base, which can significantly constrain or support the options that are available to patients. In the

field of discourse analysis in aphasia, there are several barriers that reportedly affect clinical practice (Bryant et al. 2017; Cruice et al., 2020).

It is thus important that any clinical tool is grounded in the existing research evidence but also sensitive to the needs of the intended users, SLPs working in inpatient or community settings. In the next section we outline the *discourse analysis protocol* (DAP) we created through this process of weaving together research evidence and clinical expertise.

Creating the LUNA DAP

The LUNA DAP was created in two stages. We first collected and reviewed information from two key knowledge bases: (1) clinical practice and (2) research. We then used this knowledge-gathering process to prepare for codesign sessions, in which codesigners (the academic research team, SLPs, and people with aphasia) used information extracted from the knowledge bases to make decisions about the DAP (see Cruice et al., 2021, for a full description of the LUNA codesign process). The outcome of this process was two versions of the LUNA DAP: the LUNA *Research DAP* and the LUNA *Clinical DAP*. The content of each DAP is outlined in Table 6–1. Definitions and an explanation about how to carry out these analyses come in a later section of the chapter.

Clinical Knowledge Base for the LUNA DAP

In 2019, 211 SLPs across the United Kingdom completed an online survey reporting on their regular clinical practice in sampling and analyzing discourse from people with

Table 6–1. Discourse Indicators Chosen in the LUNA Codesign Process

Indicator	Clinical Protocol	Research Protocol
Word Level		
Narrative words	X	X
Correct information units		X
Word classes		X
Type–token ratio of word classes		X
Sentence Level		
Complete utterances	X	X
Multiclause utterances		X
Predicate argument structure score		X
Discourse Superstructure Level		
Story grammar	X	X
Reference chains		X
Overall listener judgment		X

aphasia (Cruice et al., 2020). Most SLPs used standardized test picture descriptions for collecting samples and used clinical judgment to evaluate discourse ability. Few used transcription. When SLPs analyzed discourse, they considered word-finding difficulties, sentence structure, errors, word class, and communication of ideas, and they were largely confident in undertaking these analyses. Fewer SLPs analyzed story structure, cohesion, lexical diversity, morphology, and efficiency, and were significantly less confident in these analyses. The main reported barriers were time constraints, lack of expertise, lack of training, and no access to relevant resources. These survey findings highlighted a range in clinical expertise among those who participated in research, but also the substantial constraints of the practice context which needed consideration. These findings echoed previous reviews of clinical practice in what they reveal about the use of discourse analysis by clinicians internationally (Bryant et al., 2017; Frith et al., 2014).

Research Knowledge Base for the LUNA DAP

For this knowledge base, we consulted five sources: a review of the psychometrics of discourse measures (Pritchard et al., 2017); an empirical study on psychometric properties of discourse measures in aphasia (Pritchard et al., 2018); a study relating to the test-retest stability of measures of words in discourse (Boyle, 2014); and a review of spoken discourse treatment (Dipper, Marshall, Boyle, Botting, et al., 2021).

The first source revealed that psychometric data for discourse measures was sparse, and the key finding was that main concepts measures and correct information unit (CIU) measures had the strongest reported psychometric properties (Pritchard et al., 2017). Findings from the second source (Pritchard et al., 2018) indicated that story grammar, reference chains, and predicate argument structure were the strongest measures (in acceptability, reliability, and validity). The third source (Boyle, 2014) considered 25 word-based measures used to evaluate discourse (see Table 2 in Boyle [2014]), and found that only four were reliable enough for clinical decision making (# words per minute; #CIUs/minute; % of T-units with time fillers; and % of T-units with delays). In the final source, the outcome measures from 25 discourse treatment studies were categorized descriptively into whether they were standardized or not, and which linguistic level they assessed: word, sentence, or superstructure (Dipper, Marshall, Boyle, Botting, et al., 2021).

The Codesign Process

In creating the LUNA assessment and treatment package, the academic research team aimed to develop both a DAP and a treatment protocol that would be *feasible* and *acceptable* to SLPs and people with aphasia. One key means of achieving this was to involve these stakeholders in the development of LUNA so their perspectives and needs were considered from the very start. To this end, we worked with four SLPs and four people with aphasia in parallel strands of work, meeting regularly across a 6-month period. The SLP codesign group met 11 times (every 2 weeks), while the codesigners with aphasia met monthly. All sessions were conducted face to face, and the same three members of the academic research team met with both groups of codesigners. Groups were intentionally separated, as SLPs and people with aphasia were con-

tributing to different components. More information on the codesign process can be found in Cruice and colleagues (2021).

By working with SLPs and by constantly looking at discourse assessment and proposed therapy side by side in sessions, we created a program with strong links between assessment, goals, and treatment tasks. This close linkage between assessment and therapy constitutes a unique feature of LUNA. We return to the links between assessment, goals, and treatment at the end of this chapter in a section on the alignment of measurement and treatment.

Word-Level Decision Making

In the codesign sessions, we extracted and reviewed the possible word-level outcome measures from our knowledge bases. There were tensions among the competing demands of clinical value, psychometrics, acceptability to SLPs, and clinical utility. For example, CIUs were clearly used in many research studies, and according to Nicholas and Brookshire (1993), they can be applied to personal narratives. The CIU coding instructions were not considered user friendly for the average clinician and would need rewriting to make them usable. The SLP codesigners also considered the CIUs unlikely to drive clinical decision making in therapy, and did not consider them useful for outcome measurement, although this may not reflect international clinical practice. It was these tensions that ultimately motivated a decision to develop two protocols: one protocol intended for clinical use, and a second (more extensive) protocol intended only for research. The research protocol included the CIUs, but the clinical protocol did not. Finally, there was general consensus that word classes (count, type and token) were the most useful for therapy planning.

Suggested Word-Level Indicators for Assessment of Personal Narratives

- Correct information units (CIUs)
    - CIUs are "words that are intelligible in context, accurate in relation to the picture(s) or topic, and relevant to and informative about the content of the picture(s) or the topic" (Nicholas & Brookshire, 1993, p. 348).
    - We recommend counting them and then reporting them as an overall total for the discourse (#CIUs), as a percentage of the total number of all words (%CIUs), and as a measure of efficiency (CIUs per minute).
- Narrative words
    - Narrative words are a similar construct to CIUs, but their definition is different and is broader. There is more than one definition of narrative words in the research literature, but we recommend Saffran et al. (1989) for the most widely used operational definition. For the LUNA package, we created a simplified definition based on Saffran et al. (1989) but encompassing more words, as follows: narrative words are the words that remain in a discourse once the following have been removed:
        - Nonlinguistic fillers (e.g., *er, um, uh*)
        - Linguistic fillers (e.g., *yeah, well,* or *so*)
        - False starts (e.g., *diff-, er different, um different from, oh we were individuals*)
        - Repetitions (e.g, *a boat ... a boat, er ... a big boat*)
        - Extranarrative content (e.g., commentary about performance on the task, such as "*I can't think of the word.*")

- We recommend counting narrative words and then reporting this count as an overall total (#NWs), as a percentage of the total number of all words (%NWs), and as a measure of efficiency (NWs per minute).
- Word class
    - Word class refers to counts and lists of words in each lexical category; these are useful for therapy planning and for assessing treatment-related change.
- Lexical diversity
    - Type-token ratio (TTR) is one measure of lexical diversity. TTR can be a diversity measure for the whole discourse (irrespective of word class). It can also be calculated within a word class. We would recommend this calculation for nouns and verbs at minimum, because of the central role of these word classes in conveying the semantic content of a discourse. It is also possible to consider a TTR calculation for other word classes, such as adjectives and adverbs, if this was a target for improvement in treatment.

Sentence-Level Decision Making

As the team considered sentence- or utterance-level analyses, it rapidly emerged that the word-level indicators, while numerous, were relatively straightforward when compared with utterance-level analytical approaches. SLP codesigners proposed more global ratings of sentence structures and "lite" (less complex) options for clinicians unwilling and unable to complete detailed analyses. Ultimately, we agreed to consider complexity first and completeness second. The sentence level indicators eventually selected for inclusion in the LUNA DAPs are summarized below.

Suggested Sentence-Level Indicators for Assessment of Personal Narratives

- Complete utterances (C-units)
  - Utterances are defined in LUNA as a group of words which are grammatically connected to each other but not to any words outside the utterance. Saffran et al. (1989) used a similar definition and advocated for the combined use of syntactic, semantic, and prosodic indicators to make a decision about utterance boundaries. We followed this guidance.
  - C-unit: a main clause and all its dependent clauses
  - The distinction between dependent and independent clauses is crucial in finding utterance boundaries, which means that it is also important to distinguish the different types of conjunctions used to link clauses. There are coordinating conjunctions and subordinating conjunctions. The segmenting rule is to:
    - Separate utterances that are linked by a coordinating conjunction (into two utterances)
    - Keep together (as a single utterance) clauses that are joined by a subordinating conjunction
    - There is disagreement in the literature about which conjunctions are coordinating conjunctions. We took a narrow approach and included only *and, and then,* and *or* in this category.
  - Once a transcript has been divided into utterances, we recommend

coding each utterance as either *complete* or *incomplete*. The decision about completeness is both syntactic and semantic, with most emphasis on the syntax. Utterances are *incomplete* when they omit a key information-carrying word (e.g., a verb, noun, or key preposition) or phrase (e.g., a verb phrase, noun phrase, or key prepositional phrase). *Complete* utterances are those which appear to contain all necessary words OR those which omit only minor words (e.g., function words) such as determiners, auxiliary verbs, and less important prepositions (i.e., not those required by a verb).

  - We recommend counting the total number of utterances in a discourse (# utterances); counting the number of complete and incomplete utterances (#complete, #incomplete); and calculating the percentage of complete utterances (% complete). This yields a measure of completeness.
- Multiclause utterances
  - We recommend coding each utterance for complexity. We coded in a binary way (i.e., single-clause versus multiclause). It might also be useful to code utterances for how many dependent (i.e., subordinate or relative) clauses are combined with a main clause.
  - We recommend counting single- versus multiclause utterances (#single, #multi) and calculating the percentage of multiclause utterances in a discourse (% multi). This yields a measure of syntactic complexity.
- Predicate-argument structure (PAS)

- We recommend examining the PAS of each clause within an utterance.
  - A clause is defined as a syntactic unit containing both a noun phrase and a verb phrase; and as a semantic unit containing both a predicate (a verb or verb group) and arguments.
  - Arguments are the phrases needed to complete the core meaning of a predicate. For example, the verb *throw* requires [someone] to throw [something]; and the verb *put* requires [someone] to put [something] [somewhere]. It helps to think about sentence elements that you would embody if you were to gesture a sentence's meaning—each embodied element would be an argument.
  - Nonarguments (or adjuncts) are phrases containing semantic information that is not core to a verb's meaning such as place, time, measurement, or accompaniment. Note that these would not be part of a gesture or the predicate meaning.
- We recommend counting the number of predicates and arguments in the discourse (#predicates, #arguments) and then calculating a mean PAS score (= #arguments/#predicates). This yields a measure relating to semantic complexity.

Superstructure-Level Decision Making

A review of the clinical knowledge base showed that clinicians attempted to assess discourse superstructure. However, the extent to which they felt they did this

systematically or accurately varied widely. This knowledge base also revealed a misunderstanding about discourse superstructure; there was a belief that there is a single way to evaluate a person's skills at this level. In fact, just as at other levels of language, each analysis or measure evaluates a specific aspect of superstructure. For example, a measure of local coherence provides an evaluation of how well one utterance links to the next, whereas a measure of global coherence provides an evaluation of how well each utterance relates to the overall topic.

The SLP codesigners felt strongly about assessing the functional and pragmatic components of telling personal stories, but this did not feature in the research knowledge base. There was also some indication in the clinical knowledge base that SLPs undertake discourse assessment to try to evaluate functional and pragmatic aspects of discourse. Consequently, we agreed about the need for a social validity indicator at the discourse level. We decided on a listener judgment measure, selecting elements from two published papers (Cupit et al., 2010 and Jacobs, 2001) to include evaluation of effectiveness, informativeness and comfort (but exclude evaluation of grammar since we have this elsewhere in the DAP) and to allow rating on a specific scale. The discourse superstructure indicators eventually selected for inclusion in the LUNA DAPs are summarized below.

Suggested Superstructure-Level Indicators for Assessment of Personal Narratives

- Story grammar
  - Story grammar is a superstructure measure that identifies story elements from a predetermined set

that is expected to occur at either the beginning, middle, or end of a discourse. There are various versions of the set of story grammar elements in the aphasia literature. In LUNA we use the following nine elements:

- Beginning: abstract, time, location, participants
- Middle: initiating/complicating event, events
- End: evaluation, result/resolution, coda/conclusion

Definitions and examples of these elements are included on the companion website.

- We recommend marking each of the nine elements as either present or absent to provide a measure of overall superstructure skill and to identify targets for treatment (#SG elements present). This simple present/absent scoring may not be sensitive enough to measure post-treatment change, however. More work needs to be done on the psychometrics of this analysis before a recommendation can be made for outcome measurement.
- Reference chains
  - Reference chains are chains of words in disparate places across a discourse that refer to the same person, place, or thing. We recommend confining identification to only those chains where the first referent is a noun (or noun phrase) and the others are pronouns.
  - We recommend counting complete versus incomplete reference chains (#complete, #incomplete) and calculating the percentage of complete reference chains in a discourse (% complete). This yields a measure

of cohesion, which other authors consider to be micro- or macrostructure (see Chapter 1).

- Overall listener judgment
  - We recommend including a socially valid measure of listener judgement, where listeners are asked to rate on a scale the effectiveness and informativeness of a discourse as well as the overall listening comfort. Raters can include family members, SLPs, or naïve listeners.

Conceptualizing and Framing the Discourse Measures

An agreed theoretical framework for guiding discourse analysis is important. First, it helps us to more fully specify the key linguistic levels that we believe to be inherent in discourse production, allowing for further refinement of analytic methods in this area. Second, a framework helps us to navigate the multiplicity of discourse measures. As the sections above demonstrate, there are currently multiple ways to assess spoken discourse in the aphasia evidence base, and more than 500 ways to calculate assessment outcome scores. The unified theoretical framework outlined in Dipper, Marshall, Boyle, Hersh, et al. (2021) is intended to be routinely used to guide either assessment or treatment choices. To create it, we integrated key linguistic theories into four components: pragmatics, macrostructure[1] planning, propositional, and linguistic (Box 6–1). These components consist of groups of related skills that can be distinguished from the skills in other components. They have been drawn from the theoretical literature and can be used to

---

[1]In this paper, we refer to superstructure and macrolinguistic aspects with the term *macrostructure planning*

> **BOX 6–1. Four Key Components Underpinning Discourse Production**
>
> 1. *Pragmatics:* The skills in this component provide an overall influence on spoken discourse. The speaker makes decisions about linguistic structure, content, and form based on environmental, interpersonal, and interactional factors. In brief, the skills in this component are required for planning and monitoring the *interactional purpose* of the discourse. In the LUNA framework, the components sit inside one another to indicate that each has the potential to influence another, with feedback possible both upward and downward.
>
> 2. *Macrostructure Planning:* This component unites the skills needed for the creation of macrolinguistic coherence and superstructure. The processing needed here will involve online structural decisions (for example, in response to pragmatic factors or linguistic difficulties) as well as the use of familiar templates.
>
> 3. *Propositional:* This component is a prelinguistic component that feeds into linguistic processing. It pares down the macro plans into propositions and then sequences the propositions. The paring-down process involves creating linguistically appropriate micro plans for individual utterances.
>
> 4. *Linguistic:* This component translates each proposition into language, involving familiar linguistic skills such as lexical selection and syntax.

describe the difficulties and residual skills seen in spoken discourse, to guide discourse analysis choices, and to structure treatment for spoken discourse. The components can also be used as hypothetical processing components to guide research.

Using the Framework to Guide Discourse Analysis

In developing the two DAPs (clinical and research), we used the LUNA framework as an additional lens through which to view, consider, and select the measures. To make the decision making clear and clinically focused, we categorized measures into word, sentence, and superstructure measures during codesign. Then, as an additional filter, we mapped the selected measures onto each component of the LUNA framework to check for breadth, completeness, and overlap.

To map measures to the framework, we had to consider the concept/construct[2] as well as the skills being assessed. This distinction between concepts and related skills is not one routinely made in the aphasia literature, leading to some lack of clarity about what it is that discourse measures are

---

[2]The terms *construct* and *concept* both relate to generalizable properties, patterns, and characteristics associated with a phenomenon (in this case with spoken discourse). While there is a distinction between these terms (a concept is a precise and measurable idea used to describe a pattern or property that can be observed, whereas a construct is an abstract concept created to explain a pattern or property and hypothesized), it is not apparent or consistent in the theoretical literature relating to discourse.

measuring. For example, assessing the proportion of complete utterances produced in a discourse would determine sentence production *skill* and provide information related to the theoretical *construct* of syntax.

The connections between concepts and skills are complex, and it is difficult to uniquely assess concepts by observing a particular skill because of the interrelatedness of the concepts and the hypothesized feedback between components of the LUNA framework. For example, as we have just outlined, an assessment of the proportion of complete utterances would provide information related to the construct of syntax primarily; however, the construction of an utterance also provides information about the constructs of semantic-conceptual content, lexical-semantic content, and lexical form. Furthermore, some measures assess a theoretical construct only partially, such as correct information units (CIUs), which target informativeness in a discourse and are intended to quantitatively evaluate discourse as a function of its success in communicating information efficiently. However, the CIU score is a measure used to assess the skill of *word* production primarily and it provides information about word-level informativeness; it does not provide information about the informativeness of the discourse more broadly. In addition, there is often more than one way to measure the same, or very similar, skills. For example, sentence production skill can be assessed using the proportion of complete utterances, a mean predicate-argument structure (PAS) score, or the proportion of treated sentence structures that are produced in a discourse. Finally, there is complexity arising from a lack of specification about what skill or concept a measure is measuring and how it might relate to another measure.

Taking the selected LUNA outcome measures from the LUNA Research DAP as examples, we can illustrate how the LUNA framework helps to organize and guide discourse analysis choices and to increase some of this specification.

Linguistic component measures should evaluate the following:

- **Constructs:** cohesion, informativeness, syntax, lexical-semantic content, lexical form
- **Skills:** production of linguistic items to create reference chains/lexical cohesion; relating to topic/gist; denoting relevant semantic-conceptual content; with the correct form (syntactic, morphological, phonological)
- **Selected Research DAP measures:** narrative words, CIUs, word counts

Propositional component measures should evaluate the following:

- **Constructs:** local coherence, cohesion (planning), informativeness, semantic-conceptual content
- **Skills:** production of sentences that relate to each other, reference chains/lexical cohesion, linguistic items denoting semantic-conceptual content
- **Selected Research DAP measures:** complete utterances, multiclause utterances, PAS score

Macrostructure planning measures should evaluate the following:

- **Constructs:** macrostructure (or superstructure), topic coherence, informativeness
- **Skills:** production of specific schemas/story grammar elements and linguistic items relating to topic/gist; reference chains and cohesion planning and monitoring

■ **Selected Research DAP measures:** story grammar, reference chains

Pragmatics measures should evaluate the following

■ **Constructs:** informativeness, relevance, quantity, quality, and appropriateness
■ **Skills:** there are no specifically pragmatic skills that are commonly referred to in the discourse literature in aphasia, neither in the treatment literature or assessment literature, that we examined as part of the five sources. We can speculate here, based on the wider pragmatics literature, that the key skills relate to three main areas:
  ■ *Using* language for a particular purpose (e.g., to convince or to make someone laugh) or effect (e.g., to convey emotion or evocatively describe a scene); thinking about engaging the listener;
  ■ *Changing* language or communicative adaptation (Penn, 1999) in response to linguistic, environmental, and interpersonal factors; and
  ■ *Following* rules, which in conversation might include turn taking and in spoken narrative discourse would relate to expectations about how stories start and are otherwise structured, as well as expectations about how long you should talk and how you leave space for listener reactions or signal that you have finished.
■ **Selected Research DAP measures:** listener judgement

Being able to situate a measure in the LUNA framework reveals potential links between performance in different components. For example, the following can co-occur:

■ Word-finding difficulties indicated by a low score in a linguistic measure such as CIUs
■ Sentence level difficulties indicated by a measure that sits on the boundary between the linguistic and propositional components of discourse such as complete utterances
■ Difficulties with superstructure indicated by a measure such as story grammar
■ Difficulties in the pragmatic component, indicated by a low score on a measure of listener judgement.

The LUNA framework guides us to consider these concurrently as components of spoken discourse, rather than presenting these as the results from diverse assessments of different skills. This, in turn, motivates and structures the search for a link between them. There are various ways that these behaviours could be linked, and the particular link for an individual will be related to their profile of impairment.

Using the LUNA Framework—Example 1

The discourse of a person with anomia is characterized by difficulty with nouns and a relative absence of them. This is likely to manifest across a discourse in *microlinguistic* difficulties in word (noun) and sentence (argument nouns) production, affecting productivity, informational content, and grammatical completeness, as well as in linking meaning across adjacent sentences using nouns (cohesion). At the *macrolinguistic* level, the difficulty or absence of nouns will affect coherence (gist) and at the *superstructural* level, the noun difficulty will result in missing aspects of story content, such as missing labels for people, places, and things, and missing temporal and logical relationships between people and events. However, a different profile of impairment might pattern in similar but subtly different ways across the components of the LUNA framework as in the next example.

Using the LUNA Framework— Example 2

The discourse of a person with nonfluent (Broca's) aphasia is characterized by a lack of verbs and difficulties constructing sentences. This is likely to manifest across a discourse in *microlinguistic* difficulties in word (verb) and sentence (verb and argument phrase) production, affecting productivity, informational content, and grammatical completeness, as well as in cohesion—this time because of difficulties linking verbs and argument phrases across sentences. At the *macrolinguistic* level, the difficulty with verbs and sentences will significantly affect coherence and at the *superstructural* level, the result will be missing aspects of story content relating to events and missing temporal and logical relationships between them.

Aligning Measurement and Treatment

While the sections above are concerned with *what* we are measuring in spoken discourse, an equally important question to ask is *why* we are measuring it and what we will do with the outcome. International surveys of clinical practice in aphasia outcome measurement present a picture of evolution toward more routine use of outcome measurement, an increase in understanding its purpose, and diversification in the

constructs measured (Kiran et al., 2018). Researchers have noted a similar increase over time in the use of discourse analysis as part of outcome measurement: this is true of both *research* practice (Brady et al., 2016; Bryant et al., 2016; Dietz & Boyle, 2018) and *clinical* practice (Bryant et al., 2017; Cruice et al., 2020).

Measurement does more than just evaluate an outcome. Clinicians measure to assist in treatment planning, to monitor change, to evaluate the impact of treatment (Golper & Frattali, 2013); to diagnose; to describe the characteristics, severity, and functional impact of aphasia; and to make recommendations for intervention and other support (ASHA Aphasia Practice Portal, n.d.). Thus, clinicians use measurement to guide and to evaluate their practice, and it is integral to everything they do. For this reason, it is important that assessment, treatment, and outcome measurement should align. It is not clear, however, that such alignment is always apparent in the research evidence base. In our systematic review of spoken discourse treatment literature in aphasia (Dipper, Marshall, Boyle, Botting, et al., 2021), we found that discourse treatments have been evaluated in a wide range of ways, including measures of word, sentence, and superstructure; language ability more generally; functional communication; and impact.

Within this overall picture, there are some signs of alignment such as the finding that treatments aimed specifically at improving the words produced in discourse used outcome measures that assessed word production. But in fact, the most used measure across *all* discourse treatments was related to words, which means that treatments targeting sentences in discourse, treatments targeting superstructure, and treatments simultaneously targeting multiple levels of discourse also evaluated their effectiveness in words produced in discourse. There were other signs of misalignment, too, such as the finding that very few studies evaluated the effects of their treatment on discourse superstructure.

The LUNA framework can help to increase the assessment-treatment-outcome measurement alignment through its distinct components. Consider Examples 1 and 2 above and how they might be remediated.

Example 1 described the discourse of a person with anomia, highlighting the effects of a difficulty with nouns at multiple levels. How then might assessment and treatment be aligned for this person? The LUNA framework would suggest that assessment focused on the *Linguistic* component and primarily evaluating words used in discourse (for example, errors, omissions, and diversity) would be appropriate. The outcome of this assessment would support the clinician in planning treatment for words in discourse, both in selecting relevant treatment targets and choosing the relevant discourse or discourses to be treated. For example, the initial assessment might reveal that abstract nouns are routinely omitted from discourse, that there was little diversity in the concrete nouns produced, and that there was an associated lack of adjectives. This outcome might motivate the clinician to plan treatment activities first targeting words in isolation (i.e., targeting the *Linguistic* component) to increase diversity, using semantic or phonological strategies. Next, treatment might target the wider linguistic context using activities that require the production of nouns in noun phrases (*Linguistic* component) to support increased adjective use, and others that require the production of nouns in sentences (*Linguistic* and *Propositional* components) using color-coded sentence frames to highlight noun slots. Finally, nouns could be practiced in

discourse, which would utilize strengths in *Macrostructure Planning* and *Pragmatics* rather than directly treating skills in these components. An appropriate outcome measure for this treatment would be a measure of words in discourse, such as a noun count, CIUs, or narrative words.

If, however, the initial evaluation indicated that pronouns were a source of difficulty, the treatment plan could be tailored to reflect the fact that difficulties with pronouns would have greater effect in the *Propositional* and *Macrostructure Planning* components than the *Linguistic* component. This is because of the important role of pronouns in creating cohesion and coherence. Treatment activities could target the production of complete and clear reference chains, and the outcome of treatment could be evaluated by means of a count of complete reference chains (used in a discourse) or a rating of local coherence.

Example 2 described the discourse of a person with a nonfluent aphasia affecting verb and sentence production. It would be appropriate to focus assessment on both the *Linguistic* and *Propositional* components of the LUNA framework, evaluating words used in isolation and in sentences (for example, errors, omissions, and diversity of verbs; and completeness of sentences or PAS). The outcome of this assessment might reveal that verbs are routinely produced in isolation or with a subject noun only, and that they lack diversity (mostly event verbs, few state verbs). There could also be a paucity of adverbs and prepositions linked to the predicate-argument production difficulties. This outcome might motivate the clinician to plan treatment activities first targeting verbs in isolation (targeting the *Linguistic* component), using semantic strategies to increase diversity and to support the production of state verbs. Next, it would be important to also target the *Propositional* component with treatment activities requiring the production of verbs in sentence contexts, for example describing events using color-coded sentence frames to support the production of appropriate arguments (including noun and prepositional phrase arguments for events, and noun, preposition, and adjective phrase arguments for state verbs). Additionally, the use of these sentences could be practiced in a discourse context, linking them to elements of story grammar, and thereby also drawing on the *Macrostructure Planning* component. A relevant outcome measure for this treatment would be a *Propositional* measure such as complete utterances or PAS score.

The outcome measures highlighted in the sections above can be considered the most appropriate measures for assessing the proximal effect of treatment activity. Given the interrelatedness of the components in the LUNA framework, however, there is some rationale for also considering distal effects. For example, treatment targeting words in discourse should be primarily evaluated for its proximal effect on the *Linguistic* component but could additionally be evaluated for its distal effect on the *Propositional* component (e.g., by exploring whether increased noun production has a knock-on effect on the completeness of utterances), on the *Macrostructure Planning* component (e.g., by exploring whether increased noun production has a knock-on effect on the number of complete reference chains produced or on story grammar), and on *Pragmatics* (e.g., improved listener judgement). Although less positive, it could be just as informative to find an absence of any of these hypothesized distal improvements because it would suggest that additional treatment activities are needed to scaffold improvements from one component to the next.

Recommendations for Future Work

Future research needs to ensure that we have psychometrically robust measures available that reflect the linguistic complexity of discourse, including, at a minimum, measures of word and sentence production, superstructure, and pragmatics. This echoes and extends the recommendation made by Dietz and Boyle (2018) that consensus be reached on a set of outcome measures for discourse treatment that address micro- and macrolinguistic aspects of discourse and superstructure. We believe the best way to ensure this is to recommend alignment of measures with a processing model or theoretical framework such as the LUNA framework.

Central to the LUNA project were feasibility and acceptability, which motivate further recommendations. First, clinical feasibility should be at the forefront of future developments in discourse assessment so that clear information is provided to guide clinicians in selecting measures, such as information about which skill a measure targets and to which conceptual component of discourse this skill relates. Furthermore, a consideration of clinical usage would mean that new discourse measures are designed from the outset to be feasible and acceptable to clinicians. A final recommendation relating to acceptability is for measures to be chosen with meaningfulness for people with aphasia in mind. As an example, in partnership with the people with aphasia who acted as advisors and collaborators for the treatment phase of the LUNA project, we agreed on a set of goals for therapeutic work on personal stories. These goals indicated that LUNA treatment should have at least five beneficial effects: it should make the story (1) richer, (2) more meaningful, (3) more complete, (4) make more sense, and (5) flow more. Discourse analysis researchers would do well to target the development or refinement of measures that evaluate whether treatment does indeed have the five beneficial effects on discourse.

References

American Speech-Language-Hearing Association (ASHA). (n.d.). *Aphasia* [Practice portal]. http://www.asha.org/Practice-Portal/Clinical-Topics/Aphasia/

ASHA. (2021). *Evidence-based practice (EBP)*. https://www.asha.org/research/ebp/

Boyle, M. (2014). Test-retest stability of word retrieval in aphasic discourse. *Journal of Speech, Language, and Hearing Research, 57*, 966–978. https://doi.org/10.1044/2014_JSLHR-L-13-0171

Brady, M. C., Kelly, H., Godwin, J., Enderby, P., & Campbell, P. (2016). Speech and language therapy for aphasia following stroke. *Cochrane Database of Systematic Reviews, 6*, CD000425. https://doi.org/10.1002/14651858.CD000425.pub4

Bryant, L., Ferguson, A., & Spencer, E. (2016). Linguistic analysis of discourse in aphasia: A review of the literature. *Clinical Linguistics and Phonetics, 30*(7), 489–518. https://doi.org/10.3109/02699206.2016.1145740

Bryant, L., Spencer, E., & Ferguson, A. (2017). Clinical use of linguistic discourse analysis for the assessment of language in aphasia. *Aphasiology, 31*(10), 1105–1126. https://doi.org/10.1080/02687038.2016.1239013

Cruice, M., Aujla, S., Bannister, J., Botting, N., Boyle, M., Charles, N., . . . Dipper, L. (2021). Creating a novel approach to discourse treatment through coproduction with people with aphasia and speech and language therapists. *Aphasiology*, online. https://doi.org/10.1080/02687038.2021.1942775

Cruice, M., Botting, N., Marshall, J., Boyle, M., Hersh, D., Pritchard, M., & Dipper, L. (2020). U.K. speech and language therapists' views

and reported practices of discourse analysis in aphasia rehabilitation. *International Journal of Language and Communication Disorders, 55*(3), 417–442. https://doi.org/10.1111/1460-6984.12528

Cupit, J., Rochon, E., Leonard, C. and Laird, L. (2010). Social validation as a measure of improvement after aphasia treatment: Its usefulness and influencing factors. *Aphasiology, 24*(11), 1486–1500. https://doi.org/10.1080/02687031003615235

Dietz, A., & Boyle, M. (2018). Discourse measurement in aphasia research: Have we reached the tipping point? *Aphasiology, 32*(4), 459–464. https://doi.org/10.1080/02687038.2017.1398803

Dipper, L., Marshall, J., Boyle, M., Botting, N., Hersh, D., Pritchard, M., & Cruice, M. (2021). Treatment for improving discourse in aphasia: A systematic review and synthesis of the evidence base. *Aphasiology, 35*(9), 1125–1167. https://doi.org/10.1080/02687038.2020.1765305

Dipper, L., Marshall, J., Boyle, M., Hersh, D., Botting, N., & Cruice, M. (2021). Creating a theoretical framework to underpin discourse assessment and intervention in aphasia. *Brain Sciences, 11*(2), 183. https://doi.org/10.3390/brainsci11020183

Frith, M., Togher, L., Ferguson, A., Levick, W., & Docking, K. (2014). Assessment practices of speech-language pathologists for cognitive communication disorders following traumatic brain injury in adults: An international survey. *Brain Injury, 28*(13–14), 1657–1666. https://doi.org/10.3109/02699052.2014.947619

Golper, L. C., & Frattali, C. M. (Eds.). (2013). *Outcomes in speech-language pathology* (2nd ed.). Thieme.

Hebert, D., Lindsay, M. P., McIntyre, A., Kirton, A., Rumney, P. G., Bagg, S., . . . Glasser, E. (2016). Canadian stroke best practice recommendations: Stroke rehabilitation practice guidelines (updated 2015). *International Journal of Stroke, 11*(4), 459–484. https://doi.org/10.1177/1747493016643553

Jacobs, B. (2001). Social validity of changes in informativeness and efficiency of aphasic discourse following linguistic specific treatment

(LST). *Brain and Language, 78*(1), 115–127. https://doi.org/10.1006/brln.2001.2452

Kiran, S., Cherney, L. R., Kagan, A., Haley, K. L., Antonucci, S. M., Schwartz, M., . . . Simmons-Mackie, N. (2018). Aphasia assessments: A survey of clinical and research settings. *Aphasiology, 32*(Suppl. 1), 47–49. https://doi.org/10.1080/02687038.2018.1487923

Nicholas, L. E., & Brookshire, R. H. (1993). A system for quantifying the informativeness and efficiency of the connected speech of adults with aphasia. *Journal of Speech, Language, and Hearing Research, 36*(2), 338–350. https://doi.org/10.1044/jshr.3602.338

Penn, C. (1999). Pragmatic assessment and therapy for persons with brain damage: What have clinicians gleaned in two decades? *Brain and Language, 68*(3), 535–552. https://doi.org/10.1006/brln.1999.2127

Power, E., Thomas, E., Worrall, L., Rose, M., Togher, L., Nickels, L., . . . O'Connor, C. (2015). Development and validation of Australian aphasia rehabilitation best practice statements using the RAND/UCLA appropriateness method. *BMJ Open, 5*(7), e007641. https://doi.org/10.1136/bmjopen-2015-007641

Pritchard, M., Hilari, K., Cocks, N., & Dipper, L. (2017). Reviewing the quality of discourse information measures in aphasia. *International Journal of Language and Communication Disorders, 52*(6), 689–732. https://doi.org/10.1111/1460-6984.12318

Pritchard, M., Hilari, K., Cocks, N., & Dipper, L. (2018). Psychometric properties of discourse measures in aphasia: Acceptability, reliability, and validity. *International Journal of Language and Communication Disorders, 53*(6), 1078–1093. https://doi.org/10.1111/1460-6984.12420

Saffran, E. M., Berndt, R. S., & Schwartz, M. F. (1989). The quantitative analysis of agrammatic production: Procedure and data. *Brain and Language, 37*(3), 440–479. https://doi.org/10.1016/0093-934X(89)90030-8

Wallace, S. J., Worrall, L., Rose, T., Le Dorze, G., Cruice, M., Isaksen, J., . . . Gauvreau, C. A. (2017). Which outcomes are most important to people with aphasia and their families? An international nominal group technique study framed within the ICF. *Disability and Rehabilitation, 39*(14), 1364–1379. https://doi.org/10.1080/09638288.2016.1194899

7 Clinical Application of Conversation Analysis in Aphasia

Jamie H. Azios and Nina Simmons-Mackie

Introduction

Traditionally, assessment of aphasia has focused largely on words, sentences, and monologues such as describing a picture, retelling a story, or describing a procedure. In other words, the language of the individual with aphasia has been the focus. However, an ultimate therapy goal for most people with aphasia is to be able to engage *with others* in conversation. Conversation is the most familiar and widespread of all discourse genres. People with aphasia, like all of us, want to socialize, share information, and reveal who they are through conversation. Goodwin (2003) describes conversation as "the site where language emerges as action in the lived social world, and the place where the results of brain damage become both visible and consequential for people's lives" (p. 3). Therefore, analysis of conversational discourse is an important objective in meaningful management of aphasia. But what is required to converse? What makes a successful conversation? How is conversation different from other discourse genres? Answers to these questions are of critical importance to assessing and managing aphasia.

Understanding Conversation

An understanding of conversation is the first step toward assessing conversational discourse in aphasia (see the companion website). Some elements of conversation are obvious to all of us. For example, conversation requires interaction between two or more people. Conversation requires a cooperative give and take among participants to achieve an orderly and meaningful exchange. Even an argument requires cooperation as participants take turns and observe conversational conventions. Conversation is synchronous; that is, participants are present and engaged at the same time. Conversation entails both the exchange of messages and the management of social relationships. "Conversational situations are never just conversational. They are governed by social rules as well as conversational rules" (Bach & Harnish, 1979, p. 105). Although we typically think of conversation as spoken, multiple channels convey information and social meanings. Channels such as voice, speech, gesture, body movement, silence, and gaze are layered into an interaction to assist in the fulfillment of conversational goals.

Conversation includes obligatory as well as optional actions. For example, although turn taking is a required element of conversation, there are several methods for shifting turns and, although participant turns are not always equal, all participants have the "right" to participate and collaborate on the actual distribution and length of turns.

Obvious Elements of Conversation

- Involves two or more people
- Interactive/entails give and take
- Cooperative
- Synchronous
- Involves both message exchange and social management
- Involves multiple communication channels
- Includes obligatory as well as optional actions
- The "right" to participate is distributed across or among participants

---

In addition to the obvious elements of conversation, there are a variety of less obvious features that are essential for successful conversation. The sequential organization of conversational interaction is a key feature. Sequential organization is the way that individual utterances or actions are embedded within orderly sequences of talk (Sacks et al., 1974). Adjacency pairs are components of sequential organization. An adjacency pair is a two-part sequence in which the second utterance is dependent on the first. For example, a question calls for an answer (e.g., 1: "What is that?" 2: "A pen"); a greeting calls for a return greeting (e.g., 1: "Hi Jane." 2: "Hi"); and a conversational closure calls for a subsequent closure (e.g., 1: "Bye Claire." 2: "Bye Laura"). In other words, the first part of the adjacency pair determines what happens next. If person 1 says "Hi," and person 2 fails to return the greeting, the result is likely to be social awkwardness; the expected adjacency sequence has not been observed. There are also three-part sequences such as the familiar teaching sequence (request-response-evaluation) in which the clinician makes a request ("Tell me the name of that"), the client responds ("A coat"), and the clinician evaluates the response ("Good!").

An appreciation of conversation requires understanding the concept of preference organization, a notion closely tied to sequential organization. Preference organization is based on the principle that certain actions in conversation constrain what follows in a discourse sequence (i.e., sequential organization) and within these sequential constraints, certain actions tend to be favored or *preferred* because they promote affiliation (i.e., a positive relationship), while other actions are not favored since they are more likely to promote disaffiliation. For example, if one speaker invites the other to dinner ("Would you join me for dinner tonight?"), the next speaker might choose to agree ("Yes, I'd love to"—a preferred response) or decline the invitation ("No"—a dispreferred action). The companion website includes examples of preferred and dispreferred responses to conversational acts. Preference management is important in fostering and maintaining relationships and establishing a desired public image.

The concept of face is closely related to preference organization and is important to the social management of conversation. Face is the public image that people wish to project in a social situation. During conversation participants strive to maintain face and protect the face of others. Conversation often involves potentially face-threatening actions such as disagreements, requests, or criticisms. "The goal of face work is to maintain the 'ritual equilibrium' of everyday social life through ceremonial rules and expressions" (Treviño, 2003, p. 38). These rules and expressions might include elements such as compliments and apologies as well as less obvious practices designed to maintain face. For example, expressing disagreement might result in the speaker being evaluated as disagreeable or rude. To mitigate such face threats, speakers employ politeness strategies. The use of hedging or moving a disagreement further from the source of disagreement are typical strategies to soften a disagreement. Consider the different image projected by these two disagreements: "No, you're wrong" versus "I can see your point, but I rather disagree." The second uses an introduction that establishes common ground, and then hedges with "rather" to weaken the disagreement. Depending on the context and the goals of participants, speakers modify utterances to manage face. Imagine the difficulty encountered by people with aphasia in attempting to layer politeness strategies and face work on to the raw content of an utterance. In analyzing conversation in aphasia, it is important to remain sensitive to novel methods used to manage face.

Another key feature of conversation is the drive for progressivity; conversationalists continuously work to move the conversation forward. For example, in Western communities, if a speaker pauses for 2 or more seconds, another participant might take over talk to keep the conversation going. Repair of conversational breakdown is particularly relevant to progressivity issues in conversation. Speakers in conversation sometimes experience problems; these "trouble sources" typically entail problems in speaking, hearing, or under-

standing. When a speaker has trouble, participants strive to repair or fix the problem quickly and progress forward. When one of the participants has aphasia, repairs can be lengthy. In conversation there is a difficult trade-off between attempting to get it right and moving the conversation forward. It might be preferable for the person with aphasia to opt for an agrammatic utterance rather than interrupting progress with a slow or repaired attempt at accurate syntax. Additionally, a lengthy repair signals that something is wrong (e.g., the speaker is not fulfilling the conversational imperative; is not competent). Thus, failure to fulfill a conversational preference such as progressivity not only impedes communication, but also has implications for the person's identity and social standing.

Related to progressivity is the drive for economy or least collaborative effort (Clark & Wilkes-Gibbs, 1986). Participants in conversation prefer to progress forward with the least amount of effort. Thus, natural conversation is often not well formed; it is rife with ellipses, sentence fragments, repetitions, omissions, discourse markers ("you know," "well") and other characteristics not representative of grammatically complete utterances but that serve other purposes, such as managing the progress of discourse and reducing burden of effort.

Another important consideration in conversation is the role of context. Utterances and social actions are shaped by the immediate context and create context as conversation unfolds (Heritage, 1984). Moment-to-moment events and unfolding talk have significant influences on the conversation. Context often contributes significantly to communication in aphasia. For example, Goodwin (2003) describes a man who utters only three words yet embeds these words along with finely tuned gestures into the turns of others to create meaning that can only be understood in the immediate context.

Co-construction is an important characteristic that distinguishes conversation from monologic discourse. Co-construction refers to the joint activity by which conversational participants collaborate to create meaning. Co-construction of talk is particularly apparent in word searches as demonstrated in the following excerpt of conversation between a man with aphasia (Ed), his wife (M), and a third party (from Oelschlaeger & Damico, 2003, p. 216).

Example 7–1.

01	Ed	Well, I was a (pause) I'm the—uhm how should I say it? (pause) I'm:::
02		Can't think of the name of it.
03	M	Draftsman?
04	Ed	Draftsman.

Participation of speaking partners during word searches is a frequently observed joint action in both aphasic and standard conversation. Verbal as well as nonverbal behaviors (e.g., gaze, body lean, pauses) serve as invitations to partners to participate in word searches.

Conversational discourse requires multilevel management. Conversation is a social act embedded in a larger social situation. That is, conversational contributions not only require semantics, phonology, and syntax, but also require titrating verbal and nonverbal behaviors to prevailing social norms, the immediate context, and the speaking partner. A good example is the difference in a linguistic task requiring the retelling of a story by someone with aphasia (e.g., the *Cinderella* retell often used in aphasia research) and the telling of a story within the flow of a conversation. In a structured story retell, there is a focus on the orderly, accurate production of content. However, when a story is told in conversation, it requires careful attention to the interactional and sequential context. The potential storyteller must first establish an audience for the story and gain permission for the story to begin. This is typically accomplished with a story preface, a turn in which the speaker proposes (possibly indirectly) to tell a story. The listener then either agrees to hear the story or not. A story sequence and related actions from a typical conversation in partners without aphasia can be seen in Example 7–2.

Example 7–2 (from Hutchby & Wooffitt, 2008, p. 131).

01	Story preface	L:	Oh: .hh Yi—m— You know I—I— I'm broiling about
02			something hhhhheh ⌈heh. hhhh
03	Request to tell story	J:	⌊Wha::t.
04	Story begins	L:	Well that sa:le (0.2) At—at the vicarage.
05			(0.6)
06	Recipient accepts	J:	Oh ye:s
		L:	(story continues)

The storyteller uses multiple modalities to identify an entry moment for the story. Often this requires quickly entering the flow of talk and offering a story preface to gain permission to tell the story (line 1). The listener either requests that the speaker continue and tell the story (as in line 3 above) or declines to hear the story (e.g., changes the topic, refers to earlier talk). The story preface sets the tone and the context for the hearer's interpretation of what is to come. Then as stories unfold, listeners provide comments, questions, or acknowledgments that become part of the sequential organization of the story. Listener responses that do not demonstrate alignment or affiliation can effectively shut down the storytelling. In other words, stories in conversation typically require multiple turns and involve the listener(s) as well as the storyteller. As the story is told, the timing, word choice, intonation, accompanying gestures and body language, gaze, and other elements are carefully adjusted by teller and hearer(s) to co-construct the story *in situ*. In addition, the telling of the story is designed specifically for the current hearer(s), a characteristic called *recipient design*. If the story is retold to other listeners, it is likely that the telling will be different with elements added or changed to suit the new audience. Finally, the goal of conversational story telling is multidimensional. Storytellers not only recount events but also tell stories to complain, boast, tease, blame, explain, or justify (Schegloff, 1997).

Additional Features of Conversation

■ Sequential organization
■ Preference management
■ Face work
■ Progressivity
■ Economy (least collaborative effort)
■ Lack of linguistic well-formedness
■ Use of context
■ Co-construction
■ Multilevel management

Conversation Analysis

Assessment of conversation in aphasia is an important undertaking. A growing literature describes conversation analysis (CA) as a meaningful tool for understanding conversation in aphasia (e.g., Beeke, Maxim, et al., 2007). CA is a systematic approach to examining and understanding the workings of conversation and the resources involved in accomplishing social interaction (Goodwin & Heritage, 1990). Conversation analysts have developed a rigorous methodology for describing conversational machinery and orderliness. Naturally occurring conversation is the target of analysis, not artificial tasks such as describing a picture or a structured interview. Conversation is not judged in relation to a standard or norm since "different" or "impaired" speakers can be effective communicators and the goal is to discover what mechanics create effective communication. For example, elements such as pauses, repetitions, restarts, or filler words are not treated as problematic if they serve a functional purpose in the conversation and are not viewed by the participants as problematic.

CA conducted as research tends to be rigorous, systematic, and time consuming. As a routine clinical procedure, comprehensive CA is probably impractical. However, there are clear benefits for clinicians to gain an understanding of CA methods and learn to think like a conversation analyst while assessing and treating people with aphasia. By better understanding CA methodology, clinicians view conversation through a different lens and learn to appropriately target conversation in aphasia treatment. Therefore, the next section describes the mechanics of CA including collecting appropriate samples, making decisions regarding transcription of samples, and identifying behaviors that either enhance or degrade interactions. Figure 7–1 includes each phase of CA, including example activities that occur in each stage.

Collecting Conversation Samples

Appropriate samples for analysis should be authentic conversation. While collection strategies might vary depending on the client's goal(s), there are a few basic considerations.

A conversation sample should capture natural conversation as opposed to a structured interview or monologue. Unscripted conversation is the most revealing context. For unscripted conversations, no topics or structure are suggested; rather, participants are asked to talk as they usually do about

whatever they wish, preferably in their natural setting. However, the variability in conversations across topics, contexts, and partners is often cited as a barrier to reliable outcome measurement of conversation.

> ### Considerations for Collecting Conversation Samples
>
> - Unscripted conversation versus control methods
> - Participants (e.g., family, friends, clinician, unfamiliar partner)
> - Length of sample
> - Number of samples
> - Location of conversation (e.g., client's home, clinic, community)
> - Video recording method

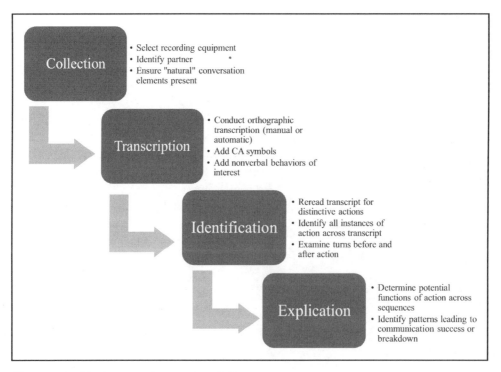

Figure 7–1. CA phases and example activities.

Therefore, a variety of methods that contribute some control have been suggested. For example, gathering multiple samples increases the likelihood of sampling representative behaviors of the individual. Employing standardized procedures for instructions, sampling, and analysis helps guard against variability and inconsistency of behaviors. Proposing specific topics of conversation (e.g., "weekend plans," "if I won the lottery") also provides some consistency across samples. Having participants watch a short video (e.g., a news clip, brief sequence from a TV series), then having participants discuss the recording is another method of partially controlling topic. Scripted conversations using standard partners and carefully designed questions and comments have also been suggested (Kagan et al., 2021).

Collecting a conversation sample between a person with aphasia and a routine communication partner may not be possible or appropriate. Not all people with aphasia have routine partners or partners may be unavailable in hospital settings. In such situations, clinicians may opt to serve as the conversation partner. This provides an opportunity to experiment with different supports such as written key words or pictographs.

Video recording of all parties in conversation is necessary for capturing multiple communication channels and collaboration involved in interaction. For example, improved use of multimodality communication after intervention would be missed if audio recording were used instead of video. Each sample should be approximately equal in length. Around 10 minutes of conversation is considered adequate. Since people with aphasia often use writing, pictures, or other resources, it is important to keep notes or collect artifacts for elements not clearly visible on the recording.

Transcription

CA in its purest form requires specific transcription procedures. Despite technological innovations, CA transcription largely remains a manual and labor-intensive process. Because the clinician or researcher is the main instrument for producing transcripts, transcription is often viewed as the first stage of data analysis. Damico and Simmons-Mackie (2002) suggest a valid, uniform, and flexible transcription process that includes multiple layers of transcription. The base layer consists of an orthographic transcription of all participants in the conversation along with descriptive symbols that have been used extensively in the CA literature. The most common system for annotating orthographic transcription includes a set of conventions first described by Gail Jefferson, one of the pioneers of CA, and is often referred to as the "Jeffersonian Transcription System" (e.g., Jefferson, 1996). Table 7–1 lists these transcription symbols. Readers interested in becoming more familiar with transcription conventions may visit the companion website.

Consider the following example adapted from Oelschlaeger and Damico (2000). Ed has moderately severe expressive aphasia and he is conversing with M, his wife. They are conversing about different items Ed has planted in his garden.

Example 7–3.

01   Ed   and there's one more there's a

02   M   okra

03   Ed   okra, that's it

A reader of this transcript could obtain a basic understanding of spoken words between Ed and M. Based on this simple transcription, it may be interpreted that M

Table 7–1. Common Symbols From Jeffersonian Transcription System

⌈ ⌊	A large left-hand bracket links an ongoing utterance with an overlapping utterance or nonverbal action point where the overlap/simultaneous nonverbal action begins.
⌉ ⌋	A large right-hand bracket marks where overlapping utterances/simultaneous nonverbal actions stop overlapping.
=	An equals sign marks where there is no interval between adjacent utterances.
(.)	A full stop in single brackets indicates an interval of less than one-tenth of a second in the stream of talk.
(0.6)	A number in single brackets indicates the length, in tenths of a second, of a pause in the talk.
oh:	A colon indicates an extension of the sound or syllable it follows (more colons prolong the stretch.
.	A full stop indicates a stopping fall in tone, not necessarily the end of a sentence.
,	A comma indicates a continuing intonation.
?	A question mark indicates a rising inflection, not necessarily a question.
!	An exclamation mark indicates an animated tone, not necessarily an exclamation.
but—	A single dash indicates a halting, abrupt cutoff to a word or part of a word.
↑↓	Marked rising and falling shifts in intonation are indicated by upward and downward pointing arrows immediately prior to the rise or fall.
<u>stress</u>	Underlining indicates emphasis.
°no°	Degree signs indicate a passage of talk that is quieter than surrounding talk.
TALK	Capital letters indicate talk delivered at a louder volume than surrounding talk.
heh	Indicates discernible aspiration or laughter (the more *h*s, the longer the aspiration/laughter).
>talk<	Less-than/greater-than signs indicate sections of an utterance delivered at a greater speed than the surrounding talk.
⌈yes ⌊*((nods))*	Italicized text in double parentheses represents a gloss or description of some nonverbal aspect of the talk and is linked to simultaneous talk with large brackets.
(dog)	Single brackets containing either a word, phrase, or syllable count (if utterance is very unclear) mark where target item(s) is/are in doubt.
→	Arrows alert the reader to talk that is discussed in the analysis.
XXX	Marks an unintelligible utterance.

"spoke for" Ed and finished his sentence. However, once CA conventions are added, readers may come to a different interpretation of the interaction:

Example 7–4.

01 Ed and there's one more (1.3)
         there's a:::::::=

02 M   =okra.

03 Ed okra, that's it

In Example 7–4, we have included (a) lapsed time, which is symbolized by the length of the pause in parentheses; (b) sound prolongation, indicated by several colons (longer colons equal longer sound); and (c) latching, which is represented with an equal sign. A latching symbol is used when one speaker's turn is immediately followed by the next speaker's turn, without any silence between the two turns. These added symbols change the clinical interpretation of the interaction. We now understand that Ed likely had a significant word-finding problem in line 1, indicated by his long pause and incomplete turn. We also can interpret the end of Ed's turn in line 1 as a *request* for M to take over his speaking turn and supply the missing word, which is indicated on the transcript by the long sound stretch of *a*. Sound stretches are often a signal that a speaker wishes to end their turn and have been defined as turn-termi-

nal items (Schegloff, 1996). M recognizes this sign and collaboratively completes Ed's turn for him, which is a type of completion strategy that the couple has discovered over the years of living with aphasia (Oelsch-laeger & Damico, 2000). The fact that she recognizes this signal so quickly is noted by the latching that occurs from line 1 to line 2. This additional descriptive information is critical to identifying potential barriers and strategies in conversation, such as how a person with aphasia overcomes a word-finding problem or how a couple negotiates a repair sequence.

An additional layer of transcription is used in CA to include nonverbal aspects of communication such as gaze or gesture. This layer of transcription is usually located on a separate transcription line. Double parentheses (( )) are used as the symbol for the analyst to enter any comments that would describe the actions of participants. Not every eye or hand movement is included in the transcript. Instead, the analyst elects to include any obvious or symbolic movement impacting interpretation of the ongoing talk. In the example below, a man with severe aphasia and apraxia of speech communicates important information to his spouse through a combination of semiotic resources (contiguous talk, drawing, and gesture). The success of this exchange can only be demonstrated through the gesture layer of this CA transcription (Example 7–5).

Example 7–5.

01 Rudy XXX I don't know XXX ⌈(here)   ⌉XXX

02   ⌊((points to paper with pen))⌋

03   ⌈°XXX XXX XXX°   ⌉⌈XXX

04   ⌊((draws box with small circles in it))⌋⌋|

05 Lila |is this the shelf?

06   ⌊((taps on Rudy's drawing))

```
07   Rudy   no (0.4) ⌈ouwlet                                    ⌉ (0.9) ⌈XXX
08                   ⌊((makes a circular shape with hands))⌋      ⌊((moves hands apart))
09                   (1.6) ⌈XXX XXX                              ⌉ ⌈(did em)
10                   ⌊((turns to wall and motions hand to wall))⌋ ⌊((pulls fist from wall))
11   Rudy   ⌈XXX XXX XXX heh heh heh °XXX XXX°
12           ⌊((points at paper))((draws circle in box))((draws wavy lines to and from box))
13   Lila   is that the cor– (0.7) the plug in?
14   Rudy   no
15   Lila   the the cord outside the (0.6) did you have something plugged in to the uh
16          outside and he ch– he pulled on ⌈↑it
17   Rudy                                    ⌊oh yeah XXX ⌈suh suh see it
18                                                      ⌊((points to paper))
```

Layers of the transcription may be done in steps, with orthographic transcription done first, followed by descriptive symbols and nonverbal actions. Researchers have begun to use automatic speech-recognition software as a first step in transcription, which appears reliable for capturing speakership, words, and pauses (Moore, 2015). Full automation of transcription, though, will likely never be attractive for the CA analyst of aphasic conversation, who would be interested in various nonverbal devices not captured in automated systems.

Analysis: Identifying Behaviors of Interest

The next step in the CA process involves a search of the transcript to identify behaviors of interest. In clinical applications of CA, these behaviors are conversational practices that are potential targets of treatment. The overarching goals of the clinician or researcher will influence this analysis but, in general, this stage should be data driven. That is, the analyst should immerse herself into the transcripts and identify a particu-

lar conversation practice that is distinctive or worthy of pursuit (Heritage, 2011). For example, lengthy or unresolved repair sequences following trouble sources could be a potential target of analysis. Once the target is identified (e.g., repair), the analyst can locate all points in a transcript where a trouble source occurs and can begin to examine the turns before and after the trouble. This part of the analysis focuses on identifying and explicating the sequential process of the practice. The analyst may ask, "What happens in the turn leading up to the trouble source?" and "What happens in the turns immediately after the trouble source?" Understanding the actions leading up to the source of trouble and what each speaker does sequentially to resolve the trouble will help identify what behaviors are similar or different across the sequences. From a clinical standpoint, this would elucidate any barriers to successfully repairing trouble or any strategies that the speakers use to help solve the problem.

In the following example adapted from Azios and colleagues (in press, 2021), Rudy is attempting to introduce a topic to his wife, Lila, but his word-finding difficulties and

Example 7–6.

01   Rudy   everyday boy ⌈XXX XXX XXX XXX   ⌉

02   ⌊*((opens hands in front of body, moves hands forward))*⌋

03   (0.4) one (.) two (.) gone *((raises arm, moves open hand quickly toward door))*

04   Lila   okay okay I don't know what buh buh buh buh buh is (.) so give me
            something (.)

05   give me some kinda clue of what this is

06   Rudy   *((puts pen to paper))* *((writes "<u>Geme</u>"))* XXX

07   Lila   (5.2) *((puts on glasses))* *((points to "<u>Geme</u>"))* Gene?=

08   Rudy   =yeah

---

unintelligible strings of speech create a trouble source (lines 1–3). Lila communicates to Rudy that she cannot understand and needs more information (lines 4–5). This prompts Rudy to repair the trouble source by writing "Geme" (line 6). While Rudy's written production is not spelled correctly, the conversational context enables Lila to correctly guess Rudy's target ("Gene"). Rudy confirms Lila's guess and the conversation progresses forward. Lila's request for a clue and Rudy's use of writing successfully and quickly resolve the trouble.

Alternative Methodology: Clinician Hacks

While traditional CA may not be realistic for the practicing clinician, many principles of analysis can be adapted so that they are feasible for clinical practice. In the following section, we discuss some alterations to CA helpful for clinicians.

Limited Transcription Analysis

Transcription of conversation provides important information about potential barriers and strengths. Unfortunately, most practicing clinicians have little time that

can be dedicated to lengthy transcriptions. In these situations, clinicians may choose to conduct automated or manual transcription of small sections of the conversation that contain conversation behaviors of interest. As discussed in previous sections, trouble sources followed by repair are common in aphasic talk. The clinician may identify all areas where trouble is occurring between a person with aphasia and a partner and transcribe the turns around the trouble source. Having a transcription of the turn prior to the trouble source, the trouble source, and the turns directly following the trouble source would provide a description of what led to the problematic turn for the person with aphasia and the layered strategies that the partner and person with aphasia used to solve the breakdown. For example, after limited transcription, a clinician may examine several trouble sources that occur in turns following the closing of one topic and that appear to signal difficulty with a person with aphasia initiating a new topic in conversation. Treatment might then focus on more effective strategies for topic initiation.

Transcriptionless Analysis

Instead of transcribing the sample, clinicians may elect to use transcriptionless methods to assess conversation (e.g., Armstrong et al., 2007). As part of the first visit and initial assessment, the clinician likely has some preliminary ideas of strategies and barriers the person with aphasia experiences in natural communication contexts. For example, when getting to know the person with aphasia and obtaining case history information, the clinician may note potential behaviors that aid in moving conversation forward (i.e., progressivity) and others that work to fix linguistic problems related to aphasia (i.e., repair). The clinician may ask herself, "Does the person with aphasia tend to gesture or write when there is a word-finding problem?" "Does he look to his wife to request help if the information is known to her?" "Does he fixate on the exact word or phrase and give up if he cannot access the word?" Once the clinician obtains the video-recorded samples, she can examine the conversation for these behaviors across a fixed time period, taking a simple tally of any facilitative or inhibitory actions of the person with aphasia or partner. This creates an inventory of strengths and weaknesses that can serve as baseline data and can also be used to create meaningful and measurable goals for the person with aphasia and potentially the partner. Another method might include brief qualitative descriptions of behaviors that help or hinder conversation (see the case example on the companion website for a checklist of conversation behaviors). These qualitative observations serve as targets of treatment and a basis for behavioral comparisons post treatment.

Application of Clinical CA to Assessment of Aphasia

When applying CA to clinical practice in aphasia, there are several general principles to consider. These include defining success in meaningful and functional change, taking a strength-based perspective, recognizing that traditional language measures often fail to capture important aspects of conversation, and appreciating the role of communication partners.

Meaningful and Functional Behavior Changes Are the Outcomes of Interest

Rather than comparing a person's communication to a norm or standard, CA teaches us to look for meaningful patterns of behavior that help or hinder interaction. By analyzing conversation and social interaction, we discover how a behavior impacts adherence to rules of social action and identify acceptable communication options. Relatedly, by avoiding a focus on standard linguistic forms, clinical assessment helps clinicians identify functionally important behaviors and capture meaningful change over time. The goal of assessment shifts from simply determining if language has improved, to determining if the **accomplishment of social action** has changed and, if so, in what way(s).

A Strength-Based Perspective

CA has enabled us to suspend notions that linguistic accuracy and completeness are integral to accomplishing social action. This strength-based perspective confirms Audrey Holland's (1977) well-known adage that people with aphasia communicate better than they speak. For example, people with agrammatic aphasia have been noted to use fronting or standard subject–verb constructions such as "I suppose" to overcome grammatical constraints caused by aphasia (Beeke, 2003). From the outside, these idiosyncratic behaviors seem unusual, but CA has revealed that these actions serve an interactional function, namely that they allow conversation to move forward so speakers can reach a mutual understanding. Fronting occurs when a turn starts with a noun or temporal phrase to introduce a topic. In the following example from Beeke and colleagues (2003, p. 89). Connie, a woman with aphasia, is chatting with her friend. They have just ended one topic and Connie opens a new topic with the following utterance.

Example 7–7.

  Connie: Last week (.) you go out?

The temporal phrase "last week" is dislocated to the left, allowing Connie to hold the turn, signal a new topic, and establish past tense without an accurately inflected verb. This method of turn management kept Connie active in the conversation without resorting to long pauses to construct a more standard grammatical turn. In traditional aphasia management, this fronting strategy might be considered a problem; from a CA perspective, it is considered a strength. People with aphasia are not always completely aware of these strategies or the consequences of their use. Thus, these actions serve as a potential untapped resource and could be exploited in therapy. They should be considered as both important targets and outcomes of strength-based interventions.

Difference Between Traditional Linguistic Tasks and Conversation

People with aphasia are able to creatively deploy all kinds of resources in conversation that are not showcased in impairment-level assessments. CA sensitizes us to the need to look at authentic conversation as significantly different from linguistic tasks. For example, Beeke, Wilkinson, et al. (2007)

provide an example of natural conversation of a man with aphasia who used alternatives to standard grammatical structures (e.g., combining talk with mime, putting unexpected elements in the initial positions of turns) to achieve successful communication. The example highlights the fact that "conversation and sentence-level tests provide complementary but *essentially different information* about grammatical ability" (p. 256; emphasis added). Similar examples pervade the CA literature suggesting that people with aphasia employ a variety of strategies for engaging in conversation that are not apparent on traditional language tasks. In other words, assessing conversation is critical to fully understanding a person's natural communication.

Role of Conversation Partners

The International Classification of Functioning, Disability, and Health (ICF) (World Health Organization, 2001) and the Living With Aphasia: Framework for Outcome Measurement (A-FROM) (Kagan et al., 2008) have helped us recognize aphasia as a socially constructed disability. Aphasia is no longer seen as a deficit within the person with aphasia; instead, it is a disability acknowledged through the interaction of the person with aphasia with others in various communication contexts. This places an explicit responsibility on the communication dyad. However, outcomes in aphasia treatment studies generally focus on the (dis)abilities of the person with aphasia and rarely account for the impact of the communication partner. An understanding of CA orients us to the role of communication partners in co-constructing conversation and highlights the significant impact that communication partners have on the communication of the person with aphasia. In other words, language is not a static ability;

one's ability to effectively use language varies with the context and communication partner. Therefore, an analyst will often need to focus directly on the partner's conversational turns to obtain a full understanding of the impact of aphasia on conversation.

Quantitative Versus Qualitative Outcomes

Capturing outcomes in conversation is not straightforward. Conversation-based outcomes must orient toward the complexity of conversation without sacrificing the rigor required for psychometrically sound measures. While many studies have elected to use a more traditional CA approach to report qualitive changes from pretreatment to post-treatment (e.g., Wilkinson et al., 2011), other studies have used a CA framework to quantify different variables that may exhibit change. For clinicians and researchers interested in taking a quantitative approach, CA can be used to operationalize and track a number of outcomes sensitive to change. The companion website includes a list of quantitative measures based on CA principles. Practitioners may also consider selecting published outcome measures based upon CA principles such as the Conversation Analysis Profile for People With Aphasia (CAPPA) (Whitworth et al., 1997) and the Profile of Word Errors and Retrieval in Speech (POWERS) (Herbert et al., 2013).

There are many aspects of conversation that could be assessed; therefore, understanding the clinical or research goal at the outset is critical to narrowing the foci and determining targets of clinical analysis. The following sections describe examples of behaviors that occur frequently in aphasic conversation and may become targets of assessment and intervention.

Variety of Speech Acts

Although not an explicit aspect of traditional CA, identification of the variety and type of speech acts often provides an excellent snapshot of a person's level of participation in conversation. Speech acts are utterances that perform a function; that is, the act is identified by its functional intent rather than the grammatical construction. For example, a question may serve as a request for information or a request for performance. The companion website provides examples of speech act labels.

Clinical analysts should obtain a gloss of utterance functions and not necessarily follow rigid rules of utterance classification as defined by speech act theorists. The idea is to determine a client's use of varied and appropriate acts in conversation and look for successful or unsuccessful patterns. The transcript in Appendix 7–1 demonstrates a practical speech act analysis in which the person with aphasia has three minimal turns and three failed self-repair attempts.

Repair

Trouble spots are frequent in aphasic conversation. Therefore, attempts at repair are initiated to fix the trouble or conversational breakdown. There are several components of repair, including the original trouble source, the indication or signal that repair is needed (either by oneself or another), and the actual repair (either by oneself or another person). In conversations involving people with and without aphasia, speakers have demonstrated a preference for self-repair over other types of repair (e.g., repairing one's own error is preferred to a partner repairing it; e.g., Schegloff et al.,1977). Identifying who signals the need for repair and who fixes the trouble is a valuable target of clinical assessment.

In addition to who performs components of a repair, the mechanics of repair are of clinical interest. There are various means of repairing a turn, and the severity of a person's aphasia may impact the speed and strategies of repair. People with aphasia who are more verbally restricted may have to rely on a combination of verbal and nonverbal resources (e.g., partial utterances, gesture, pictures, drawing, eye gaze) for self-repair, while those with milder forms of aphasia may have more verbal repair mechanisms such as self-cueing systems (e.g., spelling part of the word, circumlocution). Regardless, the length of repair, methods used to negotiate repair (e.g., verbal and/or nonverbal strategies), and overall success (i.e., the trouble is resolved) are all important components of assessment.

To assess repairs, the clinician would locate all trouble sources that occur across the conversation sample and examine if and how repair sequences are negotiated in following turns. Narrowing the analysis to focus on each trouble source and ensuing repair sequence enables the clinician to recognize patterns that may serve as intervention targets. In the examples below, we see a *qualitative* difference in the conversation when writing is used to repair a trouble source.

Example 7–8.

	Dr. M	So where do you live?
Trouble	David	U:::h mostle (.) over here ((*points to the right*))
Other repair attempt	Dr. M	Moss Park?
Self-repair attempt	David	No no (.) uh ((*points to the right*)) ba boss pa
Failure	Dr. M	I'm not getting that.

Example 7–9.

	Dr. M	So last time I wasn't sure where you lived. Can you tell me where you live?
Trouble	David	Ha hhh Over over U::h
Self-repair with writing		((*writes North*))
Success	Dr. M	Oh North York.
	David	Yeah yeah

Multimodal Communication

The use of multiple modalities (e.g., gesture, body language, gaze) is an example of efforts to communicate meaning or repair trouble. Therefore, an analysis of the frequency of multimodal strategies and the success of these for moving the conversation forward is a valid assessment target. Also important to note is the timing and strategic deployment of multimodal strategies. Some gestures may be used in the absence of speech to overcome a word-finding barrier in conversation, while others may be used in conjunction with speech as a means of repair. Consider the common clinical example of a person with aphasia who produces semantic paraphasias when attempting to verbalize numbers. Many people with aphasia will *say* an incorrect number and simultaneously gesture the correct (or intended) number. Examining how often this strategy occurs and its effectiveness in conveying meaning is critical to understanding strengths and weaknesses across language modalities.

> ### *Multimodal Strategies*
>
> Note frequency of occurrence, which speaker produces it, and its success.
>
> ■ Symbolic gesture
> ■ Pointing
> ■ Mime
> ■ Facial expressions
> ■ Writing
> ■ Drawing
> ■ Photographs/pictographs/objects
> ■ Assistive technology

Topic Management

Based on CA methods, Schegloff and Sacks (1973) have described topic initiation mechanics in standard conversation. New topics typically follow topic-ending actions such as pauses or summary remarks. Smooth introduction of a new topic tends to occur by using a cohesive device that ties the new topic semantically to the prior talk. New topics also frequently are preceded by an alerting device or topic preface such as a discontinuity marker (e.g., by the way, so, hey) to signal that the conversation is diverting to a new direction. Initiating new topics can be difficult for people with aphasia (see Leaman & Edmonds, 2020, for a review). Failure to offer new topics, abrupt topic change, or noncoherent topic initiation are often characteristic of speakers with aphasia. By reviewing samples of conversation, the clinician can identify the frequency and success of topic initiation and introduce topic management strategies as a treatment goal.

Turn Management

The organization of turn taking is fundamental to any analysis of aphasic conversation. Due to lengthy pauses or slow entry into the flow of talk, people with aphasia may have difficulty securing a turn in conversation. Likewise, partners may experience difficulty recognizing when a person with aphasia is ready to terminate a turn, which may cause periods of overlap where two speakers are talking at the same time. Examining how turns are organized and how both speakers orient to the transfer of speakership can be helpful in determining if a person with aphasia is able to successfully hold the floor to convey new ideas, elaborate on a topic, ask for a partner's opinion, and so on. Many people with aphasia develop a variety of discourse devices to help organize speakership and alert partners to important information contained in turns. For instance, people with aphasia may use gaze and nonverbal resources to alert a partner to take over the speaking floor. These actions usually serve as a means of shifting the burden of communication to the partner.

Some discourse devices for turn management are more atypical or idiosyncratic. For example, Simmons-Mackie and Damico (1996) discuss the use of the semantically meaningless word *is* (pronounced /ɪs/ with unvoiced sibilant) as an initiation marker used by a woman with aphasia to alert her listener to expect information. The same woman consistently produced *isy* (pronounced /ɪsi/ with stress on the second syllable) as a termination marker to mark the end of her own thought and signal a shift in orientation. Uncovering these individualized actions and their functions in assessment can arm the clinician with valuable information for identifying obstacles to or facilitators of effective turn management and developing goals to improve participation in conversation.

Considering Communication Partner Behaviors

Clinicians will want to pay attention to some specific partner behaviors that facilitate or hinder conversational participation of the person with aphasia. Some partner actions have been described as inhibitory and negatively impact the ability of a person with aphasia to participate in the next conversational turn. For example, questions appear to be exceptionally influential in shaping future turn sequences in aphasic conversation (Beeke et al., 2013). Test questions—questions that the asker already knows the answer to—are particularly problematic for people with aphasia, both from an interactional standpoint and for issues related to social and linguistic competence. Because of sequential dependency, test questions require the person with aphasia to provide a specific response. Test-question sequences often involve marked word search behaviors and turns are often left incomplete (Beeke et al., 2015). Moreover, test questions expose the aphasic impairment, effectively diminishing the image of the person with aphasia. Clinicians may wish to train partners to eliminate test questions from their conversations and employ supportive behaviors that give a person with aphasia the opportunity to contribute.

Another example of inhibitory partner behavior can be seen in the transcript in the speech act analysis example on the companion website. The communication partner tries to compel the person with aphasia to say what he means rather than provide communication support to progress the conversation forward. By analyzing conversation, clinicians and researchers can identify inhibitory partner behaviors and their impact on turn sequences and devise intervention to improve conversational interactions.

CA is also critical to revealing facilitative behaviors used by partners of people with aphasia. Facilitative behaviors tend to open up possibilities for the next turn of a person with aphasia or provide some level of support that would enable greater participation in conversation. Questions, when used appropriately, can be incredibly supportive for future turns of persons with aphasia. For example, asking yes/no questions can help people with marked aphasia initiate topics and hold the speaking floor during group conversations (Archer et al., 2021). Clinicians and researchers interested in assessing how well people with aphasia can participate in group conversations may begin CA with identification and comparison of sequences that involve group mechanics such as sequential actions surrounding topic initiation and floor transfer. Comparisons across these sequences may reveal partner actions, leading to improved topic initiation or general participation.

Conclusion

This overview of CA in aphasia has introduced the mechanics of CA and described a variety of behaviors observed in conversation with a person with aphasia. For those who are interested in delving deeper into CA, there are texts that address CA methods and issues (e.g., Heritage, 2011; Hutchby & Wooffitt,

2008), and an ever-increasing number of excellent articles describing CA findings in aphasia. Armed with an understanding of CA, clinicians will better understand conversation in aphasia, capture socially valid assessment of communication, and contribute to functional and meaningful intervention to improve social interaction and conversation.

References

Archer, B., Azios, J. H., Gulick, N., & Tetnowski, J. (2021). Facilitating participation in conversation groups for aphasia. *Aphasiology*, *35*(6), 764–782. https://doi.org/10.1080/02687038.2 020.1812030

Armstrong, L., Brady, M., Mackenzie, C., & Norrie, J. (2007). Transcription-less analysis of aphasic discourse: A clinician's dream or a possibility? *Aphasiology*, *21*(3–4), 355–374. https://doi.org/10.1080/0268703060091 1310

Azios, J., Archer, B., & Lee, J. B. (2021). Detecting behavioural change in conversation: Procedures and preliminary data. *Aphasiology*, 35(7), 961–983. https://doi.org/10.1080/0268 7038.2020.1812031

Azios, J., Archer, B., & Lee, J. B. (in press). Understanding mechanisms of change after conversation-focused therapy in aphasia: A conversation analysis investigation. *Journal of Interactional Research in Communication Disorders*.

Bach, K., & Harnish, R. (1979). *Linguistic communication and speech acts*. MIT Press.

Beeke, S. (2003). "I suppose" as a resource for the construction of turns at talk in agrammatic aphasia. *Clinical Linguistics and Phonetics*, *17*(4–5), 291–298. https://doi.org/10.1080/ 0269920031000080055

Beeke, S., Beckley, F., Best, W., Johnson, F., Edwards, S., & Maxim, J. (2013). Extended turn construction and test question sequences in the conversations of three speakers with agrammatic aphasia. *Clinical Linguistics and Phonetics*, *27*(10–11), 784–804. https://doi.org/10.3109/02699206.2013.808 267

Beeke, S., Beckley, F., Johnson, F., Heilemann, C., Edwards, S., Maxim, J., & Best, W. (2015). Conversation-focused aphasia therapy: Investigating the adoption of strategies by people with agrammatism. *Aphasiology*, *29*(3), 355–377. https://doi.org/10.1080/02687038.2014 .881459

Beeke, S., Maxim, J., & Wilkinson, R. (2003). Exploring aphasic grammar 1: A single case analysis of conversation. *Clinical Linguistics and Phonetics*, *17*(2), 81–107. https://doi.org/ 10.1080/0269920031000061795

Beeke, S., Maxim, J., & Wilkinson, R. (2007). Using conversation analysis to assess and treat people with aphasia. *Seminars in Speech and Language*, *28*(2), 136–147. https://doi .org/10.1055/s-2007-970571

Beeke, S., Wilkinson, R., & Maxim, J. (2007). Grammar without sentence structure: A conversation analytic investigation of agrammatism. *Aphasiology*, *21*(3–4), 256–282. https://doi.org/10.1080/0268703060091 1344

Clark, H., & Wilkes-Gibbs, D. (1986). Referring as a collaborative process. *Cognition*, *22*(1), 1–39. https://doi.org/10.1016/0010-0277(86) 90010-7

Damico, J. S., & Simmons-Mackie, N. (2002). The base layer and the gaze/gesture layer of transcription. *Clinical Linguistics and Phonetics*, *16*(5), 317–327. https://doi.org/10.1080/ 02699200210135857

Goodwin, C. (2003). Conversational frameworks for accomplishment of meaning in aphasia. In C. Goodwin (Ed.), *Conversation and brain damage* (pp. 90–116). Oxford University Press.

Goodwin, C., & Heritage, J. (1990). Conversation analysis. *Annual Review of Anthropology*, *19*(1), 283–307. https://www.jstor.org/stable/ 2155967

Herbert, R., Best, W., Hickin, J., Howard, D., & Osborne, F. (2013). *POWERS: Profile of Word Errors and Retrieval in Speech: An assessment tool for use with people with communication impairment.* J & R Press.

Heritage, J. (1984). *Garfinkel and ethnomethodology.* Prentice-Hall.

Heritage, J. (2011). Conversation analysis: Practices and methods. In D. Silverman (Ed.), *Qualitative research: Issues of theory, method and practice* (3rd ed., pp. 208–230). Sage Publications.

Holland, A. (1977). Some practical considerations in aphasia rehabilitation. In M. Sullivan & M. Kommers (Eds.), *Rationale for adult aphasia therapy* (pp. 167–180). University of Nebraska Press.

Hutchby, I., & Wooffitt, R. (2008). *Conversation analysis* (2nd ed.). Polity Press.

Jefferson, G. (1996). A case of transcriptional stereotyping. *Journal of Pragmatics, 26*(2), 159–170. https://doi.org/10.1016/0378-2166(96)00010-0

Kagan, A., Simmons-Mackie, N., Rowland, A., Huijbregts, M., Shumway, E., McEwen, S., & Sharp, S. (2008). Counting what counts: A framework for capturing real-life outcomes of aphasia intervention. *Aphasiology, 22*(3), 258–280. https://doi.org/10.1080/02687030701282595

Kagan, A., Simmons-Mackie, N., Shumway, E., Victor, J. C., & Chan, L. (2021). Development and evaluation of the Basic Outcome Measure Protocol for Aphasia (BOMPA). *International Journal of Speech-Language Pathology, 23*(3), 258–264. https://doi.org/10.1080/17549507.2020.1784278

Leaman, M., & Edmonds, L. (2020). "By the way" . . . How people with aphasia and their communication partners initiate new topics of conversation. *American Journal of Speech-Language Pathology, 29,* 375–392. https://doi.org/10.1044/2019_AJSLP-CAC48-18-0198

Moore, R. J. (2015). Automated transcription and conversation analysis. *Research on Language and Social Interaction, 48*(3), 253–270. https://doi.org/10.1080/08351813.2015.1058600

Oelschlaeger, M. L., & Damico, J. S. (2000). Partnership in conversation: A study of word search strategies. *Journal of Communication Disorders, 33*(3), 205–225. https://doi.org/10.1016/S0021-9924(00)00019-8

Oelschlaeger, M., & Damico, J. (2003). Word searches in aphasia: A study of collaborative responses of communicative partners. In C. Goodwin (Ed.), *Conversation and brain damage* (pp. 211–230). Oxford University Press.

Sacks, H., Schegloff, E., & Jefferson, G. (1974). A simplest systematics for the organization of turn taking for conversation. *Language,* 50, 696–735. https://doi.org/10.2307/412243

Schegloff, E. A. (1996). Turn organization: One intersection of grammar and interaction. In E. Ochs, E. A. Schegloff, & S. Thompson (Eds.), *Interaction and grammar* (pp. 52–133). Cambridge University Press.

Schegloff, E. A. (1997). "Narrative analysis" 30 years later. *Journal of Narrative and Life History, 7*(1–4), 97–106. https://doi.org/10.1075/jnlh.7.11nar

Schegloff, E. A., Jefferson, G., & Sacks, H. (1977). The preference for self-correction in the organization of repair in conversation. *Language, 53*(2), 361–382. https://doi.org/10.2307/413107

Schegloff, E. A., & Sacks, H. (1973). Opening up closings. *Semiotica,* 8, 289–327. https://doi.org/10.1515/semi.1973.8.4.289

Simmons-Mackie, N., & Damico, J. S. (1996). The contribution of discourse markers to communicative competence in aphasia. *American Journal of Speech-Language Pathology, 5*(1), 37–43. https://doi.org/10.1044/1058-0360.0501.37

Treviño, A. J. (2003). Introduction: Erving Goffman and the interactional order. In A. J. Treviño (Ed.), *Goffman's legacy* (pp. 1–49). Rowman & Littlefield Publishers.

Whitworth, A., Perkins, L., & Lesser, R. (1997). *Conversation Analysis Profile for People With Aphasia (CAPPA).* Whurr.

Wilkinson, R., Lock, S., Bryan, K., & Sage, K. (2011). Interaction-focused intervention for acquired language disorders: Facilitating mu-tual adaptation in couples where one partner has aphasia. *International Journal of Speech-Language Pathology, 13*(1), 74–87.

https://doi.org/10.3109/17549507.2011.55
1140

World Health Organization. (2001). *World Health
Organization: International Classification of
Functioning, Disability, and Health (ICF).*

APPENDIX 7-1

Example of a Clinical Speech Act Analysis

A married couple is discussing a video recording about computer use in the classroom. The sequence represents repeated "trouble" in the talk of the person with aphasia with the wife asking clarification questions to signal her inability to understand. Note the three minimal turns ("right") and three failed self-repair attempts by the person with aphasia. Transcript from unpublished data used with permission of Roberta J. Elman. (See Table A7–1 on the following page.)

Table A7–1. Example of a Clinical Speech Act Analysis

Speech Act	Speaker	Transcription
Apologize	PWA	((yawns)) cuse me.
Assert	Wife	Well,well nowadays kids, not even kids, even adults, everybody needs to kinda get familiar with the computers.
Assert		so uh because everything you do now is basically connected to the computer
Self-repeat		basically connected to the computer.
Agree	PWA	((nods)) right.
Assert	Wife	xxx back you can, they have now where you can stay home and you can uh uh log on from the telephone to hook up to the computer to do a lot of things.
Assert Self-repair attempt	PWA	um um um ((coughs)) um (..) computer I take in ss um (Child's name) it corner computer. I take and . . .
Clarification question (trouble signal)	Wife	(Child's name) gonna take the computer?
Respond/agree	PWA	right.
Clarification question (trouble signal)	Wife	That's what you sayin?
Respond/agree	PWA	right.
Assert/predict		and later on (Child's name) can um school (Child's name) can ah . . .
Clarification question (trouble signal)	Wife	(Child's name) can what?
Assert Self-repair attempt	PWA	um later on (.) and . . .
Reject/give up		I don't know.
Assert/disagree	Wife	yeah you do know.
Direct/urge		you have to say what you mean.
Self-repair attempt Assert/predict	PWA	((sniffs)) ((wipes face)) hm ((sniffs)) later on (Child's name) can . . .
Reject/give up		um I don't know.
Assert/evaluate	Wife	you always say you don't know.

8 Cross-Cultural Perspectives on Conversational Assessment and Treatment in Aphasia: Learnings From a First Nations Context

Elizabeth Armstrong, Tara Lewis, Alice Robins,
Ian Malcolm, and Natalie Ciccone

Introduction

Many speech-language pathologists (SLPs) routinely work with clients and families who come from cultures other than their own. For a discipline that focuses on communication, the implications of assessing an individual's communication skills and offering relevant treatments in this context pose numerous challenges. Culture and language are inextricably interwoven. Worldview[1] and life experience shape all aspects of both the structure of language and language use, and language also shapes worldview[1] and life experience (Halliday, 1985; Malinowski, 2002). While translation of wording from one language to another (where possible) may play a key part in successful cross-cultural communication between two speakers, many other components are involved.

Speakers need to understand each other's nonverbal communication strategies, know the pragmatic rules of the other's language, and be critically conscious of differing worldviews. From this knowledge, they must also be able to create a safe environment in which both feel enabled to enter into a meaningful and reciprocal interaction. However, the situation becomes even more complex when one person (in this case, the SLP) is in the relative position of power as the expert—consistent with Western hegemonic ontologies (Moreton-Robinson, 2006; Nelson, 2007)—and assumes the role of assessing the adequacy of the other's communication skills. The SLP (in Western contexts, typically white) is socially empowered because of the structural locality of the position of expert. SLPs in this context are socially situated in a power relation where whiteness remains

---

[1]Palmer (1996) discusses worldview at some length, relating it to "culturally defined imagery" and suggests "a concept of worldview that highlights the framework of tradition without arguing that it is all there is, or that all traditions are old, unchanging and shared by all within a culture . . ." (p. 117).

invisible, natural, normal, and unmarked, and it is from this position that others' conversational skills are understood and assessed.

Culture and Conversation

To date, cross-linguistic/cross-cultural work in aphasiology has largely compared manifestations of aphasia in different languages from a syntactic perspective (e.g., Bastiaanse & Edwards, 2004; Lee & Faroqi-Shah, 2021). Studies have also involved translation of largely English-based standardized tests into other languages (see Fyndanisa et al., 2017, for a recent overview). The use of interpreters in cross-linguistic assessment using standardized psycholinguistic test batteries has also been explored (Huang et al., 2019). Less attention has been paid to the cultural context of the person with aphasia and the potential implications of this for language use in everyday conversational interactions. It is crucial to note that with practitioners from the dominant culture typically providing services in many countries, the notion of worldview is rarely considered. Practice subsequently maintains the dominant epistemology and ontology with Western notions of normal interactions and interactions skills often forming the basis for clinical judgements.

The more recent development of conversational assessment and treatment techniques in aphasiology has encouraged SLPs to systematically observe the dyadic nature of their clients' communication skills in real-life interactions or rate specific abilities of speakers with aphasia to engage in generic interactional skills. These include tasks such as talking on the phone or making an appointment via simulated conversa-

tional settings within the clinic environment (e.g., the Communication Activities of Daily Living assessment [CADL3]; Holland et al., 2018). This differs from a more traditional impairment-based approach that typically relies on assessments of decontextualized language skills such as the person's ability to name a picture or describe a picture sequence (e.g., Western Aphasia Battery-Revised; Kertesz, 2006). Direct facilitation of interactional skills has been extended to involve training communication partners to assist people with aphasia to participate in conversations (for overview, see Simmons-Mackie et al., 2016).

Challenges involved in conversational assessment and treatment include ensuring that conversational samples are representative of the client's conversational skills in authentic everyday interactions while considering the impact different conversational partners, interaction contexts, conversational topics, genres, and modes of communication may have on the individual's skills (see Chapter 7). Variation is expected, and without obtaining a representative sample, clinicians risk either underestimating or overestimating a person with aphasia's communication abilities.

Attempting to assess the conversational skills of someone from a culture that is different from one's own presents numerous critical issues for consideration. Notions of conversational assessment in the speech-language pathology context are typically underpinned by "a Western cultural system of classification and representation, by views about human nature, human morality and virtue, by conceptions of space and time, by conceptions of gender and race" (Tuhiwai Smith, 2012, p. 46). A lack of awareness or reflection on this positioning often results in 'othering' of cultures other than the Western dominant culture and a further positioning of the potentially benign concept of 'difference' as being exotic or even primitive and less than (Moreton-Robinson, 2006; Tuhiwai Smith, 2012). A lack of awareness of differences in worldview, cultural protocols, and linguistic conventions may lead the clinician to make assumptions about appropriate ways of interacting with the client. These assumptions may not align with the discourse rules in the client's language or culture (e.g., interviews involving a question/answer format; topics explored, such as health and family, that may not be appropriate depending on the clinician's and client's age or gender). Variations from dominant culture languages and dialects can also cause confusion for an uninformed clinician and lead to misdiagnosis of disorder versus difference. The use of code switching during conversations may also complicate the clinical assessment if the clinician is not aware of the linguistic codes the speaker has access to.

To date, such cross-cultural issues related to conversational assessment and treatment in acquired communication disorders have rarely been addressed. Again, it is also important to reflect on notions of cultural difference and on attempts to navigate cultural difference between a clinician and client in a clinical context. Being in the role of expert immediately places the clinician in a position of cultural dominance, employing or even attempting to adjust his or her own cultural frameworks to accommodate the client. While this presents an ongoing challenge, it is through awareness of this positioning, open two-way discussion, and learning that professional development can take place and SLPs can truly begin to address concerns of their clients.

This chapter discusses the challenges of cross-cultural conversational assessment, with particular reference to the Australian Aboriginal/First Nations context. Aboriginal Australians with acquired communication disorders are particularly poorly represented in rehabilitation services (Armstrong et al., 2015; Armstrong, Coffin, et al., 2019), suggesting a cultural mismatch between what is needed and what is being offered. In Australia, shortcomings in mainstream health systems regarding their ability to provide culturally appropriate and accessible services to First Nations peoples have been repeatedly reported, with Aboriginal people reporting ongoing difficulties in accessing services (Durey et al., 2016; Gilroy et al., 2013, 2016). In the brain injury rehabilitation context, many have reported managing largely on their own after discharge from the hospital, with breakdown in communication between non-Aboriginal health staff and Aboriginal patients and families often cited as core to the problem (Armstrong, Coffin, et al., 2019). Communication is the core business of SLPs, and clinical interactions and assessment sessions are some of the key initial points of contact for people after brain injury. The importance of conversational interactions and assessments should not be underestimated—either in their significance for diagnosis of any communication difficulties occurring as a result of the brain damage, or for establishing important relationships that may lay a successful foundation to support and facilitate the person's recovery and rehabilitation journey. Principles derived from discussion of this context have relevance not only for practices involving indigenous/First Nations peoples internationally but also for cross-cultural conversational assessment and treatment practices generally. With multilingual, multicultural caseloads growing globally (Centeno et al., 2020), cross-cultural practice is now a critical part of speech-language pathology.

The Field of Cultural Linguistics

In line with the challenges outlined above, the field of cultural linguistics offers some insights that may be helpful to clinicians. Cultural linguistics is concerned with understanding differences and similarities between languages at all levels, including phonology, syntax, semantics, pragmatics, and how the languages position their speakers in social organization (Palmer, 1996; Sharifian, 2017). As culture and language are inextricably interwoven, the nature of linguistic patterns can vary considerably across cultural contexts, with languages both reflecting and creating patterns of meaning-making and conceptualizations that are relevant to different cultures. These align with different purposes for communication, foregrounding of different meanings, sociopolitical influences, and different social and worldviews. At a relatively transparent level, vocabulary can reflect different perceptions of the world by speakers from different cultures. However, the challenges in looking for literal translations of words from one language to another demonstrate the differing underlying conceptualizations that may be involved across languages and cultures where there are often no equivalents.

Pragmatic behaviors also vary across languages and cultures. For example, what is considered polite to say in one culture might be considered impolite in another. Silence during interactions may signify different things in different cultures. However, it is not merely a matter of the behavior observed, but what underlies that behavior in cultural schema. Sharifian (2017) discusses cultural schemas as a subclass of cognitive schemas that have been culturally constructed and encompass both

lexical and pragmatic meanings based on knowledge and views of the world that are shared by a speech community. The following quote (Collard et al., 2000, as cited in Malcolm, 2018) provides an example of a cultural schema related to how interactions can unfold—in this case, a quote from an Aboriginal academic at an Australian university describing how conversations take place in her home environment:

> . . . interacting in my family often involves a lot of talking at once. In Standard English that's actually seen as being really really quite rude and we tend not to talk over people. And you certainly don't get five people . . . all talking at once, often having two or three different conversations going, and as a participant you're involved in all of those conversations happening at one time. I mean everyone's talking at once. (p. 130)

When considering conversational interactions, cultural linguists are not only interested in vocabulary and grammatical structures constituting talk, but also underlying conceptualizations and how these are realized in everyday conversations. Conversations are not simply the venue for putting phonological, vocabulary, and grammatical skills into practice; they are organized so that these components merge in particular ways so as to produce meaningful interactions between members of the speech community who share a particular language or dialect.

The relevance of cultural linguistics to the assessment of communication skills is obvious in this multicultural, multilingual world. Any person making judgements about another speaker's skills must be familiar with the rules of that person's language and underlying cultural schema. Any judgements or recommendations made by clinicians about the need for a speaker to regain particular communication skills or change modes of interacting must be based on comprehensive understandings of these rules and not on the clinician's own linguistic and cultural schema and associated assumptions. The evidence base for making such recommendations should be interrogated for relevance to the language and culture at hand, rather than assumptions made about particular behaviors observed or tested, regardless of cultural context.

Clinicians do not have to learn about all languages and cultures but must be aware of concepts such as worldview and cultural assumptions affecting their perceptions. In addition, they have to be prepared to seek knowledge from cultural brokers or other cultural and linguistic experts to inform their practice. Personal and cultural identity are intricately connected to language use; hence, entering the world of language use is a sensitive area in which to operate. It is against this backdrop—relevant to all cross-cultural speech and language pathology practice—that the current chapter explores a particular context that encompasses the intersection of linguistic, cultural, social, and historical influences that have shaped and continue to shape the lives of one of the oldest cultures in the world.

The Aboriginal and Torres Strait Islander Context Within Australia

Australia's First Nations peoples comprise two distinct heritages: Aboriginal peoples and Torres Strait Islanders. Some individuals identify with both heritages, and within these two groups there is great diversity. At the time of the British invasion in 1788, there were 250 Aboriginal languages spoken in Australia (Department of Communications, Information, Technology and the Arts, 2005). Since that time, and due to subsequent colonial laws and policies that directly impacted culture, language and kinship within Aboriginal and Torres Strait Islander communities (e.g., Aborigines Protection Act 1909 and subsequent amendments until 1969), the number has now dropped to 140. Of these, approximately 10 to 12 are the primary languages spoken at home (Australian Bureau of Statistics, 2016). However, preservation and revitalization initiatives of Aboriginal languages are currently underway and are increasing in number (e.g., Bracknell, 2020).

While philosophical approaches often seem far removed from clinical practice, culture runs deep. To provide services that are culturally secure and appropriate, significant attention needs to be paid to underlying philosophies of services and theoretical frameworks. The ongoing nature of invasion continues to impact First Nations peoples today, with differences in life expectancy and other social outcomes well documented and undisputed (Australian Institute of Health and Welfare, 2020). With growing Aboriginal leadership at the highest levels of policy making, health service provision, and academic scholarship, the context is changing; however, change remains slow (Lowitja Institute, 2021). Aboriginal scholars such as Chelsea Watego (Watego et al., 2021) advocate for reconceptualization of traditionally accepted notions of health and health research, which emanate largely from Anglo-American traditions, and draw on Rigney's Indigenism (Rigney, 1999) and critical race theory to suggest new ways forward that address current health and social concerns from an Indigenous perspective.

As noted above, the focus on providing appropriate services is on increasing accessibility for Aboriginal peoples who are currently significantly underrepresented in mainstream rehabilitation services (Armstrong, Coffin, et al., 2019; Fitts et al., 2019). Culturally inappropriate assessment practices, including use of inappropriate assessment tools, poor intercultural communication practices, and lack of knowledge of cultural and linguistic norms of many non-Aboriginal clinicians, all potentially contribute to this situation (Armstrong et al., 2017; Bohanna et al., 2019; Hersh et al., 2015).

The same principles that apply to the use of different languages by the clinician and the client also apply to different dialects. While there may often be superficial similarities between dialects in phonology and grammar, significantly different underlying semantic systems, conceptualizations, and cultural schema may exist. Approximately 10% of Aboriginal Australians speak an Indigenous language at home (Australian Bureau of Statistics, 2016), with many speakers being fluent in more than one language. However, the majority of Aboriginal Australians speak a dialect of English called Australian Aboriginal English (AAE), Aboriginal English, or Home Language, and many code switch between this and the Standard Australian English (SAE) dialect used specifically for academic, and sometimes employment and social, purposes depending on context.

Features of AAE/Home Language to Consider

AAE/Home Language is a "range of varieties of English spoken by Aboriginal and Torres Strait Islander people . . . which differ in systematic ways from Standard Australian English at all levels of linguistic structure and which are used for distinc-tive speech acts, speech events and genres" (Malcolm, 1995, as cited in Malcolm et al., 1999, p. 11). Louro and Collard (2021) note that there are differences in AAE across Australia, with so-called light varieties being closest to SAE dialect while the heavy varieties are closer to Kriol, a language spoken in Northern Australia. As has been widely noted, identity is notably carried in a speaker's first language (Geia et al., 2013) and, as a variety of English, AAE constitutes the first language for many Aboriginal Australians. Modifications to adopted English made by Aboriginal speakers over time have emanated from linguistic (Malcolm, 2021), social (Malcolm, 2017) and cognitive (Malcolm, 2017; Sharifian, 2017) origins.

Rather than being a lesser or substandard version of English, AAE constitutes a dialect in its own right, of the same standing as SAE and other variations of English, and has maintained the cultural identity of its speakers while adopting forms from standard English as well. It retains a different underlying semantic system and retains concepts, phonology, and grammatical features from traditional Aboriginal languages that are crucial to such maintenance.

Malcolm (2017, 2018) describes a number of cultural conceptualizations underlying AAE that form the basis for linguistic patterns observed. These include speakers of AAE and traditional Aboriginal languages being environmentally attuned, with the relevance of country central to their discourse (Malcolm, 2018). Observations of events and embodiment of meaning (e.g., repetition of verbs for emphasis of extent of something—*Next day we bin walking walking walking)* are also common features (Malcolm, 2018). Other features include marking manner adverbials explicitly—*e just got up quick way; we went Ceduna way* (Malcolm, 2018).

AAE discourse also often has the potential for multilevel interpretation, incorporating spiritual dimensions that may not be accessible or obvious to the non-AAE speaker. For example, a story told by an AAE speaker may have completely different connotations for another AAE speaker (related to spiritual beliefs) than for an SAE speaker.

It is beyond the scope of this chapter to provide an overview of AAE that encompasses all levels of language. Readers are referred to other sources that provide such overviews of AAE and that will be helpful in identifying specific features that will assist with assessment (e.g., Butcher, 2008; Malcolm, 2018). We focus here on aspects of AAE that can serve as examples of features that may more generally challenge non-Aboriginal, Western assumptions regarding communicative interactions upon which much aphasia assessment and intervention practices are currently based. While many of the examples cited are more in line with the pragmatic level of language evidence in conversation, the instantiation of many of these through particular lexical and grammatic patterns should also be noted.

Particular features of AAE that have been noted from an interactional perspective are listed in the box below. Distinctive features related to a variety of Aboriginal languages are also described elsewhere and should be referenced by clinicians for broader insight into Aboriginal discourse (e.g., Mushin & Baker, 2008).

Of particular interest when looking at conversational behaviors are Walsh's maxims (Walsh, 2009), written in response to Grice's (1975) conversational maxims, which are used extensively to discuss conversational principles in many contexts. Grice's maxims have been discussed and criticized for being Anglo-centric and have been revised by others to be more applicable to a range of languages and cultures (e.g., Clyne, 1995). Walsh (2009) suggests six conversational maxims for traditional Aboriginal languages that also have relevance to AAE: autonomy, intentional vagueness, epistemic discretion, traditional ascription, broadcast address, and open-endedness. When contrasted with Grice's maxims, these highlight potential challenges for the current aphasiology context, which is still largely based on Western frameworks such as Grice's.

Interactional Features of AAE Discourse (Malcolm, 2018)

- Discomfort with individualization (i.e., greater comfort with group rather than dyadic conversations)
- Reluctance to speak on behalf of others without authorization
- Reluctance to respond to direct questions
- Special vocabularies and constraints with respect to addressing certain kin
- Gratuitous concurrence (i.e., set responses to satisfy the questioner)

- Alternative cultural conceptualizations: affecting interpretation of SAE entailed in AAE utterances
- Respectful avoidance of eye contact
- Inexplicitness (i.e., assumption of social/environmental relevance)
- Dependence on embodiment (i.e., unfamiliarity with abstraction)
- Silence (valued as respectful behavior)

> ### Conversational Maxims for Traditional Aboriginal Languages (Walsh, 2009)
>
> - Autonomy: Speak for yourself, do not speak for others
> - Intentional vagueness: Be vague; this often results in situations where people are communicating primarily through inferences, while the actual talk, although sometimes quite minimal and even vague, is communicatively very rich in signal to message ratio
> - Epistemic discretion: Speak of what you know, unless your age is inappropriate and/or your gender
>
> is inappropriate, and/or there are others who should speak instead
> - Traditional ascription: Speak of traditional matters preferably when your statement can be ascribed to earlier, reliable sources
> - Broadcast address: Speak to no one in particular (i.e., everyone in general)
> - Open-endedness: Speak in such a way that other points of view are given space, as well as other discursive turns

Aphasia Context in Conversational Assessment and Treatment

While some general principles have been considered, when working cross-culturally clinicians must be sure not to overgeneralize, to consider individual and regional diversity, and to reflect on their own worldviews and professional frameworks. However, there are numerous implications of the above features that are specifically relevant to the aphasia context when considering both assessment and treatment focused on conversation. While many of these will appear as challenges in a cross-cultural context, it is also worth remembering the value in utilizing a conversational framework.

Language and Dialect Carry Identity

A basic notion that should underpin clinical speech-language pathology practice is acknowledgment that language and dialect carry cultural identity. Hence, it is crucial that any clinical advice provided does not interfere with or run counterintuitively to cultural norms. Advice regarding facilitation of communication between the person with aphasia and family and community members should be closely navigated with those family and community members and other Aboriginal colleagues or advisers. While treatments involving manipulation or practice of linguistic forms also obviously require close expert attention from speakers of a particular language or dialect, navigation around pragmatics, interactions, conversations, and yarns (discussed later in this chapter) is even more sensitive as these are essential for social connection and maintenance of cultural identity. The term *navigation* is used here to reflect the exploratory process required in cross-cultural assessment, with the clinician working closely with the client, family, interpreters (as needed), and cultural brokers to ensure that assessment methods are appropriate and that interpretations are accurate and relevant to the client.

Navigation Surrounding Assessment

The importance of involving family in navigations around assessment and treatment surrounding conversations has been advocated in aphasiology for a number of years. For example, rather than promoting a generic toolkit of tips for assisting a person with aphasia in conversations, the conversation analysis framework promotes the idea of negotiating what works and doesn't work for individual dyads (e.g., a person with aphasia and their partner, sibling, child). Strategies are made explicit to both communication partners, and therapy consists of assisting them in using those strategies they find helpful even more often and more consistently (see Chapter 7; Beeke et al., 2015). Such an approach is even more important when working cross-culturally.

In the Aboriginal context, it is very important to frame assessments and therapeutic conversations not around preconceived notions of pragmatic appropriateness, but more on schemas and discourse principles involved in AAE, with close reference to family input. For example, talk considered to be tangential by a non-Aboriginal clinician may not be tangential when considered from an Aboriginal discourse strategy perspective (Bessarab & Ng'andu, 2010; Walsh, 2009). Research papers in the traumatic brain injury literature continue to suggest that social communication problems are often manifested in the following ways: "poor eye contact, impaired initiation of conversation, poor topic maintenance, verbosity, difficulties adapting conversation to the needs of the listener and lack of conversation cohesion" (Finch et al., 2017). Some of these features described as pathological may not be considered in this way by speakers from Aboriginal and other non-Western backgrounds. For example, some traditional Aboriginal groups may regard lack of eye contact as a sign of respect. The concept of cohesion is very much based on a framework of explicit connectivity within a discourse—again, not a feature of traditional Aboriginal languages or AAE, which tend to be on the implicit end of the continuum due to shared community understandings and the lack of need for extended explicitness or detail (Malcolm, 2018). From a practical perspective, obtaining family opinions as to whether the person has changed from before their brain injury is crucial. For example, does the person talk more, talk less, become confused when telling a story, give too much detail, too little detail, or use language or a manner of interacting that appears to be lacking in respect for elders?

Partner Training and Conversational Therapies

In the Aboriginal context, what is currently termed *communication partner training* (Simmons-Mackie et al., 2016) could incorporate a wider range of people than is often targeted, including extended family members and relevant community contacts. For example, a spouse, child, or sibling of the person with aphasia is most routinely approached currently in a clinical setting, whereas for an Aboriginal person with aphasia, an extended family member may be the carer or another individual most involved with the person with aphasia. Social networks may include elders or family members who may not immediately be perceived by the non-Aboriginal clinician as the key partner; this must be explored in depth to find out who the key communication partners are. Kinship and social structures may also influence who is most appropriate to be involved in communication partner training discussions. Rather than a dyad-based intervention, a family-based intervention might be more appropriate. It is very important to ask who are the appropriate people to be speaking to about treatment, then ask those particular people—is X (the person with aphasia) different from before, and how? (Douglas et al., 2000). Asking the person themselves how they are feeling about their communication and what changes they have noticed is also crucial.

The clinician needs to be open to developing different notions of strategies with the variety of partners involved. For example, ways of guessing and cueing behaviors often discussed in relation to aphasic conversations may be quite different in Aboriginal discourse, with different methods potentially used for different people depending on community status (e.g., elder), age (child with parent), or gender. Use of humor, notions of shame, yarning strategies (discussed below), and the role of silence may be issues worth considering, given their significance in Aboriginal discourse and culture (Malcolm, 2018). It is crucial that Western maxims such as succinctness are not proposed as goals in conversations unless identified as an issue with family or the person themselves. Conversational discourse in AAE is not typically a linear, succinct form of conversation in the Western sense, hence different ways of approaching and facilitating conversation will be employed. It is important to negotiate strategies in a two-way fashion rather than presenting previously identified notions of conversational strategies from the aphasia evidence base to date.

Group talk is a particular context that should also be considered, seeing as conversational groups often constitute an option

for people with aphasia in current practice (Simmons-Mackie & Holland, 2011; Archer et al., 2021). What might be considered easy or difficult tasks for Aboriginal people with aphasia may be different from non-Aboriginal people. For example, group talk may be more familiar or important to Aboriginal people with aphasia for whom large family gatherings may be more the norm, but facilitation and participation strategies and communication roles may be different. The notion of group support (i.e., meeting with people with whom one is not familiar but may simply share the same condition such as aphasia) may also be considered differently by Aboriginal people, although some Aboriginal people with brain injury have expressed benefits obtained through meeting other Aboriginal people who have had similar experiences (Armstrong, Coffin, et al., 2019).

Yarning as Conversation

A yarning framework is increasingly being advocated to create a more culturally safe environment for Aboriginal clients. Bessarab and Ng'andu's (2010) definition of yarning relates to the undertaking of a conversation between two people, which is a dialogical process that is reciprocal and mutual (p. 38). They note that storytelling constitutes the majority of yarning conversations based on an Aboriginal oral tradition for passing on knowledge and culture across generations through stories (Wingard & Lester, 2001).

Lin and colleagues (2016) embrace a clinical context for health professionals working with Aboriginal clients in the form of clinical yarning. Their purpose was to provide both Aboriginal and non-Aboriginal clinicians (especially the latter) with a way of having conversations within a clinical environment that were meaningful to Aboriginal clients and more in line with the pragmatic rules of Aboriginal discourse rather than structured in a Western medical mode that often rely on a question-answer format and potentially inhibit Aboriginal clients' interactions with the clinician.

In such a framework, the conversation goes both ways and flows smoothly through the clinician and client sharing information about themselves; hence participants are crucial determiners of how the interaction will unfold. The importance of rapport building, establishing meaningful relationships and the social yarn cannot be over-stated. The tone of voice is also important so that the interactions are non-confrontational.

Lin et al. (2016) describe three types of yarning: social, diagnostic, and management yarns. The social yarn sets the scene for the clinical interaction. It is client centered, with the clinician creating space for the client to share their health story within the context of their everyday life. When the clinician also shares some personal details, the dyad establishes some common ground in important life components such as family and country (where each is from), and the client is able to lead the yarn in many respects, with the client's life story, experiences valued, and health issue(s) being seen within that context by the clinician. The diagnostic yarn continues as an unfolding story rather than the more typical clinical question-and-answer case history-taking process. The management yarn is again a collaborative process, with the clinician exploring further what the client understands about his or her condition, often explaining further through stories and metaphors, and again listening to the relevant goals and contexts of the client. Examples of the different types of yarns are available in Lin et al. (2016).

This framework has been applied to working with children in the speech-language pathology context (Lewis et al., 2017) and more recently in the adult context (Ciccone, Armstrong, Hersh, et al., 2019; Ciccone, Armstrong, Adams, et al., 2019). In both contexts, the principle of reciprocity applies (Bessarab & Ng'andu, 2010; Geia et al., 2013), where a two-way sharing of stories and information is essential. Lewis and colleagues (2017) have especially focused on yarning as an assessment framework (see Box). While her work primarily involves children, the principles involved relate equally to working with adults. Lewis notes that as yarning is a central form of Aboriginal discourse, it is essential that the clinician engages with this form of discourse so as to "ensure the strengths of Aboriginal children are validated and respected in a way that minimises misdiagnosis" (p. 16). She has developed an assessment tool called the Gumerri Assessment, which is a strengths-based approach to assessing children's communication skills that incorporates principles of yarning throughout. Lewis emphasizes that yarning is more than having a conversation or establishing rapport:

> Engaging in assessment yarning provides clinical insight into the centrality of the client and their family's journey. Assessment yarning enables clinicians to really 'see' the client in their 'humanness' within their context and to potentially disrupt any preconceived notions about the client. (p. 16)

Assessment Yarning

There are five important questions for the clinician to ask about assessment yarning (Lewis et al., 2017). These are also relevant to conversational interactions within the aphasia context.

- Is the yarn reciprocal?
- Is the yarn meaningful?
- Is a deep relational connection being formed?
- Is the aim of yarning to support learning through teaching?
- Am I listening for the meanings and information being conveyed through yarning?

Quotes From Yarning Together and Wangi Studies

"You have both made her talk a lot more. It's the stuff you got her to talk about as well. Like you talked about racism and sport and stuff like that. It sort of made her think . . . it's the subjects you guys have given her to think about has opened up the mind and the language as well."
(Parent of a participant—Ciccone, Armstrong, Adams, et al., 2019)

"Things that are relevant today so when you recover you can go back into the real world."
(Participant with aphasia referring to topics covered in treatment—Ciccone, Armstrong, Adams, et al., 2019)

"It's something they're interested in. Something they want to talk about, something that they're possibly passionate about . . . the first couple you're getting to know someone and they're not as open. But then you can see someone opening up."
(Aboriginal Coworker—Ciccone, Armstrong, Hersh, et al., 2019, p. 312)

Ciccone and colleagues trialed a yarning-based treatment with adults with acquired communication disorders in the Wangi (talking) study (Ciccone, Armstrong, Hersh, et al., 2019) and the more recent Yarning Together study (Ciccone, Armstrong, Adams, et al., 2019). Within both studies, yarning was used as the basis of the treatment and sessions were provided cojointly by a speech-language pathologist and Aboriginal coworker. Within the sessions, the conversations were based on topics of interest to those with the communication disorders, with participants encouraged to lead the direction of conversation within and across sessions. The participants, Aboriginal coworker and speech-language pathologist, were equal partners in the conversations with the Aboriginal coworker and speech-language pathologist encouraged to share their own stories to build a collaborative and shared yarn. Both studies yielded positive responses from the Aboriginal clients and their families (see box), with the conclusion that the model was both feasible and acceptable.

Cultural Security: What Does a Culturally Secure Clinical Environment Look Like?

One of the overriding issues that arises in cross-cultural practice is the limited understanding of cultural capabilities applied by SLPs in creating culturally safe and secure services for First Nations clients (Armstrong, Carmody, et al., 2019; Brewer et al., 2019; Hersh et al., 2015; Lewis et al., 2017; Pillay & Kathard, 2015). The terms *cultural safety* and *cultural security* are often used interchangeably, although the latter aims to emphasize the importance of institutional practices as well as individual clinical practices. However, both involve a context in which services are provided that both acknowledge and respect clients' cultural knowledges, values, and attitudes and ensure these are not violated in any way in how the service is structured or carried out (Coffin, 2007).

In the Australian context, there are a relatively small number of SLPs who identify as Aboriginal and/or Torres Strait Islander. In an ideal clinical scenario, Aboriginal SLPs would deliver health care services to their own communities, which is critical to the provision of culturally safe services and can ultimately improve overall health outcomes (Australian Government, 2016). It's important to acknowledge this shortfall and that clinicians working with Aboriginal and/or Torres Strait Islander people would likely be from a non-Aboriginal background. Given the diversity of Aboriginal peoples across Australia, the variety of Home Languages, and increasing but still limited input at the professional learning stages during university education, it is highly likely that non-Aboriginal clinicians would have very limited knowledge or experience in working with people from an Aboriginal background. In this instance, they should work closely with an Aboriginal health worker and a respected community person who can provide additional support as needed. Local interpreting services should be accessed as needed.

It is essential that clinicians provide culturally safe, secure, and responsive services to ensure First Nations peoples and communities have access to safe and culturally appropriate services. The importance of developing deep and meaningful relationships and applying culturally secure practice for SLPs working with Aboriginal peoples is well documented (Armstrong, Carmody, et al., 2019; Hersh et al., 2015). It is vital that clinicians understand the impact of colonization, intergenerational trauma, and the personal, lived experiences for First Nations peoples, considering the associated stress and anxiety of attending a hospital or traditional health setting. It is also essential that clinicians are critically conscious of the intersectionality of race and racism within the speech-language pathology profession and the role we continue to play in empowering a racialized ideology of First Nation communication capabilities.

Employing the principles of clinical yarning as outlined above is increasingly being recommended when working with Aboriginal and Torres Strait Islander peoples. This approach is essentially two-way in nature and involves avoiding the use of direct and closed questions, which may make the interaction feel like an interrogation or interview instead of a collaborative consultation. Armstrong, Carmody, et al. (2019) provide further details on clear principles of practice for clinicians to adhere to in both pediatric and adult settings.

Clinicians need to acknowledge and understand extended kinship systems because they may be expected to work with extended family members. These family members should be welcomed and included in sessions as much as they feel comfortable. Family can provide valuable information on whether the client is presenting with a communication difference due to Home Language or with a communication disorder.

Summary and Conclusions

An increasing focus on discourse and conversational interactions in speech-language pathology clinical practice and research has seen numerous approaches to assessment and treatment adopted. In this chapter we have presented challenges to clinicians and researchers working in a cross-cultural context specifically focused on conversational frameworks and have provided some suggestions for beginning to address these challenges. While acknowledging the importance of frameworks, we have highlighted the importance of culture when working on conversation—both of which are intrinsically linked to a person's individual as well as community identity. Unpacking discourse through its component parts may be valid for some purposes and can certainly contribute to theoretical hypotheses about impairments to an extent. However, this can only work if the clinician or researcher understands the interaction between culture and language, the framework they are using for analysis and its inherent cultural bias, and their own cultural and linguistic assumptions. It is also important to emphasize that meanings are conveyed between people based on deep cultural understandings and that analyzing what are often surface-level linguistic features may not do justice to understanding interactional communication strengths and weaknesses.

We have raised the importance of these issues as well as potential ways forward that include reflections on one's own worldview and associated assumptions, and how these affect approaches to conversational assessment and treatments; use of a cultural linguistic framework that can assist clinicians in being aware of and exploring potential cross-cultural differences in interactional styles of communication; the role of yarning as a framework for pursuing conversational treatments with people with aphasia; and ways of ensuring cultural security of services. As everyday conversation has become increasingly significant in the aphasiology literature and in clinical practice, an understanding of cross-cultural implications of assessment and treatment practices becomes increasingly important.

We have presented these insights from the context of Australian First Nations peoples from which we believe there is much to be learned about cross-cultural practice in speech-language pathology and aphasiology. Principles involved relate to cross-cultural practice in general, as well as ethical implications and responsibilities for clinicians and researchers alike (Brewer et al., 2019; Centeno et al., 2020; Lewis et al., 2017; Penn et al., 2017; Watego et al., 2021).

Language is more than words and more than a process that occurs between the ears within the individual's brain; it encompasses culture, identity, and social relationships, and is co-constructed between speakers. As such, assessment and intervention processes in speech-language pathology and aphasiology need to continue to expand their application of sociolinguistic frameworks, incorporating increasing reference to research emanating from the perspectives and philosophical approaches of First Nations peoples and from non-Western standpoints. Looking holistically, it is extremely important for clinicians and researchers to combine knowledge of linguistic and pragmatic features of interactions with notions of cultural security. The Aboriginal and Torres Strait Islander cultural context in Australia has provided an example of the challenges and nuances of cross-cultural speech-language pathology practice related to assessment and treatment practices within the aphasia context, with particular focus on conversational frameworks. While the issues raised are context specific in some respects, the principles can be applied to multiple cultural contexts.

References

Aborigines Protection Act 1909. NSW Government Legislation. https://www.legislation.nsw.gov.au/view/pdf/asmade/act-1909-25

Archer, B., Azios, J. H., Gulick, N., & Tetnowski, J. (2021). Facilitating participation in conversation groups for aphasia. *Aphasiology, 35*(6), 764–782. https://doi.org/10.1080/02687038.2020.1812030

Armstrong, E., Carmody, A., Robins, A., & Lewis, T. (2019). Assessment and outcome measures for Aboriginal Australians with communication disorders. *Journal of Clinical Practice in Speech-Language Pathology, 21*(2), 50–57. https://speechpathologyaustralia.cld.bz/JCPSLP-Vol-21-No-2-2019-DIGITAL-Edition/4

Armstrong, E., Coffin, C., Hersh, D., Katzenellenbogen, J. M., Thompson, S. C., Ciccone, N., . . . McAllister, M. (2019, online). "You felt like a prisoner in your own self, trapped": The experiences of Aboriginal people with acquired communication disorders. *Disability and Rehabilitation, 43*(13), 1903–1916. https://doi.org/10.1080/09638288.2019.1686073

Armstrong, E., Hersh, D., Hayward, C., & Fraser, J. (2015). Communication disorders after stroke in Aboriginal Australians. *Disability and Rehabilitation, 37*(16), 1462–1469. https://doi.org/10.3109/09638288.2014.972581

Armstrong, E., McKay, G., & Hersh, D. (2017). Assessment and treatment of aphasia in Aboriginal Australians: Linguistic and cultural issues. *Journal of Clinical Practice in Speech-Language Pathology, 19* (1), 27–34. https://speechpathologyaustralia.cld.bz/JCPSLP-Vol-19-No-1-March-2017/29

Australian Bureau of Statistics. (2016). *Estimates of Aboriginal and Torres Strait Islander Australians.* ABS Cat. No. 3238.0.55.001 2016

Australian Government. (2016). *National Framework for Health Services for Aboriginal and Torres Strait Islander Children and Families.* https://www.catsinam.org.au/static/uploads/files/national-framework-for-health-services-for-aboriginal-and-torres-strait-islander.pdf

Australian Institute of Health and Welfare. (2020). *Australia's health 2020 data insights.* Australia's health series no. 17. Cat. no. AUS 231. AIHW.

Bastiaanse, R., & Edwards, S. (2004). Word order and finiteness in Dutch and English Broca's and Wernicke's aphasia. *Brain and Language, 89*(1), 91–107. https://doi.org/10.1016/S0093-934X(03)00306-7

Beeke, S., Beckley, F., Johnson, F., Heilemann, C., Edwards, S., Maxim, J., & Best, W. (2015). Conversation-focused aphasia therapy: Investigating the adoption of strategies by people with agrammatism. *Aphasiology, 29*(3), 355–377. https://doi.org/10.1080/02687038.2014.881459

Bessarab, D., & Ng'andu, B. (2010). Yarning about yarning as a legitimate method in Indigenous research. *International Journal of Critical Indigenous Studies, 3*(1), 37–50. http://hdl.handle.net/20.500.11937/37083

Bohanna, I., Fitts, M., Bird, K., Fleming, J., Gilroy, J., Clough, A., . . . Potter, M. (2019). The potential of a narrative and creative arts approach to enhance transition outcomes for Indigenous Australians following traumatic brain injury. *Brain Impairment, 20*(2), 160–170. https://doi.org/10.1017/BrImp.2019.25

Bracknell, C. (2020). Rebuilding as research: Noongar song, language and ways of knowing. *Journal of Australian Studies, 44*(2), 210–223. https://doi.org/10.1080/14443058.2020.1746380

Brewer, K., Lewis, T., Bond, C., Armstrong, E., Hill, A. E., Nelson, A., & Coffin, J. (2019). Maintaining cultural integrity in Aboriginal and Māori qualitative research. In L. McAllister & R. Lyons (Eds.), *Qualitative research in communication disorders: An introduction for students and clinicians.* J & R Press.

Butcher, A. (2008). Linguistic aspects of Australian Aboriginal English. *Clinical Linguistics and Phonetics, 22*(8), 625–642. https://doi.org/10.1080/02699200802223535

Centeno, J., Kiran, S., & Armstrong, E. (2020). Editorial: Aphasia management in growing multiethnic populations. *Aphasiology*, *34*(11), 1314–1318. https://doi.org/10.1080/026870 38.2020.1781420

Ciccone, N., Armstrong, E., Adams, M., Bessarab, D., Hersh, D., McAllister, M., . . . Coffin, J. (2019, May 2–4). *Yarning together: Developing a culturally secure rehabilitation approach for Aboriginal Australians after brain injury* [Conference presentation]. Australasian Society for the Study of Brain Impairment/New Zealand Rehabilitation Association Inaugural Trans-Tasman Conference, Wellington, New Zealand.

Ciccone, N., Armstrong, E., Hersh, D., Adams, M., & McAllister, M. (2019). The Wangi (talking) project: A feasibility study of a rehabilitation model for Aboriginal people with acquired communication disorders after stroke. *International Journal of Speech-Language Pathology*, *21*, 305–316. https://doi.org/10.1080/17549507.2019.1595146

Clyne, M. (1995). *Cross-cultural communication at work: Cultural values in discourse*. Cambridge University Press.

Coffin, J. (2007). Rising to the challenge in Aboriginal health by creating cultural security. *Aboriginal and Islander Health Worker Journal*, *31*(3), 22–24. https://search.informit.org/doi/10.3316/informit.955665869609324

Collard, S., Fatnowna, S., Oxenham, D., Roberts, J., & Rodriguez, L. (2000). Styles, appropriateness and usage of Aboriginal English. *Asian Englishes*, *3*(2), 82–97.

Department of Communications, Information, Technology, and the Arts. (2005). *National Indigenous languages survey report 2005*. http://www.fatsilc.org.au/images/pdfs/NILS-Report-2005.pdf

Douglas, J., O'Flaherty, C., & Snow, P. (2000). Measuring perception of communicative ability: The development and evaluation of the La Trobe Communication Questionnaire. *Aphasiology*, *14*, 251–268. https://doi.org/10.1080/026870300401469

Durey, A., McEvoy, S., Swift-Otero, V., Taylor, K., Katzenellenbogen, J., & Bessarab, D. (2016). Improving healthcare for Aboriginal Australians through effective engagement between community and health services. *BMC Health Services Research.*, *16*(1), 224. https://doi.org/10.1186/s12913-016-1497-0

Finch, E., Cornwell, P., Copley, A., Doig, E., & Fleming, J. (2017). Remediation of social communication impairments following traumatic brain injury using metacognitive strategy intervention: A pilot study. *Brain Injury*, *31*(13–14), 1830–1839. https://doi.org/10.1080/02699052.2017.1346284

Fitts, M. S., Bird, K., Gilroy, J., Fleming, J., Clough, A. R., Esterman, A., . . . Bohanna, I. (2019). A qualitative study on the transition support needs of Indigenous Australians following traumatic brain injury. *Brain Impairment*, *20*(2), 137–159. https://doi.org/10.1017/BrImp.2019.24

Fyndanisa, V., Linda, M., Varlokostac, S., Kambanaros, M., Sorolie, E., Cederf, K., . . . Howard, D. (2017). Cross-linguistic adaptations of The Comprehensive Aphasia Test: Challenges and solutions. *Clinical Linguistics and Phonetics*, *31* (7–9), 697–710. https://doi.org/10.1080/02699206.2017.1310299

Geia, L., Hayes, B., & Usher, K. (2013). Yarning/Aboriginal storytelling: Towards an understanding of an Indigenous perspective and its implications for research practice. *Contemporary Nurse*, *46*(1), 13–17. https://doi.org/10.5172/conu.2013.46.1.13

Gilroy, J., Donelly, M., Colmar, S., & Parmenter, T. (2013). Conceptual framework for policy and research development with Indigenous people with disabilities. *Australian Aboriginal Studies.*, *2*, 42–58.

Gilroy, J., Donelly, M., Colmar, S., & Parmenter, T. (2016). Twelve factors that influence participation of Aboriginal people in disability services. *Australian Indigenous Health Bulletin*, *16*(1), 1–9. https://healthbulletin.org.au/wp-content/uploads/2016/03/bulletin_original_articles_Gilroy.pdf

Grice, P. (1975). Logic and conversation. In P. Cole & J. Morgan (Eds.), *Syntax and semantics 3: Speech acts* (pp. 41–58). Academic Press.

Halliday, M. A. K. (1985). Context of situation. In M. A. K. Halliday & R. Hasan (Eds.), *Lan-*

guage, context, and text: Aspects of language in a social-semiotic perspective (pp. 3–14). Deakin University Press.

Hersh, D., Armstrong, E., Panak, V., & Coombes, J. (2015). Speech-language pathology practices with Indigenous Australians with acquired communication disorders. *International Journal of Speech-Language Pathology, 17*(1), 74–85. https://doi.org/10.3109/17549507.2014.923510

Holland, A. L., Fromm, D., & Wozniak, L. (2018). CADL–3: *Communication activities of daily living*. Pro-Ed.

Huang, A. J. R., Siyambalapitiya, S., & Cornwell, P. (2019). Speech pathologists and professional interpreters managing culturally and linguistically diverse adults with communication disorders: A systematic review. *International Journal of Language and Communication Disorders, 54*(5), 689–704. https://doi.org/10.1111/1460-6984.12475

Kertesz, A. (2006). *Western Aphasia Battery–Revised*. Pearson.

Konigsberg, P., & Collard, G. (2002). *Ways of being, ways of talk*. Education Department of Western Australia.

Geia, L., Hayes, B., & Usher, K. (2013 Lee, S., & Faroqi-Shah, Y. (2021). Performance of Korean-English bilinguals on an adaptation of the screening bilingual aphasia test. *International Journal of Language and Communication Disorders, 56*(4), 719–738. https://doi.org/10.1111/1460-6984.12623

Lewis, T., Hill, A. E., Bond, C., & Nelson, A. (2017). Yarning: assessing proppa ways. *Journal of Clinical Practice in Speech-Language Pathology, 19*(1), 14–18. https://speechpathologyaustralia.cld.bz/JCPSLP-Vol-19-No-1-March-2017/16

Lin, I., Green, C., & Bessarab, D. (2016). "Yarn with me": Applying clinical yarning to improve clinician-patient communication in Aboriginal health care. *Australian Journal of Primary Health, 22*(5), 377–382. https://doi.org/10.1071/PY16051

Louro, C. R., & Collard, G. (2021). Australian Aboriginal English: Linguistic and sociolinguistic perspectives. *Language and Linguistics Compass, 15*(5),1–12. https://doi.org/10.1111/lnc3.12415

Lowitja Institute. (2021). *Close the Gap Campaign Report 2021: Leadership and legacy through crises: Keeping our mob safe*. Lowitja Institute. https://humanrights.gov.au/our-work/aboriginal-and-torres-strait-islander-social-justice/publications

Malcolm, I. G. (1995). *Language and communication enhancement for two-way education. Report to the Department of Employment, Education and Training*. Centre for Applied Language Research, Edith Cowan University.

Malcolm, I. G. (2017). Embedding cultural conceptualization within an adopted language: the English of Aboriginal Australia. *The International Journal of Language and Culture, 4*(2), 149–169. https://doi.org/10.1075/ijolc.4.2.02mal

Malcolm, I. G. (2018). *Australian Aboriginal English: Change and continuity in an adopted language*. de Gruyter Mouton. (e-book)

Malcolm, I. G. (2021). Australian Aboriginal English and linguistic inquiry. In M. Sadeghpour & F. Sharifian (Eds.), *Cultural linguistics and world Englishes* (pp. 15–36). Springer.

Malcolm, I., Haig, Y., Konigsberg, P., Rochecouste, J., Collard, G., Hill, A., & Cahill, R. (1999). *Towards more user-friendly education for speakers of Aboriginal English*. Edith Cowan University. Research Online. https://ro.ecu.edu.au/ecuworks/7175

Malinowski, B. (2002). *The language of magic and gardening: Vol. 2. Coral gardens and their magic*. Routledge. (Original work published 1935).

Moreton-Robinson, A. (2006). Towards a new research agenda? Foucault, whiteness and Indigenous sovereignty. *Journal of Sociology, 42*(4), 383–395. https://doi.org/10.1177%2F1440783306069995

Mushin, I., & Baker, B. (Eds.). (2008). *Discourse and grammar in Australian languages*. John Benjamins.

Nelson, A. (2007). Seeing white: A critical exploration of occupational therapy with Indigenous Australian people. *Occupational Therapy International, 14*(4), 237–255. https://doi.org/10.1002/oti.236

Palmer, G. (1996). *Toward a theory of cultural linguistics*. University of Austin Press. http://

ebookcentral.proquest.com/lib/ecu/detail
.action?docID=622234

Penn, C., Armstrong, E., Brewer, K., Purves, B., McAllister, M., Hersh, D., . . . Lewis, A. (2017). Decolonizing speech-language pathology practice in acquired neurogenic disorders. *SIG 2 Perspectives on Neurophysiology and Neurogenic Speech and Language Disorders, 2*(3), 91–99.

Pillay, M., & Kathard, H. (2015). Decolonizing health professionals' education: Audiology and speech therapy in South Africa. *African Journal of Rhetoric, 7*, 193–227. https://journals.co.za/doi/10.10520/EJC172807

Rigney, L. I. (1999). Internationalization of an Indigenous anticolonial cultural critique of research methodologies: A guide to Indigenist research methodology and its principles. *Wíčazo Ša Review, 14*(2), 109–121. https://doi.org/10.2307/1409555

Sharifian, F. (2017). *Cultural linguistics: Cultural conceptualisations and language.* John Benjamins.

Simmons-Mackie, N., & Holland, A. L. (2011). Aphasia centers in North America: A survey. *Seminars in Speech and Language, 32*(3), 203–215. https://doi.org/10.1055/s-0031-1286175

Simmons-Mackie, N., Raymer, A., & Cherney, L. (2016). Communication partner training in aphasia: An updated systematic review. *Archives of Physical Medicine and Rehabilitation, 97*(12), 2202–2221. https://doi.org/10.1016/j.apmr.2016.03.023

Tuhiwai Smith, L. (2012). *Decolonizing methodologies: Research and Indigenous peoples.* Zed Books.

Walsh, M. (2009, July 12–17). *Some neo-Gricean maxims for Aboriginal Australia* [Conference presentation]. International Pragmatics Association Conference, Melbourne, Australia.

Watego, C., Whop, L. J., Singh, D., Mukandi, B., Macoun, A., Newhouse, G., . . . Brough, M. (2021). Black to the future: Making the case for Indigenist health humanities. *International Journal of Environmental Research and Public Health, 18*, 8704. https://doi.org/10.3390/ijerph18168704

Wingard, B., & Lester, J. (2001). *Telling our stories in ways that make us stronger.* Dulwich Centre Publications.

SECTION III
Discourse of People With Cognitive Communication Disorders

Leanne Togher, Topic Chair

Cognitive communication disorders (CCDs) comprise a unique set of communication difficulties that can arise from a range of neurological insults including traumatic brain injury (TBI) and right hemisphere damage (RHD) associated with stroke or other causes, such as brain tumor. CCDs are ubiquitous for people with moderate to severe TBI; in fact, it is reported to be present for approximately 70% of this group (MacDonald, 2017). CCDs arise from the neurological disruption of the complex interplay of language, which is viewed as a cognitive function; other cognitive functions such as attention, memory, information processing, and executive functioning; and the sociocultural context within which interactions occur. CCDs typically lead to difficulty with conversational discourse, which has been described as occurring across a spectrum ranging from deficient and impoverished output to excessive talkativeness with poor turn taking and repetitiveness (Snow, Douglas, & Ponsford, 1998).

Communication underpins our capacity to engage in everyday activities, such as talking with friends and families, following instructions in the workplace, making appointments, and planning our future. As such, the ability to engage in the discourse genres that enact these scenarios is central to our success in navigating daily life activities. Communication can be described as the currency of social life. The difficulty for a person with CCD, however, whether it be from TBI or RHD, is that access to these discourse genres is impaired or interrupted, and this can have significant detrimental impacts on a person's ability to work, study, and maintain and develop social relationships. Words often used to describe CCDs in everyday terms include "subtle communication deficits," "personality change," "not the same person as before the injury"; in worst-case scenarios, a person may be described as "difficult," "offensive," "awkward," and/or "insensitive." Capturing the nature of these difficulties has posed significant challenges to clinicians and researchers. However, there has been considerable progress made in the conceptualization of CCDs (MacDonald, 2017; McDonald et al., 2012).

CCDs were initially viewed as interplay between cognition and language so that the term *cognitive-language disorder* described cognitive problems impacting upon language processing (Hagen, 1984; Kennedy & DeRuyter, 1991). For example, Hagen suggested that the impairments of attention, memory, sequencing, categorization, and associative abilities were the result of an impaired capacity to organize and structure incoming information, emotional reactions, and the flow of thought. Such impairments, Hagen argued, caused a disorganization of language processes. Cognitive disorganization was reflected through language use characterized by irrelevant utterances that may not make sense, difficulty inhibiting inappropriate utterances, word-finding difficulties, and problems ordering words and propositions. A decade later, the term *cognitive-communication disorder* was coined by Leila Hartley and others and is now the common term used clinically, in research, and in policy documents (Hartley, 1995). For example, the Canadian College of Audiologists and Speech-Language Pathologists of Ontario (CASLPO)'s (2015) definition of CCDs states the person has difficulties with listening, speaking, reading, written expression, or social interaction that occur due to underlying problems with cognitive skills such as attention, memory, organization, reasoning, social cognition, or executive functions (CASLPO, 2015).

The focus on the relationship between cognition and communication originally arose from an examination of the underlying pathophysiology of TBI, which commonly results in multifocal cerebral damage with a preponderance of injury to the frontal lobes. Cognition can be broadly described as "mental activities or operations involved in taking in, interpreting, encoding, storing, retrieving and making use of knowledge or information and generating a response" (Ylvisaker & Szekeres, 1994, p. 548). Examples of cognitive processes attributed to the frontal lobes include attention to stimuli, remembering and learning, organizing

information, reasoning, and problem solving. In addition to specific cognitive processes, the frontal lobes appear to mediate executive control of thought and behavior. Such executive functions include goal setting, behavior planning and sequencing, goal-oriented behavior initiation, and evaluation of behavior (Lezak, 1993).

Serendipitously, in the late 1980s and early 1990s, theoretical advances in the field of discourse assessment for people with TBI were emerging at the same time as insights into CCDs. Discourse was defined at the time as a unit of language that conveys a message (Ulatowska & Bond Chapman, 1989). There are different types of discourse tasks that have been referred to as different discourse *genres*. A genre is a particular text type that has its own structure, sequence, and purpose. Some types of discourse genres include narrative (recounting a story), procedural (a set of instructions for doing something), expository (giving an opinion or discussing a topic in detail), and conversation. The use of discourse genres, including narrative and conversation, sheds light on the communication difficulties of people with TBI rather than relying on standardized tests developed for aphasia. Discourse analyses represented a watershed in the characterization of this population.

Developments in discourse analyses to study CCD populations were situated within a proliferation of interest across several disciplines including sociology (Hymes, 1986; Labov, 1970), psychology (Mandler & Johnson, 1977), artificial intelligence (Schank & Abelson, 1977), and linguistics (Grimes, 1975; van Dijk, 1977). Techniques in discourse analyses for CCD populations were derived from both the psycholinguistic and sociolinguistic perspectives. The psycholinguistic analyses include measures of syntax (Chapman et al., 1992; Glosser & Deser, 1990; Liles et al., 1989), productivity (Hartley & Jensen, 1991; Mentis & Prutting,

1987) and content (Hartley & Jensen, 1991). Conversely, sociolinguistic techniques include cohesion analysis (Coelho et al., 1991a; McDonald, 1993; Mentis & Prutting, 1987), analysis of coherence (Chapman et al., 1992; McDonald, 1993), analysis of topic (Mentis & Prutting, 1991), and compensatory strategies (Penn & Cleary, 1988). This foundational work underpins and is built upon by the four chapters reported in this section on CCDs and discourse assessment.

Considerable advances have been made to our conceptualizations of the discourse of people with CCDs since the publication of the Cherney et al. (1998) landmark book. Since the dawn of the new millennium and the new century, there has been an array of advances so that clinicians and researchers can ask clinically relevant questions and find the answers in a person's discourse. Using discourse measures to predict outcomes and measure recovery following TBI has progressed significantly over the past decade. For example, in Elbourn et al.'s chapter on discourse recovery of people with TBI across the continuum (see Chapter 9), you will find the answers to the following questions:

■ Can we determine indicators of recovery by studying a person's discourse while they are in post-traumatic amnesia?
■ Which features of a person's discourse will predict their outcomes 12 months postinjury?
■ Which discourse genres are sensitive to measuring change over time?
■ As a busy clinician working with people with TBI, what tips are there to help me include discourse analysis in my clinical practice?

While recovery of language function is common below the sentence level, it has been frequently observed that people with TBI do not perform well in connected speech tasks, leading to the discovery that the hallmark feature of TBI is impaired conversation (Coelho et al., 1991b). Assessing conversation of people with TBI is a challenging endeavor, given the complexity of everyday interactions and the diverse purposes for which we are conversing. A significant clinical challenge is the impracticality of conducting transcription during a busy clinical day while at the same time measuring how people are conversing with a range of communication partners in a clinically replicable and reliable manner. Keegan et al. (see Chapter 10) provide clarity with regards to these issues by offering the reader a suite of assessment tools that do not require transcription and that have been well tested and validated. In Chapter 10, the reader will find answers to the following clinical questions:

■ If I want to assess a person's conversational skills, what assessment tools are available to me?
■ How do I assess the interactions of people during group sessions?
■ How do I measure the person with TBI's perception of their own conversational skills, and that of their significant other?
■ What theoretical perspectives are commonly used to assess conversations of people with TBI?
■ How do I measure progress when working with a patient to improve their conversational skills?

Cognitive communication disorders are not limited to people with brain damage arising from TBI. Right hemisphere damage (RHD) following a focal stroke can also lead to cognitive communication disorders, which can be difficult to diagnose and are often missed in clinical practice. CCDs associated with RHD are a specialized area of investigation that has expanded steadily over the past 20 years. Stockbridge et al. (see Chapter 11) describe both expressive and receptive studies undertaken of RHD discourse. The study of discourse comprehension in RHD participants has led to theories of discourse processing, such as the Bilateral Activation, Inhibition, and Selection (BAIS) model (Jung-Beeman, 2005) and the Structure-Building Framework (Gernsbacher et al., 1990), which, in turn, have informed clinical practice such as the development of Contextual Constraint Treatment (Blake et al., 2015). Our understanding of expressive discourse difficulties following RHD has been enhanced by discourse analysis techniques such as coherence analysis, cohesion analysis, story grammar analysis and the use of discourse task stimuli which are sensitive to RHD discourse deficits. Chapter 11 will help the clinician answer the following questions:

- Which discourse analyses are most sensitive to the nuanced difficulties that can occur following RHD?
- What are the most sensitive stimuli I can use to evaluate the discourse of a person with RHD?
- What is the gold-standard approach I should use to examine communication skills after RHD?

The new millennium has led to significant advances in technology, which have already impacted clinical practice, including the analysis of discourse for populations with CCDs. The pandemic has highlighted how valuable telehealth has become as a model of clinical care for people with acquired communication disorders following TBI and stroke. Technology offers other advantages, including rapid speech-to-text transcription, the use of artificial intelligence to code and parse discourse, and the development of novel discourse assessment methods that can fast track assess-

ment results. Rietdijk and Meulenbroek (see Chapter 12) provide the clinician with an overview of telepractice, including how to plan a telepractice discourse assessment, how to choose validated discourse measures, and how to use technology to collect and analyze data. Meulenbroek's Voicemail Elicitation Task is an exciting example of how technology can provide a one-stop shop for the busy clinician with automated discourse data collection and rapid analysis (Meulenbroek & Cherney, 2019). Rietdijk and Meulenbroek's chapter answers the following clinical questions:

- How do I plan for a telepractice discourse assessment?
- Which CCD measures have been validated for telepractice?
- How do I use technology to collect and analyze discourse data?
- What readily available technology is available to help me provide feedback to my patient regarding their intonation?
- Which technology can help with examining written discourse of people with CCDs, including social media posts?
- How can I use technology to measure discourse change over time for a person with CCDs?
- Which technologies are showing promise for clinical practice in the future?

The study of discourse in CCD populations has grown exponentially over the past 20 years. There have been advances in the theoretical underpinnings of how cognition and language include *sensory and cognitive prerequisites*, such as sensation and perception, social cognition, and memory functioning, as well as how *metapragmatic skills* address self-awareness and strategy use. The *sociocultural context* within which discourse is occurring has also expanded (McDonald et al., 2012). The goals of clinical discourse analysis with individuals with CCDs are to diagnose changes to communication ability during personally relevant everyday activities; reliably measure those changes; develop a treatment plan using sensitive goal-setting approaches; track discourse recovery over time; and integrate this with a treatment program that focuses on life outcomes. The four chapters in this CCD topic section cover all these issues and provide the clinician and clinical researcher with practical, feasible solutions to key clinical questions as outlined above.

References

Blake, M. L., Tompkins, C. A., Scharp, V. L., Meigh, K. M., & Wambaugh, J. (2015). Contextual Constraint Treatment for coarse coding deficit in adults with right hemisphere brain damage: Generalisation to narrative discourse comprehension. *Neuropsychological Rehabilitation*, *25*(1), 15–52. https://doi.org/10.1080/09602011.2014.932290

CASLPO. (2015). *Practice standards and guidelines for acquired cognitive communication disorders*. College of Audiologists and Speech-Language Pathologists of Ontario. http://www.caslpo.com/sites/default/uploads/files/PSG_EN_Acquired_Cognitive_Communication_Disorders.pdf

Chapman, S. B., Culhane, K. A., Levin, H. S., Harward, H., Mendelsohn, D., Ewing-Cobbs, L., . . . Bruce, D. (1992). Narrative discourse after closed head injury in children and adolescents. *Brain and Language*, *43*, 42–65. https://doi.org/10.1016/0093-934X(92)90020-F

Coelho, C., Liles, B. Z., & Duffy, R. J. (1991a). Discourse analysis with closed head injured adults: Evidence for differing patterns of deficits. *Archives of Physical Medicine and Rehabilitation*, *72*, 465–468. Retrieved through Archives of Physical Medicine and Rehabilitation home page.

Coelho, C., Liles, B. Z., & Duffy, R. J. (1991b). Analysis of conversational discourse in head-injured adults. *Journal of Head Trauma Rehabilitation*, *6*(2), 92–98. https://doi.org/10.1097/00001199-199106000-00011

Gernsbacher, M. A., Varner, K. R., & Faust, M. E. (1990). Investigating differences in general comprehension skill. *Journal of Experimental Psychology: Learning, Memory, and Cognition*, *16*(3), 430. https://doi.org/10.1037/0278-7393.16.3.430

Glosser, G., & Deser, T. (1990). Patterns of discourse production among neurological patients with fluent language disorders. *Brain and Language*, *40*, 67–88. https://doi.org/10.1016/0093-934x(91)90117-j.

Grimes, J. (1975). *The thread of discourse*. The Hague: Mouton.

Hagen, C. (1984). Language disorders in head trauma. In A. Holland (Ed.), *Language disorders in adults* (pp. 245–281). College Hill Press.

Hartley, L. (1995). *Cognitive-communicative abilities following brain injury: A functional approach*. Singular Publishing.

Hartley, L., & Jensen, P. (1991). Narrative and procedural discourse after closed head injury. *Brain Injury*, *5* (3), 267–285. https://doi.org/10.3109/02699059109008097

Hymes, D. (1986). Models of the interaction of language and social life. In J. J. Gumperz & D. Hymes (Eds.), *Directions in sociolinguistics. The ethnography of communication* (pp. 35–71). Basil Blackwell.

Jung-Beeman, M. (2005). Bilateral brain processes for comprehending natural language. *Trends in Cognitive Sciences*, *9*(11), 512–518. https://doi.org/10.1016/j.tics.2005.09.009

Kennedy, M. R. T., & DeRuyter, F. (1991). Cognitive and language bases for communication disorders. In D. R. Beukelman & K. M. Yorkston (Eds.), *Communication disorders following traumatic brain injury : Management of cognitive, language and motor impairments* (pp. 123–190). Pro-Ed.

Labov, W. (1970). The study of language in its social context. *Studium Generale*, *23*, 30–87. https://doi.org/10.1515/9783111417509-004

Lezak, M. D. (1993). Newer contributions to the neuropsychological assessment of executive functions. *Journal of Head Trauma Rehabilitation*, *8*(1), 24–31. https://doi.org/10.1097/00001199-199303000-00004

Liles, B. Z., Coelho, C. A., Duffy, R. J., & Zalagens, M. R. (1989). Effects of elicitation procedures on the narratives of normal and closed head-injured adults. *Journal of Speech and Hearing Disorders, 54*, 356–366. https://doi.org/10.1044/jshd.5403.356

MacDonald, S. (2017). Introducing the model of cognitive-communication competence: A model to guide evidence-based communication interventions after brain injury. *Brain Injury, 31*(13–14), 1760–1780. https://doi.org/10.1080/02699052.2017.1379613

Mandler, J. A., & Johnson, N. S. (1977). Remebrance of things parsed: Story structure and recall. *Cognitive Psychology, 9*, 111–151. https://doi.org/10.1016/0010-0285(77)90006-8

McDonald, S. (1993). Pragmatic skills after closed head injury: Ability to meet the informational needs of the listener. *Brain and Language, 44 (1)*, 28–46. https://doi.org/10.1006/brln.1993.1003

McDonald, S., Turkstra, L. S., & Togher, L. (2012). Pragmatic language impairment after brain injury: Social implications and treatment models. In *Developmental social neuroscience and childhood brain insult: Theory and practice* (pp. 325–349). Guilford Press.

Mentis, M., & Prutting, C. A. (1987). Cohesion in the discourse of normal and head-injured adults. *Journal of Speech and Hearing Research, 30*, 88–98. https://doi.org/10.1044/jshr.3001.88

Mentis, M., & Prutting, C. A. (1991). Analysis of topic as illustrated in a head-injured and a normal adult. *Journal of Speech and Hearing Research, 34*, 583–595. https://doi.org/10.1044/jshr.3403.583

Meulenbroek, P., & Cherney, L. R. (2019). The voicemail elicitation task: Functional workplace langauge assessment for persons with traumatic brain injury. *Journal of Speech, Language, and Hearing Research, 62*, 3367–3380. https://doi.org/10.1044/2019_JSLHR-L-18-0466

Penn, C., & Cleary, J. (1988). Compensatory strategies in the language of closed head injured patients. *Brain Injury, 2*(1), 3–17. https://doi.org/10.3109/02699058809150928

Schank, R., & Abelson, R. (1977). *Scripts, plans, goals and understanding*. Lawrence Erlbaum.

Snow, P., Douglas, J., & Ponsford, J. (1998). Conversational discourse abilities following severe traumatic brain injury: A follow-up study. *Brain Injury, 12*(11), 911–935. https://psycnet.apa.org/doi/10.1080/026990598121981

Ulatowska, H. K., & Bond Chapman, S. (1989). Discourse considerations for aphasia management. *Seminars in Speech and Language: Aphasia and Pragmatics, 10*(4), 298–314. Thieme Medical Publishers. doi:10.1055/s-2008-1064270

van Dijk, T. A. (1977). *Text and context: Explorations in the semantics and pragmatics of discourse*. Longman.

Ylvisaker, M., & Szekeres, S. F. (1994). Communication disorders associated with closed head injury. In R. Chapey (Ed.), *Language intervention strategies in adult aphasia* (3rd ed., pp. 546–568). Williams & Wilkins.

9 Discourse Assessment Across the Recovery Continuum of Traumatic Brain Injury

Elise Elbourn, Joanne Steel, and Elizabeth Spencer

Introduction

In this chapter we examine discourse assessment across the recovery continuum following traumatic brain injury (TBI). The chapter begins by outlining the phases of recovery from TBI and illustrates how spoken discourse manifests across these phases. Considerations for discourse recovery are highlighted with reference to evidence-based clinical practice guidelines, protocols for discourse assessment, and discourse sampling. These guidelines are consistent with those developed by an international group of researchers and clinicians for cognitive rehabilitation following TBI, known as INCOG (Togher et al., 2014). We describe the communication patterns observed at various recovery phases and offer worked examples of analyses including story grammar and main concept analysis. The chapter concludes with a discussion regarding clinical application and tips for the busy clinician evaluating discourse over time.

Recovery Continuum of TBI

Spoken discourse abilities are closely tied to the phase of recovery following a TBI. The process of recovery from a TBI follows a predictable pattern of cognitive and behavioral phases, which is more protracted in those with moderate and severe injuries compared to mild TBI. The Ranchos Los Amigos Scale–Revised (RLAS-R; Box 9–1) (Hagen et al., 1979; Lin & Wroten, 2020) is a widely accepted rating scale that describes these phases of cognitive recovery after TBI.

During RLAS phases I–III, spoken discourse is minimal. Communication assessment involves observational tools of behaviors (Smith et al., 2001), such as the Western Neurosensory Stimulation Profile (WNSSP; Ansell & Keenan, 1989) or the Wessex Head Injury Matrix (WHIM; Shiel et al., 2000).

Post-traumatic amnesia (PTA; Box 9–2) corresponds with RLAS stages IV–VI and may last from a few minutes to months. PTA refers to a transient period of disordered consciousness, characterized by

BOX 9–1. The Ranchos Los Amigos Scale–Revised (RLAS-R) *(Hagen et al., 1979; Lin & Wroten, 2020)*

Phases I–III (I: No response, II: Generalized response, and III: Localized response) include functioning that requires total assistance such as a coma or minimally conscious state.

Phases IV–VI (IV: Confused-agitated, V: Confused-inappropriate, and VI: Confused-appropriate) are characterized by confusion and the need for moderate to maximum assistance with daily functioning.

Phases VII–X (VII: Automatic-appropriate; VIII: Purposeful-appropriate with standby assistance; IX: Purposeful-appropriate-standby assistance on request, and X: Purposeful-appropriate-modified independent) represent a gradual improvement from requiring minimal assistance to modified independence with daily functioning.

BOX 9–2. Example of Discourse During Post-Traumatic Amnesia (PTA)

PTA is a transient period of disordered consciousness, characterized by cognitive and behavioral disturbance and confusion (Sherer et al., 2005).

Discourse from a 47-year-old male with PTA:

"Oh it's been natural sort of thing, like getting the paper, [hactic] sort of thing um, sort of [newme] bout me brain sort of thing, and I'll say oh, y—well that was 6 weeks ago you know, that was only, that was only 1 or 2 days sort of thing, not a week sort of thing, was one of them things I sort of forgotten about sort of thing um, one of them things I don't really need to recover at the moment sort of thing d—, just as long as I can get out, so I can get out and get a thingo at home."

cognitive and behavioral disturbance and confusion (Sherer et al., 2005). Measuring the duration and symptom severity of PTA is considered critical for determining the patient's evolving level of consciousness. PTA length is also indicative of injury severity and outcome (Nakase-Richardson et al., 2009). Therefore, recovery over this period is closely monitored. PTA has been established to be a multifactorial condition (Sherer et al., 2020), including disturbances in attentional, perceptual, and neurobe-havioral processes and sleep-wake cycle disruptions (Weir et al., 2006). Individuals commonly present with delusions, confabulation, agitation (McKay et al., 2020), and communication impairments (Steel et al., 2017a, 2017b). It is possible to detect early signs of persisting cognitive communication disorder while the patient is in PTA (Steel et al., 2017a).

During later phases of recovery, including RLAS phases VII–X, individuals with TBI can engage in a range of spoken dis-

course tasks such as conversation, narrative, or procedural discourse. While improvements may be observed from the PTA stage, many individuals will have persisting difficulties with productivity, accuracy, and clarity in spoken discourse (Elbourn, Kenny, Power, Honan, et al., 2019a). Discourse patterns such as the impoverished profile, the inefficient profile, and the confused profile (Hartley & Jensen, 1992) may emerge during this phase (Box 9–3).

BOX 9–3. Characteristics of Discourse Profiles
(Hartley & Jensen, 1992)

Impoverished profile: marked reduction in productivity and content; brief utterances with nonspecific vocabulary and silent pauses

Inefficient profile: increased productivity in verbal output; irrelevant and excessive detail and verbal mazes

Confused profile: inaccuracy of content; high number of verbal mazes; confabulation and ambiguous pronouns

---

Considerations for Longitudinal Discourse Assessment

Longitudinal assessment and intervention for spoken discourse after TBI should be approached within a multidisciplinary context. The INCOG clinical practice guidelines for cognitive rehabilitation offer evidence-based guidelines for multidisciplinary clinical care that can be applied across the spectrum of recovery.

BOX 9–4. INCOG

The INCOG clinical practice guidelines were developed by a group of international experts and offer evidence-based recommendations for cognitive assessment and rehabilitation. The recommendations comprise five parts:

Part I: Post-Traumatic Amnesia/Delirium

Part II: Attention and Information Processing Speed

Part III: Executive Function and Self-Awareness

Part IV: Cognitive Communication

Part V: Memory

The evidence-based guidelines for cognitive rehabilitation, Part I: PTA/Delirium (INCOG-I) recommend that SLPs work with patients on communication and swallowing throughout PTA (Ponsford et al., 2014). Spoken discourse assessment can be particularly valuable when "establish(ing) most reliable means of communication" (p. 312) and " . . . optimiz(ing) clarity of communication between the injured individual and others" (p. 313). Other research has determined that it is feasible to commence systematic cognitive communication and discourse assessment from early contact with the patient in the acute stage (Smith et al., 2001; Steel et al., 2017a, 2017b; Taylor et al., 2007). Discourse treatment is also inherent within recommendations from the Cognitive Communication (INCOG-IV) Guidelines. For example, rehearsing communication skills in real contexts requires spoken discourse (Togher et al., 2014).

Discourse assessment for TBI recovery is largely conceptualized into two distinct categories: conversational or dialogic discourse, and monologic discourse (Coelho et al., 2005; Coelho, 2007). As previously outlined in Chapter 1, analyses for monologic discourse can also be categorized into three levels: microlinguistic analysis (e.g., productivity, cohesive adequacy), macrolinguistic analysis (e.g., main concept analysis, coherence), and superstructural analysis (e.g., story grammar) (Coelho et al., 2005; Coelho, 2007; Nicholas & Brookshire, 1993). Identifying which analyses are most suited to each phase of recovery and determining which measures are most sensitive for measuring recovery can be challenging. In this chapter we offer some suggestions for potential approaches to spoken discourse assessment across the recovery journey. The TBIBank Discourse Protocol (Box 9–5) is a versatile tool for assessing spoken discourse across the spectrum of TBI recovery. An overview of the range of measures that have been utilized specifically in the context of TBI recovery is also outlined in Table 9–1. More details on the discourse studies are available on the companion website.

> ### BOX 9–5. TBIBank Discourse Protocol
>
> The protocol contains four sections with approximate administration times ranging from 10–30 minutes:
>
> Section I: Free Speech Samples (Brain Injury Story and Coping, Important Event)
>
> Section II: Picture Descriptions (Broken Window, Refused Umbrella, Cat Rescue)
>
> Section III: Story Narrative (Cinderella)
>
> Section IV: Procedure (Sandwich)
>
> All printed materials are available from https://tbi.talkbank.org/protocol/pictures/. Computerized language analysis (CLAN) can be completed with the EVAL command in the CLAN program (see Chapter 17). Alternatively, noncomputerized analyses are illustrated in the next section.

Discourse Sampling for Recovery After TBI

Another important consideration for spoken discourse recovery is the ability to detect reliable change. Spencer et al. (2020) identified the length of a discourse sample as a variable that is known to affect the stability and therefore usefulness of discourse analyses. Following a TBI, discourse samples can be collected at various time points to measure for meaningful change as a result of spontaneous improvement or as a response to intervention. Often this would be done before treatment, immediately post-treatment, and at follow-up (e.g., 1 to 6 months post-treatment). Spencer et al. (2020) proposed a way that variability could be considered and accounted for in discourse analysis. This utilizes a statistical measure called the Reliable Change Index (RCI; Box 9–6), which is a measure that indicates the likely range of change in scores for a measure taken at two time points. Overall, clinicians need to be able to determine if the change they are observing is due to true changes in the measures used at the different times. Using the reliable change tool and estimating appropriate sample sizes

Table 9–1. Recommended Measures for Spoken Discourse Assessment

Level	Task	Analysis Type—Description	Purpose/Rationale
Microlinguistic	• Personal narrative • Injury story • Important event • Picture sequence narrative: Refused Umbrella, Broken Window, Flowerpot Incident	• Productivity • Words per C-unit • Mean length of utterance or average number of words per C-unit (excludes mazes) • Maze words as a percentage of total words • Ratio of maze words to total words • Errors • Number of errors (including omitted words, omitted bound morphemes, semantic and phonemic paraphasias) as a percentage of total words	Amount and complexity of verbal output: • To observe demonstration of increased cognitive ability and alertness • To assess the patient's ability to initiate and elaborate on ideas, demonstrate clarity of thinking • To evaluate the complexity of spoken output: looking at clause length and complexity, elaboration • To observe fluency or efficiency of verbal output: can indicate word-finding difficulty, slowed cognitive processing • To determine the impact of cognitive factors on communication
Superstructural	Picture sequence narrative: Refused Umbrella, Broken Window, Flowerpot Incident	• Content and organization • Percentage of correct story grammar elements (scored according to Snow & Powell [2002] scoring schema) • Qualitative description/observation on content of sample produced	Organizational and conceptual aspects of spoken discourse: • To examine the ability to organize thoughts • To determine the ability to interpret main point of visual stimulus • To allow the SLP to hypothesize reasons for performance on testing (e.g., behavioral, emotional, perceptual issues present on testing day)
Conversation	Conversation: Can be sampled during multidisciplinary team activities, throughout swallowing assessments, during informal conversations	• Pragmatics and social communication • Profile of Pragmatic Impairment in Conversation • Measure of Cognitive Linguistic Abilities Family Rating Scale	Interactive aspects of communication: • To evaluate the patient's awareness of communication partner, pragmatic aspects of communication • To provide quantifiable measures of family perception of improvements over time

Note: C-unit = communication unit.

159

would help support clinical decision making and appropriate management across the continuum of care.

Early Recovery

This period after a moderate or severe TBI can be a challenging time for the patient, family, and staff working with the patient. At this early stage, the patient may be engaging in unusual and distressing communication interactions. As the patient recovers consciousness, this communication can include confabulatory, perseverative, disinhibited language, with a range of other expressive and receptive language, cognitive communication, and social communication impairments (Steel et al., 2015). Staff and family may struggle to manage the patient's consistent, problematic communication behaviors (Nielsen et al., 2020), indicating the need for support of a speech-language pathologist (SLP).

For SLPs, of particular interest during this recovery stage is the resolution of the *language of confusion* (Groher, 1977), a term that refers here to communication issues

that are directly related to PTA. Measuring the patient's confused discourse during PTA provides insight into cognitive and neurobehavioral status, which helps the multidisciplinary team's understanding of the patient's recovery process. Critically, samples of connected speech offer the SLP and team a descriptive view of the disordered thought processes that are present during PTA. Measuring the resolution of this confused language allows insight into the clearing of generalized cognitive disruption. In this way, discourse measures can be useful to monitor recovery and support the clinical picture of emergence from PTA. A language sample from an individual emerging from confusion (173 days after injury) appears in the next box. Compare this language sample with the earlier sample from the same individual at 40 days after injury, shown in Box 9–2 titled "Example of Discourse During Post-Traumatic Amnesia."

Research into early communication recovery by Steel et al. (2017a) found that patients' discourse was comparatively more perseverative, tangential, and disorganized and lower on relevant information during PTA than after PTA emergence. Patients also had increased difficulty with more complex cognitive communication tasks, such as comprehension of passives sentences, idioms, and verbal fluency. These cognitive communication impairments during PTA were likely exacerbated by attention, memory, and orientation disruption related to this stage. While communication change over time may be gradual, it is still possible to monitor these changes with quantitative discourse measures of narrative organization such as story grammar.

Story grammar analysis captures the logical sequencing of elements in a well-developed narrative and reflects capacity to reconstruct and share experiences with others. Key elements include the setting,

an initiating event, an internal response, a plan, an attempt, direct consequences, and the resolution (Snow & Powell, 2005). In the scoring schema, each element is scored out of 2. For example, in the Flowerpot Incident, the target utterance for the setting is, "There is a man walking along the street with his dog" (Snow & Powell, 2005, pp. 252–253). If there is no mention of the dog or no pronoun referent, this is scored *1*. An omission of the setting would result in *0*. See Snow and Powell (2005) for detailed examples of scoring.

In Boxes 9–8 and 9–9, the participant is telling the story of the Flowerpot Incident on two occasions: during PTA and at 3 months after PTA emergence. The latter story is more organized, more complete, and contains more story grammar elements.

Goals of discourse assessment during this early phase of recovery inform resolution of PTA and confusion, assist in developing strategies to optimize patient-staff

---

BOX 9–8. *Flowerpot Incident, Test Time 1 (PTA)*

Element	Sample	Score
The setting		0
An initiating event	So, it's showing that some guy's had a flowerpot dropped on his head That's a building.	2
An internal response	Basically it looks like he's got really upset about it,	2
A plan		0
An attempt	and then he went inside, and knocked on the door,	1
Direct consequences	and there was some nice [laugh] old lady who he decided to [unintelligible] round it	1
Resolution		0
	Total story grammar score: 6/14 = 43%	

BOX 9–9. Flowerpot Incident, Test Time 2 (Post-PTA)

Element	Sample	Score
The setting	Okay so there is a man walking down the street with his dog.	2
An initiating event	Um, as he's walking a flowerpot drops from above his head, um, knock him on his head and knocking his hat off.	2
An internal response	Um the man gets very angry and starts waving his cane at the owner of the balcony,	2
A plan		0
An attempt	um, he promptly takes his dog and heads inside, marches up the stairs, and bangs [hardly] on her door with his cane.	2
Direct consequences	Um, the nice old lady comes out, I think she's holding a bone, gives the dog a nice little pat, um and the man is quite taken by her, p, f— somehow, um and the dog grabs the bone and runs down the stairs, by the looks of it. Um and the dog grabs the bone and runs down the stairs, by the looks of it.	2
Resolution	And the man promptly gives the lady a kiss on the hand, so a possible romance is blooming, with um the lump on his head. So it seems to be very fortuitous occasion.	2

Total story grammar score: 12/14 = 86%

interactions, and aid prediction of cognitive communication outcomes (Steel et al., 2017b). Management considerations may include regular documentation of communication function that may occur weekly (e.g. Nakase-Thompson et al., 2004), every 2 days (Sherer et al., 2009), or daily (Stuss et al., 1999; Wilson et al., 1999). Communication assessment has been found to be feasible up to three times a week with a short discourse protocol (Steel et al., 2017a) and depending on individual and service factors.

As the patient in PTA may present with changing communication presentation daily or even hourly, static testing using extended, formal test batteries is generally unsuitable. Lengthy testing is unlikely to be tolerated due to the attentional and behavioral impairments associated with PTA. Standardized language and cognitive communication tests may fail to capture the overall contextual impacts of agitation level, alertness, mood, and attentional issues during testing. In the acute setting, the patient's performance may also be affected by sleep disruption, pain, and medication. For these reasons, regular spoken discourse assessment is a particularly useful method for monitoring communication, allowing the clinician to see if language and cognitive communication errors are transient or appear steady throughout PTA. For example, the SLP can elicit short discourse samples from a picture sequence task three times weekly for those patients with slow-resolving PTA. This type of task may be tolerated by the patient in PTA whereas other measures would not. These repeated measures can reveal changes in discourse that would not be evident in published cognitive communication tests, which would not be practical to administer repeatedly.

In addition to monitoring resolution of confusion, this process also allows for identification of communication impairments that are relatively stable and that may persist after PTA ends. Discourse measures that have been identified as particularly informative in the early phases of recovery include narrative tasks from the TBIBank protocol (personal narrative: injury story, important event; picture sequence narratives; procedural narratives) with microlinguistic, macrolinguistic, and superstructural analyses (Steel et al., 2017a, 2017b). Suggested clinical measures, tasks, and analysis levels are further described in Table 9–1, as well as on the companion website.

Mid-Recovery

During the middle stage of recovery after a TBI, individuals may show improved interest and ability to engage in discourse-level communication. Conversations with familiar conversation partners at this stage may be focused on the impacts of injury, rehabilitation progress, connection with social networks, and future plans (Brassel et al., 2016). Communication skills will reflect improved orientation and capacity to lay down new memories, resulting in resolution of con-

fused language and improved ability to recall conversations. However, discourse difficulties will continue to be evident (Elbourn, Kenny, Power, Honan, et al., 2019a).

The individual may show some emerging awareness of superficial discourse difficulties such as word-retrieval challenges but may not have a full appreciation of their discourse impairments (Douglas et al., 2007). This can present a challenge for engagement in rehabilitation. Individuals may appear to have low tolerance for lengthy conversations and topics of conversation will often be egocentric (Byom & Turkstra, 2012). Individuals in this stage often rely on skilled communication partners to support effective discourse. In this phase, family and friends may have improved capacity to be involved in the care of the affected individual and may be interested in discussions relating to prognosis and how they can best support the individual (Guldager et al., 2019). Discourse skills at this stage have a strong association with later psychosocial outcomes (Elbourn, Kenny, Power, & Togher, 2019b).

Goals of discourse assessment during mid-recovery may include establishing a diagnosis, identifying communicative strengths and weaknesses, determining a baseline of functioning, and determining performance in everyday communication situations. Management considerations may include ongoing and dynamic assessment to track improvements in discourse and guide treatment decisions. Clinicians may consider re-evaluating discourse communication skills at least every 3 months or following a period of treatment (Elbourn, Kenny, Power, Honan, et al., 2019a).

Discourse tasks that have been evaluated for use in the middle phases of recovery include conversational and monologic discourse tasks incorporating narratives, procedure, and picture description genres.

As conversational analysis measures are addressed in Chapters 4, 7, and 10, this section focuses on monologic measures. Various monologic discourse tasks offer valuable information about discourse-level communication at this stage of recovery. A macrostructural analysis on a simple procedural task (e.g., essential steps), making a sandwich, differentiated 47 individuals with severe TBI from a matched control sample at 3 and 6 months postinjury. However, this measure was not sufficiently sensitive for detecting change between 3 and 6 months (Stubbs et al., 2018). Macrostructural analysis in the form of story completeness was also effective in differentiating 42 individuals with severe TBI from a matched control sample at 3 and 6 months postinjury on the Cat story narrative retell but was similarly not sensitive to change over time (Power et al., 2020).

One measure that is sensitive for measuring discourse changes over time is the Cinderella narrative retell with main concept analysis (Elbourn, Kenny, Power, Honan, et al., 2019a). Main concept analysis (MCA) evaluates an individual's accuracy and completeness when communicating ideas (Nicholas & Brookshire, 1993; Richardson & Dalton, 2016) (see Box 9–10 on MCA). In a study tracking 57 participants with moderate to severe TBI every 3 months across the first year of recovery after their injury, the main concept analysis was effective for differentiating individuals with TBI from controls and capturing change across 3-month intervals (Elbourn, Kenny, Power, Honan, et al., 2019a). Boxes 9–11 and 9–12 illustrate the language changes of the same individual retelling the Cinderella story at 3 and 12 months postinjury as measured by the MCA.

BOX 9–10. *Main Concept Analysis (MCA)*

MCA evaluates accuracy and completeness of a person's ability to convey the general gist or idea of a discourse (Nicholas & Brookshire, 1993 Richardson & Dalton, 2016). The Cinderella narrative has 34 main concepts. Each concept is assigned a score out of 3, resulting in a total score out of 102. A score below 45 indicates an impairment. Severity ranges are as follows: Mild (25–44), Moderate (6–24), and Severe (0–5). The scoring criteria are:

■ Accurate—Complete (3): Every essential element of the main concept produced. No essential elements are incorrect.

■ Accurate—Incomplete (2): No incorrect content but missing at least one essential element.

■ Inaccurate—Complete (2): Contains at least one incorrect piece of information but includes all essential elements.

■ Inaccurate—Incomplete (1): Corresponds with a concept but is missing at least one essential element and at least one incorrect element.

■ Absent (0): None of the essential information is given.

BOX 9–11. *Cinderella Retell (3 months)*

Sample	Element	Coding (Score)
Once upon a time um two stepsisters come to stay with them with um Cinderella	2	Inaccurate—Complete (2)
Um and they were mean um um	3	Inaccurate—Complete (2)
Cinderella wants to go to the ball	9	Inaccurate—Complete (2)
So she um so a fairy godmother comes and um	14	Accurate—Complete (3)
She can go there until 12 o'clock and and then the her um everything turns into a pumpkin um	18	Inaccurate—Incomplete (1)
But she doesn't tell Prince Charming who she going to the ball with um	—	
Prince Charming then goes over to see her afterwards and	—	
And they live happily ever after	34	Accurate—Complete (3)

Total Score = 13/102 (Moderate impairment)

BOX 9–12. *Cinderella Retell (12 months)*

Sample	Element	Coding (Score)
Once upon a time there was a (.) this man that meets a lady and they get married	1	Inaccurate—Complete (2)
And she has two little daughters and the guy also has one daughter himself	—	
The two the two sisters from the mother don't like the the one from the dad and they always give her hell ah	3	Inaccurate—Incomplete (1)
Then they grow up and the prince of the land wants to have a ball	7	Accurate—Complete (3)
So he has a ball and sends out invitations and invites the girls to the ah ball	8	Accurate—Complete (3)

Sample	Element	Coding (Score)
And the two older sisters don't like that very much	—	
So they are getting dressed or getting ready to do dressed for the	—	
Ball and ah the two sisters see what the Cinderella is gonna wear and they rip it	11	Inaccurate—Complete (2)
So she's got nothing now to wear now to the ball and then um	—	
Fairy godmother comes along and gives her a new dress to wear and some shoes and stuff	14 16	Accurate—Complete (3) Inaccurate—Complete (2)
And turns a pumpkin into a carriage ah so she can get there.	15	Accurate—Complete (3)
So she goes there and she dances with the ah prince	17 19	Inaccurate—Complete (2) Accurate—Complete (3)
But she has to be out of there by midnight, otherwise she turns in a pumpkin. Her carriage turns back into a pumpkin	18	Accurate—Complete (3)
So as she, as, as the clock strikes 12,	21	Accurate—Complete (3)
she is running out the door and she she, one of her slippers falls off.	22 23	Accurate—Complete (3) Inaccurate—Complete (2)
So she goes home and she gets home in time (.) just	26	Accurate—Complete (3)
And then the prince wants to find her again and the only way to find her is through the slipper	27	Accurate—Complete (3)
So he gets everyone to try on the slipper to find out who he was dancing with.and the sisters try it on and they're too big	29 30	Accurate—Complete (3) Inaccurate—Incomplete (1)
And they, he gets Cinderella to try it on and it fits perfectly	31 32	Accurate—Complete (3) Accurate—Complete (3)
And he knows that, she is the one so he they live happily ever after.	34	Inaccurate—Complete (2)

Total Score = 53/102 (Within normal range)

Later Recovery

During the later phases of recovery, discourse deficits often persist but may show subtle improvements that reflect improved self-awareness of discourse challenges. The individual may take on some responsibility for managing compensatory supports in discourse such as utilizing a memory aid or scaffold and may show improved responsiveness to their communication partner's needs. An individual at this stage will often still benefit from supports such as additional time and occasional prompts from the communication partner. The individual may be reintegrating back into the community and may identify new challenges as they engage in a wider range of more complex discourse activities. Such activities may include conversations with multiple speakers and work-related tasks. In both instances, language skills essential for social interactions such as use of politeness markers are required (Meulenbroek et al., 2016). Family and friends may begin to feel the burden of persisting discourse impairments at this stage and social networks may diminish (Galski et al., 1998).

Goals of discourse assessment may include evaluating performance in varied everyday communication situations (e.g., varied communication partners, contexts, and genres) and monitoring for long-term changes in communication. Management considerations may include ongoing and dynamic assessment. As a guide, clinicians should consider re-evaluating discourse communication skills at least every 6 or 12 months to ensure that any decline in communication skills (Snow et al., 1998) can be identified and addressed or any potential further improvements in communication can be supported.

Discourse assessment tasks that have been examined in this phase have typically been explored as outcome measures in the context of treatment studies. The adapted Kagan rating scales are a sensitive measure for evaluating discourse-level changes following communication partner training (Mann et al., 2015; Togher et al., 2010). Story grammar measures and the Assessment Battery for Communication (Angeleri et al., 2008), which includes a discourse scale, have also been reported to demonstrate changes in discourse in response to narrative-based treatments (Angeleri et al., 2008; Cannizzaro & Coelho, 2002; Steel et al., 2021). The *Cinderella* narrative with main concept analysis was found to be effective in evaluating discourse changes up to 1 year following injury (Elbourn, Kenny, Power, Honan, et al., 2019a).

Clinical Application of Longitudinal Discourse Assessment

One of the key considerations during the early and middle stages of recovery will be time available for discourse assessment (Bryant et al., 2017), particularly with methods involving transcription. There are many workplace- and/or patient-related factors affecting how long the SLP has for assessment. SLPs have previously reported the low priority on their caseload of patients who are in PTA, a push to discharge patients from service, and patient medical status as barriers to assessment during PTA (Steel et al., 2016). While assessing patients during PTA can be challenging, this low priority is concerning, with some patients being transferred to other settings without communication being evaluated (Steel et al., 2016). It is important to document types of cognitive communication impairment and severity of symptoms throughout the recovery process, as these have been related to outcome and quality of life (LeBlanc et al., 2014). In-depth analysis of discourse production daily would be unnecessary and inappropriate. However, there are relatively quick discourse measures that can be conducted regularly with patients and that do not require extensive time in sampling, transcription, or analysis, nor extensive training to implement. A number of approaches are described below that may be relevant across the continuum of recovery, followed by suggestions for targeting specific areas for investigation, dependent on the individual's presentation (Box 9–13).

Conclusion

The rate and nature of cognitive communication recovery following TBI can vary considerably among individuals. However, clinicians can support this process by understanding the optimal methods for evaluating discourse across the recovery continuum. Discourse tools such as

---

BOX 9–13. Discourse Procedures: Tips for the Busy Clinician

Sampling: Administering the full TBIBank protocol will take between 10 minutes (impoverished profile) and 30 minutes (inefficient profiles). If you suspect the patient is inefficient, you may want to select fewer tasks with known sensitivity (e.g., *Cinderella* story).

Transcription: Dictation software may speed up transcription for non-dysarthric speech. When checking your transcript, playing back at half speed or double speed can assist. Also, consider the use of allied health assistants or other external services for transcription. Check that confidential or identifying data is removed.

Questions to guide analysis:

- How much is the patient saying and how accurate is this linguistically?—Productivity
- Is the patient able to identify the main points of a narrative?—Main concept analysis

- Is the patient able to tell a logical and organized story?—Story grammar analysis

Analysis: Automated analysis programs (e.g., CLAN or Systematic Analysis of Language Transcripts [SALT])

Quick productivity analysis: Enter the sample into an online text analyzer (e.g., https://www.online-utility.org/text/analyzer.jsp) or SALT for some gross measures of productivity. Example for Box 9–11 (3 months): 88 words; 52 unique words were produced; *um* was the most frequently used word at 11%. Example for Box 9–12 (12 months): 314 words; 135 unique words were produced; *and* and *the* were the most frequently used words.

Note: This should be supplemented with a reliable and valid linguistic analysis across a range of genres and levels of analysis, as described in the text and outlined in Table 9–1. Further details on supplementary assessments are included on the companion website.

the TBIBank protocol have flexibility over the recovery continuum, can detect subtle changes over time, and can interact with computerized programs to support efficiency of best practice. Clinicians should facilitate evidence-based discussions with the individual, their family, and the clinical team around prognosis for cognitive communication recovery and use this to guide future planning of services and supports. Clinicians are encouraged to advocate for person-centered service models that support best practice and facilitate lifelong service models that can optimize outcomes for these individuals and their families.

References

Angeleri, R., Bosco, F. M., Zettin, M., Sacco, K., Colle, L., & Bara, B. G. (2008). Communicative impairment in traumatic brain injury: A complete pragmatic assessment. *Brain and Language, 107*(3), 229–245. https://doi.org/10.1016/j.bandl.2008.01.002

Ansell, B. J., & Keenan, J. E. (1989). The Western Neuro Sensory Stimulation Profile: A tool for assessing slow-to-recover head-injured patients. *Archives of Physical Medicine and Rehabilitation, 70*(2), 104–108.

Brassel, S., Kenny, B., Power, E., Elbourn, E., McDonald, S., Tate, R., . . . Togher, L. (2016). Conversational topics discussed by individuals with severe traumatic brain injury and their communication partners during sub-acute recovery. *Brain Injury, 30*(11), 1329–1342. https://doi.org/10.1080/02699052.2016.1187288

Bryant, L., Spencer, E., & Ferguson, A. (2017). Clinical use of linguistic discourse analysis for the assessment of language in aphasia. *Aphasiology, 31*(10), 1105–1126. https://doi.org/10.1080/02687038.2016.1239013

Byom, L. J., & Turkstra, L. (2012). Effects of social cognitive demand on theory of mind in conversations of adults with traumatic brain injury: Social cognition in conversa-tion following TBI. *International Journal of Language and Communication Disorders, 47*(3), 310–321. https://doi.org/10.1111/j.1460-6984.2011.00102.x

Cannizzaro, M. S., & Coelho, C. A. (2002). Treatment of story grammar following traumatic brain injury: A pilot study [Case reports]. *Brain Injury, 16*(12), 1065–1073. https://doi.org/10.1080/02699050210155230

Coelho, C., Ylvisaker, M., & Turkstra, L. S. (2005). Nonstandardized assessment approaches for individuals with traumatic brain injuries. *Seminars in Speech and Language, 26*(4), 223–241. https://doi.org/10.1055/s-2005-922102

Coelho, C. A. (2007). Management of discourse deficits following traumatic brain injury: Progress, caveats, and needs. *Seminars in Speech and Language, 28*(2), 122–135. https://doi.org/10.1055/s-2007-970570

Douglas, J. M., Bracy, C. A., & Snow, P. C. (2007). Measuring perceived communicative ability after traumatic brain injury: Reliability and validity of the La Trobe Communication Questionnaire. *The Journal of Head Trauma Rehabilitation, 22*(1), 31–38. https://doi.org/10.1097/00001199-200701000-00004

Elbourn, E., Kenny, B., Power, E., Honan, C., McDonald, S., Tate, R., . . . Togher, L. (2019a). Discourse recovery after severe traumatic brain injury: Exploring the first year. *Brain Injury, 33*(2), 143–159. https://doi.org/10.1080/02699052.2018.1539246

Elbourn, E., Kenny, B., Power, E., & Togher, L. (2019b). Psychosocial outcomes of severe traumatic brain injury in relation to discourse recovery: A longitudinal study up to 1 year postinjury. *American Journal of Speech-Language Pathology, 28*(4), 1463–1478. https://doi.org/10.1044/2019_AJSLP-18-0204

Galski, T., Tompkins, C., & Johnston, M. V. (1998). Competence in discourse as a measure of social integration and quality of life in persons with traumatic brain injury. *Brain Injury, 12*(9), 769–782. https://doi.org/10.1080/026990598122160

Groher, M. (1977). Language and memory disorders following closed head trauma. *Journal of Speech and Hearing Research, 20*(2), 212–223. https://doi.org/10.1044/jshr.2002.212

Guldager, R., Willis, K., Larsen, K., & Poulsen, I. (2019). Relatives' strategies in subacute brain injury rehabilitation: The warrior, the observer and the hesitant. *Journal of Clinical Nursing, 28*(1–2), 289–299. https://doi.org/10.1111/jocn.14598

Hagen, C., Malkmus, D., & Durham, P. (1979). *Levels of cognitive functioning: Rehabilitation of the head injured adult.* Comprehensive Physical Management: Professional Staff Association of Rancho Los Amigos National Rehabilitation Center.

Hartley, L. L., & Jensen, P. J. (1992). Three discourse profiles of closed-head-injury speakers: Theoretical and clinical implications. *Brain Injury, 6*(3), 271–281. https://doi.org/10.3109/02699059209029669

LeBlanc, J., de Guise, E., Champoux, M. C., Couturier, C., Lamoureux, J., Marcoux, J., . . . Feyz, M. (2014). Early conversational discourse abilities following traumatic brain injury: An acute predictive study. *Brain Injury, 28*(7), 951–958. https://doi.org/10.3109/02699052.2014.888760

Lin, K., & Wroten, M. (2020). *Ranchos Los Amigos.* StatPearls Publishing. http://europepmc.org/abstract/MED/28846341

Mann, K., Power, E., Barnes, S., & Togher, L. (2015). Questioning in conversations before and after communication partner training for individuals with traumatic brain injury. *Aphasiology, 29*(9), 1082–1109. https://doi.org/10.1080/02687038.2015.1035226

McKay, A., Love, J., Trevena-Peters, J., Gracey, J., & Ponsford, J. (2020). The relationship between agitation and impairments of orientation and memory during the PTA period after traumatic brain injury. *Neuropsychological Rehabilitation, 30*(4), 579–590. https://doi.org/10.1080/09602011.2018.1479276

Meulenbroek, P., Bowers, B., & Turkstra, L. (2016). Characterizing common workplace communication skills for disorders associated with traumatic brain injury: A qualitative study. *Journal of Vocational Rehabilitation, 44*(1), 15. https://doi.org/10.3233/JVR-150777

Nakase-Richardson, R., Sepehri, A., Sherer, M., Yablon, S. A., Evans, C., & Mani, T. (2009). Classification schema of post-traumatic amnesia duration-based injury severity relative to 1-year outcome: Analysis of individuals with moderate and severe traumatic brain injury. *Archives of Physical Medicine and Rehabilitation, 90*(1), 17–19. https://doi.org/10.1016/j.apmr.2008.06.030

Nakase-Thompson, R., Sherer, M., Yablon, S. A., Nick, T. G., & Trzepacz, P. T. (2004). Acute confusion following traumatic brain injury. *Brain Injury, 18*(2), 131–142. https://doi.org/10.1080/0269905031000149542

Nicholas, L. E., & Brookshire, R. H. (1993). A system for quantifying the informativeness and efficiency of the connected speech of adults with aphasia. *Journal of Speech, Language, and Hearing Research, 36*(2), 338–350. https://doi.org/10.1044/jshr.3602.338

Nielsen, A. I., Power, E., & Jensen, L. R. (2020). Communication with patients in post-traumatic confusional state: Perception of rehabilitation staff. *Brain Injury, 34*(4), 447–455. https://doi.org/10.1080/02699052.2020.1725839

Ponsford, J., Bayley, M., Wiseman-Hakes, C., Togher, L., Velikonja, D., McIntyre, A., . . . Tate, R. (2014). INCOG recommendations for management of cognition following traumatic brain injury, part II: Attention and information processing speed. *Journal of Head Trauma Rehabilitation, 29*(4), 321–337. https://doi.org/10.1097/htr.0000000000000072

Power, E., Weir, S., Richardson, J., Fromm, D., Forbes, M., MacWhinney, B., & Togher, L. (2020). Patterns of narrative discourse in early recovery following severe traumatic brain injury. *Brain Injury, 34*(1), 98–109. https://doi.org/10.1080/02699052.2019.1682192

Richardson, J. D., & Dalton, S. G. (2016). Main concepts for three different discourse tasks in a large non-clinical sample. *Aphasiology, 30*(1), 45–73. https://doi.org/10.1080/02687038.2015.1057891

Sherer, M., Katz, D. I., Bodien, Y. G., Arciniegas, D. B., Block, C., Blum, S., . . . Yablon, S. A. (2020). Post-traumatic confusional state: A case definition and diagnostic criteria. *Archives of Physical Medicine and Rehabilita-*

tion, *101*(11), 2041–2050. https://doi.org/10 .1016/j.apmr.2020.06.021

Sherer, M., Nakase-Thompson, R., Yablon, S. A., & Gontkovsky, S. T. (2005). Multidimensional assessment of acute confusion after traumatic brain injury. *Archives of Physical Medicine and Rehabilitation*, *86*(5), 896–904. https://doi.org/10.1016/j.apmr.2004.09.029

Sherer, M., Yablon, S. A., & Nakase-Richardson, R. (2009). Patterns of recovery of post-traumatic confusional state in neurorehabilitation admissions after traumatic brain injury. *Archives of Physical Medicine and Rehabilitation*, *90*(10), 1749–1754. https://doi.org/10.10 16/j.apmr.2009.05.011

Shiel, A., Horn, S., Wilson, B., Watson, M., Campbell, M., & McLellan, D. (2000). The Wessex Head Injury Matrix (WHIM) main scale: A preliminary report on a scale to assess and monitor patient recovery after severe head injury. *Clinical Rehabilitation*, *14*(4), 408–416. https://doi.org/10.1191/0269215500cr326oa

Smith, V. H., Taylor, C. M., Lammi, M. H., & Tate, R. L. (2001). Recovery profiles of cognitive-sensory modalities in patients in the minimally conscious state following traumatic brain injury. *Brain Impairment*, *2*(1), 29–38. https://doi.org/10.1375/brim.2.1.29

Snow, P., Douglas, J. M., & Ponsford, J. (1998). Conversational discourse abilities following severe traumatic brain injury: A follow-up study. *Brain Injury*, *12*(11), 911–935. https:// doi.org/10.1080/026990598121981

Snow, P. C., & Powell, M. B. (2005). What's the story? An exploration of narrative language abilities in male juvenile offenders. *Psychology, Crime & Law*, *11*(3), 239–253. https://doi .org/10.1080/1068316042000209323

Spencer, E., Bryant, L., & Colyvas, K. (2020). Minimizing variability in language sampling analysis: A practical way to calculate text length and time variability and measure reliable change when assessing clients. *Topics in Language Disorders*, *40*(2), 166–181. https:// doi.org/10.1097/TLD.0000000000000212

Steel, J., Elbourn, E., & Togher, L. (2021). Narrative discourse intervention after traumatic brain injury: A systematic review of the literature. *Topics in Language Disorders*, *41*(1),

47–72. https://doi.org/10.1097/TLD.000000 0000000241

Steel, J., Ferguson, A., Spencer, E., & Togher, L. (2016). Speech-language pathologists' perspectives on cognitive communication assessment during post-traumatic amnesia. *Brain Injury*, *30*(9), 1131–1142. https://doi. org/10.1080/02699052.2016.1174785

Steel, J., Ferguson, A., Spencer, E., & Togher, L. (2017a). Language and cognitive communication disorder during post-traumatic amnesia: profiles of recovery after TBI from three cases. *Brain Injury*, *31*(13–14), 1889–1902. https:// doi.org/10.1080/02699052.2017.1373200

Steel, J., Ferguson, A., Spencer, E., & Togher, L. (2017b). Social communication assessment during post-traumatic amnesia and the post-acute period after traumatic brain injury. *Brain Injury*, *31*(10), 1320–1330. https://doi .org/10.1080/02699052.2017.1332385

Stubbs, E., Togher, L., Kenny, B., Fromm, D., Forbes, M., MacWhinney, B., . . . Power, E. (2018). Procedural discourse performance in adults with severe traumatic brain injury at 3 and 6 months post-injury. *Brain Injury*, *32*(2), 167–181. https://doi.org/10.1080/02699052.2 017.1291989

Stuss, D. T., Binns, M. A., Carruth, F. G., Levine, B., Brandys, C. E., Moulton, R. J., & Schwartz, M. L. (1999). The acute period of recovery from traumatic brain injury: Post-traumatic amnesia or post-traumatic confusional state? *Journal of Neurosurgery*, *90*(4), 635–643. https://doi.org/10.3171/jns.1999.90.4.0635

Taylor, C. M., Aird, V. H., Tate, R. L., & Lammi, M. H. (2007). Sequence of recovery during the course of emergence from the minimally conscious state. *Archives of Physical Medicine and Rehabilitation*, *88*(4), 521–525. https:// doi.org/10.1016/j.apmr.2007.01.013

Togher, L., Power, E., Tate, R., McDonald, S., & Rietdijk, R. (2010). Measuring the social interactions of people with traumatic brain injury and their communication partners: The adapted Kagan scales. *Aphasiology*, *24*(6–8), 914–927. https://doi.org/10.1080/ 02687030903422478

Togher, L., Wiseman-Hakes, C., Douglas, J. M., Stergiou-Kita, M., Ponsford, J. L., Teasell, R.,

& Turkstra, L. S. (2014). INCOG recommendations for management of cognition following traumatic brain injury, part IV: Cognitive communication. *The Journal of Head Trauma Rehabilitation, 29*(4), 353–368. http://doi.org/10.1097/HTR.0000000000000071

Weir, N., Doig, E. J., Fleming, J. M., Wiemers, A., & Zemljic, C. (2006). Objective and behavioral assessment of the emergence from post-traumatic amnesia (PTA). *Brain Injury, 20*(9), 927–935. https://doi.org/10.1080/02699050600832684

Wilson, B. A., Evans, J. J., Emslie, H., Balleny, H., Watson, P. C., & Baddeley, A. D. (1999). Measuring recovery from post-traumatic amnesia. *Brain Injury, 13*(7), 505–520. https://doi.org/10.1080/026990599121412

10 Assessing Conversation After Traumatic Brain Injury

Louise C. Keegan, Nicholas Behn, Emma Power, Susan Howell, and Rachael Rietdijk

Introduction

The majority of everyday interactions take the form of conversation, and yet, for individuals with traumatic brain injury (TBI), evaluation seldom involves an assessment of conversational skills. This chapter is designed to serve as a resource for assessment of conversation, outlining the range of tools that can assist with the assessment of both dyadic and group conversations. An assessment of conversation can allow a clinician to obtain an authentic representation of how an individual communicates in everyday settings.

Most often, client aspirations are related to improving their social and conversational interaction abilities. Frith et al. (2014) found that it was more likely for clinicians to complete and score standardized norm-referenced assessments that examine specific language and cognitive communicative skills of their clients rather than complete an assessment of pragmatic skills or discourse. A comprehensive assessment of conversation abilities may be a more efficient use of clinician and client time, as it can more directly address client objectives.

For example, an understanding of social and pragmatic difficulties in group settings may provide more relevant information for an intervention approach that improves quality of life than an assessment of generative naming or story retelling skills. Thus, it is important that clinicians take the time to carefully examine the conversation skills of individuals with TBI. Additionally, it is important that conversation assessment be completed "at the level of participation in everyday social life" (Togher et al., 2014, p. 361) due to the concomitant difficulties (physical, emotional, behavioral, and cognitive) that can impact the way in which individuals with TBI communicate and the social opportunities in which they participate.

Context for Conversation

The environment, the goals and demands of the interaction, and the conversation partner(s) all influence and are influenced by cognitive communication factors (MacDonald, 2017). Hence, contextual demands can have a profound influence on the conversational abilities of individuals with cognitive communication difficulties. The relationships between communication partners, responses of a communication partner, and even the social and cultural roles that communication partners assume can impact conversational outcomes (Keegan & Müller, in press). Therefore, it is not surprising that communication partner training for those who interact with individuals with cognitive communication difficulties demonstrates significantly improved outcomes (Behn et al., 2012; Behn et al., 2021; Rietdijk et al., 2020; Togher et al., 2004; Togher et al., 2013). Measurement of the outcomes of social communication skills training (either via groups or individually) is recommended as per current international guidelines "in real world environments during meaningful activities" (International Cognitive Rehabilitation Group [INCOG] Cognitive Communication recommendation #7, Togher et al., 2014, p. 361). Therefore, the measurement of discourse in different types of conversations is a critical element of the rehabilitation approach to communication difficulties after TBI. These contextual influences and the complex nature of conversation can preclude the use of a standardized norm-referenced assessment. However, there are a variety of protocols and methods available, and these are outlined in the following sections.

Collecting a Conversational Sample

The process of collecting a sample starts with determining the context or contexts of interest. Once that has been established, a sample of an authentic, meaningful conversation should be collected. The TBIBank protocol (https://tbi.talkbank.org) includes some conversational discourse tasks (e.g.,

recounting the brain injury story, discussion of an important event) and can serve as a starting point for assessment of conversation (see also Chapter 17). However, group and dyadic conversations that are characteristic of the individual's typical interactions will provide the clinician with data that is most representative of their everyday communication. Most recommendations suggest obtaining a conversational sample that is between 5 and 15 minutes long (Iwashita & Sohlberg, 2019; Prutting & Kirchner, 1987). It is also recommended that the conversational sample be audio and video recorded so that it can be carefully reviewed for both verbal and nonverbal communicative actions.

Approaches for Assessment of Conversation

Rating Scales

There are several rating scales that are available to assist clinicians in analyzing the recorded conversation sample. These scales are usually brief, clinician-friendly tools that can be administered during the observation of a conversational sample. The following section provides an overview of these scales and describes their clinical feasibility and practicality; this information is summarized in Table 10–1. Brief psychometric data regarding these rating scales are referenced in Table 10–1 and presented in more detail on the companion website.

Pragmatic Protocol

The Pragmatic Protocol was designed for application with both developmental and acquired communication disorder diagnoses, and is applicable to clients across the life

Table 10–1. Rating Scale Summary

Tool	Focus	Brief Description	Potential Clinical Application	Typically Applied to Groups/Dyads	Transcription Requirement	Psychometric Data	Training Requirements
CPS	Pragmatic communication skills	13 pragmatic behaviors rated on a 1–5 Likert scale	Outcome measurement	Group	No	Nil	No training required
CRS	Quality of spontaneous conversation	6 communicative behaviors rated on a 1–9 Likert scale	Outcome measurement	Dyad	No	Selected—reliability and validity	45-minute training
BRISS–R	Social communication skills	6 scales rate social behavior on a 7-point Likert scale	Profiling and outcome measurement	Dyad	No	Selected—reliability and validity	Lengthy training (6–28 hours reported) with variable results
Adapted Kagan scales	Participation of the person with TBI and support provided by the communication partner	Scales of participation and support rated on a 0–4, 9-point Likert rating scale.	Goal setting and outcome measurement for CPT interventions	Dyad	No	Selected—reliability	Lengthy training (14+ hours) to achieve reliability
Global Impression scales	Overall quality of conversation of a dyad	Four scales of conversation quality rated on a 0–4, 9-point Likert rating scale	Goal setting and outcome measurement for CPT interventions	Dyad	No	Selected—reliability	Lengthy training (11+ hours) to achieve reliability
PPIC	Pragmatic communication skills	84 specific behavior items (SBI) to rate communication behavior frequencies and 10 feature summary scales (FSS)	Profiling and outcome measurement	Dyad	No	Selected—reliability and validity	2 hours

continues

Table 10–1. *continued*

Tool	Focus	Brief Description	Potential Clinical Application	Typically Applied to Groups/Dyads	Transcription Requirement	Psychometric Data	Training Requirements
PRS	Pragmatic communication skills	16 behaviors categorized as nonverbal, propositional, or interactional	Clinically feasible outcome measurement	Dyad	No	More substantive—reliability and validity	No training time specified (rating a practice video with .8 agreement)
INT	Group interactional participation	7 item coding system recording verbal/nonverbal initiations and response frequencies	Profiling, goal setting, and outcome measurement	Group	No	Selected—reliability	Approx. 2 hours
Pragmatic Protocol	Speech acts—appropriate or inappropriate	30 pragmatic parameters	Providing a clinical indicator of pragmatic skills	Dyad	No	Selected—reliability and validity	8–10 hours of training
Topic Analysis	Topic management	Data is categorized according to parameters of topic initiation and maintenance, including topic changes and disruptions.	Identifying patterns and problems in topic management	Dyad and monologue	Yes	Selected—reliability	None reported
Clinical Discourse Analysis	Frequency of discourse errors in conversation	17 parameters organized into four categories (quantity, quality, relation, and manner). The modified version has 14 parameters.	Quantifying and describing discourse errors and identifying patterns of difficulty	Dyad	Yes	Selected—reliability	None reported

span (Prutting & Kirchner, 1983). This scale draws on Searle's (1969) speech act theory and examines the communicative acts of the individual within seven different categories: speech acts, topic, turn taking, lexical selection/use across speech acts, stylistic variations, intelligibility and prosodics, and kinesics and proxemics (see Cherney et al., 1998, Exhibit 7–1, p. 129). Milton, Prutting, and Binder (1984) first applied the scale to individuals with brain injury to emphasize its utility in identifying the social language difficulties that are sometimes overlooked in standardized assessment with this population; it has since been frequently applied by others (e.g., Cannizzaro et al., 2011; Penn & Cleary; 1988; Williamson & Isaki, 2015). The protocol recommends that the rating be completed during 15 minutes of spontaneous conversation with a familiar partner.

> ### BOX 10–1. The Communication Performance Scale (CPS)
>
> The CPS examines the following communication skills:
>
> - Intelligibility of speech
> - Prosody/rate
> - Body posture
> - Facial expression
> - Lexical selection
> - Syntax
> - Cohesiveness
> - Language use
>   - Topic
>   - Initiation of conversation
>   - Repair
>   - Interruption
>   - Listening

Communication Performance Scale

The Communication Performance Scale (CPS; Ehrlich & Sipes, 1985) was adapted from the Pragmatic Protocol (Box 10–1). The scale assesses pragmatic communication skills that are rated by a clinician for appropriateness on a 5-point rating scale. The total score ranges from 13 to 65, where a higher score indicates more appropriate communication skills. The individual scale items have been shown to demonstrate significant change from pre- to post-treatment for a group treatment involving six people with brain injury (Ehrlich & Sipes, 1985), and the total score has shown significant change following a group treatment for six adolescents with brain injury (Wiseman-Hakes et al., 1998).

Conversational Rating Scale

The Conversational Rating Scale (CRS; Ehrlich & Barry, 1989) contains six items

that rate the quality of spontaneous conversation for people with brain injury (i.e., intelligibility of speech, eye gaze, sentence formulation, coherence of narrative, topic, and initiation of communication). Each item is rated by the clinician on a 9-point scale that ranges from 1 (*most severe impairment*) to 9 (*no difficulty*). Five points along this scale (i.e., 1, 3, 5, 7, and 9) are defined in more detail to enable more precise ratings (see Cherney et al., 1998, Exhibit 7–1, p. 128).

Behaviorally Referenced Rating of Intermediate Social Skills–Revised

The Behaviorally Referenced Rating System of Intermediate Social Skills–Revised (BRISS-R; Farrell et al., 1985) comprises six social behavior rating scales. These scales are typically used to evaluate social behavior from a filmed interaction. Four scales evaluate the person's communication capability in language (vocabulary, grammar, and syntax), speech delivery (fluency, rate, voice quality, and speech mannerisms), conversational structure (conversation fluency and topic changes), and conversational content (topic interest and topic substance). Two scales, the Personal Conversational Style Scale (PCSS) and the Person-Directed Behavior Scale (PDBS), evaluate more adaptive capabilities and social behavior when communicating with others. The PCSS examines self-disclosure, use of humor, and social manners. The PDBS rates the use of reinforcers, self-centered behavior, and partner involvement. Behaviors are rated on a Likert scale from 1 (*very inappropriate*) to 7 (*very appropriate*). Behavioral descriptors are included to aid scoring (e.g., on the PCSS social manners subscale, "derogatory comments some of the time" scores 2; on the PDBS self-centered behavior subscale,

"talked about self some of the time" scores 5). The BRISS-R has been used to evaluate social behavior in research studies involving people with TBI (Flanagan et al., 1995; Marsh & Knight, 1991; McDonald & Flanagan, 2004; McDonald et al., 2008).

Profile of Pragmatic Impairment in Communication

The Profile of Pragmatic Impairment in Communication (PPIC; Linscott et al., 1996) is a rating scale to assess the presence and frequency of 84 social communication behaviors specific to TBI. Frequencies are recorded on a 4-point Likert scale from 0 (*not at all*) to 3 (*nearly always/always*). These 84 behaviors are organized across 10 subscales listed in Box 10–2. A feature summary scale (FSS) for each of the 10 subscales generates a summary rating using a

---

BOX 10–2. The Profile of Pragmatic Impairment in Communication (PPIC)

The PPIC documents the presence and frequency of various social communication behaviors organized within 10 subscales:

- Literal Content (encompassing use of logical, understandable, and coherent language)
- General Participation (where the contribution is both organized and sensitive to the interests of the communication partner)
- Quantity (where the amount shared meets the needs or understanding of the other person)
- Quality (where the person's contribution is both honest and factual)
- Internal Relations (where the

person's contribution is organized, relevant, and related)
- External Relations (where the person's comments are related to other people's preceding contributions)
- Clarity of Expression (clear and concise delivery)
- Social Style (that is appropriate to the context and the relationship)
- Subject Matter (that is socially, culturally, and/or morally relevant and appropriate)
- Aesthetics (encompassing additional features that add meaning, emphasis, or variety through speech style, body language, or proxemics appropriate to the context)

6-point Likert scale (where 0 is *normal* and 5 is *severely impaired*). A manual for training, administration, and scoring is available (Linscott et al., 2018). The PPIC has been used in research studies to measure change from video-recorded conversation samples between a person with TBI and an unfamiliar neurotypical communication partner (Braden et al., 2010; Dahlberg et al., 2007; Finch et al., 2017).

Global Impression Scales

The Global Impression scales (Bond & Godfrey, 1997) evaluate four dimensions of conversation: appropriateness, effortfulness, interestingness, and rewardingness. These dimensions are evaluated using 9-point rating scales ranging from 0 (e.g., *not at all appropriate*) to 8 (e.g., *very appropriate*) based on observation of a dyadic conversation (see companion website). The focus of rating is the quality of the conversation as a whole rather than on the individual contributions of each speaker. As such, it has potential for use in goal setting, monitoring of progress, and evaluation of outcomes for social communication interventions involving joint training of both the person with TBI and their communication partner. These scales have not been frequently used in interventional research but have been demonstrated as a sensitive outcome measure in several small clinical trials (Behn et al., 2012; Behn et al., 2019a).

Adapted Kagan Scales

The Adapted Kagan Scales (available in Togher et al., 2010) were based on a tool originally developed to evaluate the conversations of people with aphasia (Kagan et al., 2004) and comprise the Adapted Measure of Participation in Conversation (Adapted MPC) and the Adapted Measure of Support in Conversation (Adapted MSC) (see companion website). The original MPC and MSC scales are 9-point Likert scales, presented as a range of 0 to 4 with 0.5 levels for ease of scoring. The scale ranges from 0 (*no participation*) to 2 (*adequate participation*) to 4 (*full participation in conversation*). The Adapted MPC relates to the participation of the person with TBI and includes two scales, Interaction and Transaction. The Adapted MSC relates to the support provided by the communication partner and includes two scales, Acknowledge Competence and Reveal Competence. The unique value of these scales is the specific consideration of the role of the communication partner in facilitating or inhibiting the participation of the person with TBI, which means these scales are an informative outcome measure for communication partner training (CPT) interventions. The sensitivity of these scales to demonstrating the outcomes of intervention has been demonstrated in clinical trials of CPT (Behn et al., 2012; Rietdijk et al., 2020; Togher et al., 2013) and in group-based communication skills treatment (Behn et al., 2019a). The scales have been recommended for use in TBI research (Honan et al., 2019). The application of these scales is demonstrated in the companion website.

Pragmatic Rating Scale

The Pragmatic Rating Scale (PRS) was developed by MacLennan and colleagues (2002), and a modified PRS is available in Iwashita and Sohlberg (2019). This scale consists of 16 items divided into three subscales that include nonverbal communication (e.g., intelligibility, gesture, facial expression), propositional communication (e.g., cohesion, initiation, verbosity), and interactional communication (repair, feedback, responsiveness). It is recommended that ratings be applied to a dyadic conversation 12 to 20 minutes in length. The PRS was designed so it can be quickly learned by clinicians and scored while observing or collecting the conversational sample.

Interactional Network Tool

The Interactional Network Tool (INT; Howell, 2018) is a digital measure designed to evaluate group communication behavior (http://www.interactionalnetworks.org). It provides a means to directly assess change in interactional participation in groups, drawing on social network theories and analysis methods in its design (Scott, 2017; Wasserman & Faust, 1994) to create visual representations of group interaction patterns (Figure 10–1). These visualizations are derived from quantitative data and provide qualitative insights into adaptive behavior between group participants. Communication behaviors are coded from a filmed interaction and organized into higher-order initiations and response categories

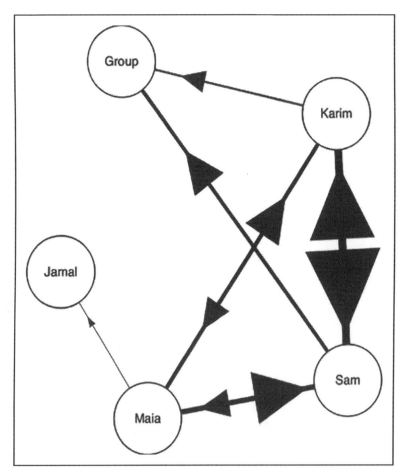

Figure 10–1. INT visualization example. The figure shows an interaction that largely involves Karim, Sam, and Maia. The thickness of the lines and arrows show that Karim and Sam interact frequently with each other and with the whole group. Jamal is a conversation isolate.

drawn from models of discourse analysis (Coulthard, 1984; Eggins & Slade, 1997). Initiation and response measures have previously been employed in conversational discourse studies of individuals with TBI (Coelho et al., 1991; Coelho et al., 2002); these deficits have been shown to undermine conversational effectiveness.

Howell, Beeke, et al. (2021) and Howell, Varley, et al. (2021) tested the feasibility of this measurement approach comparing interaction outcomes for people with acquired brain injury. Following a peer-led group intervention and a staff-led activity group, the coding system was modified to examine seven interaction types (Box 10–3). The behavioral frequency data generated from the refined coding system provide a quantitative profile of the connections between people. The visual representations show a qualitative view of their interactive relationships.

BOX 10–3. The Interactional Network Tool (INT): Seven Interaction Types

- Linguistic initiation to one other
- Linguistic initiation to group
- Linguistic response (e.g., 1–3 include verbal, writing, signing, or AAC responses)
- Nonlinguistic initiation (e.g., point, reach, gesture, draw, facial expression, eye gaze)
- Nonlinguistic response (e.g., point, reach, gesture, head shake/nod, draw, facial expression)
- Other voiced response
- Response to eye gaze

The visualization in Figure 10–1 shows a group of four participants. As the number of interactions grow, the lines connecting the participants increase in thickness and color density. The arrows show the direction of initiations and responses. Group is also included to distinguish between interactions between participants and the group as a whole. This visualization may be used to provide concrete feedback for participants and set goals (e.g., to be more inclusive or less dominant). The INT shows how people communicate and cue each other to communicate. It does not provide a qualitative analysis of the conversational content. Measuring outcomes in group interaction is a new field of investigation, and the INT brings a novel focus by capturing interactional connections between group participants.

Discourse Analysis Methods

Topic Analysis

Topic analysis was introduced as a method for examining the patterns and problems in topic management (Bedrosian 1985, 1993; Mentis & Prutting, 1991). Mentis and Prutting (1991) used topic analysis to examine the monologues and conversations of people with TBI, while Bedrosian (1985, 1993) used topic analysis for examining the conversations of people with intellectual disabilities with a peer, adult significant other, and a peer and clinician. In topic analysis, language samples (conversation and/or monologues) are video recorded, transcribed, and analyzed. There are differences between the studies in the parameters analyzed; however, they both broadly focus on topic initiation and maintenance including any topic changes or disruptions that may occur. Bedrosian (1993) suggests that the topic analysis framework is used as a guide to understand topic management skills, rather than conducting a lengthy analysis of the transcribed sample. The Mentis and Prutting (1991) topic analysis, used to successfully describe the differences in topic management for a person with TBI and a control, is available in Cherney et al. (1998, Exhibit 7–3, p. 137). It has been applied to examine changes in topic choices over time, 3 to 6 months post TBI (Brassel et al., 2016), and to identify specific topics of interest for further analysis (Keegan et al., 2017).

Clinical Discourse Analysis

Clinical discourse analysis (CDA) can be used as an in-depth method of analysis for errors in conversation (Damico, 1991). Originally used for children with language disabilities, the analysis is based on 17 parameters structured using Grice's (1975) conversational maxims: quantity, quality, manner, and relation. A sample of conversation is videotaped and transcribed, with the frequency of discourse errors recorded for each parameter. Four overall measures are obtained, including: total utterances, total discourse errors (e.g., information redundancy, message inaccuracy, topic maintenance difficulty, turn-taking difficulty), total utterances containing errors, and percentage of utterances containing errors. Questions that guide the clinician in identifying such discourse errors are presented in Exhibit 7–1 (Cherney et al., 1998, p. 127). For people with TBI, a modified version of this analysis (CDA-M) can be used (Snow et al., 1997; Snow et al., 1998). The modified version is a frequency count of discourse errors in all parameters except for nonspecific vocabulary, linguistic nonfluency, and revision; people with TBI, orthopedic controls, and university students all made errors across these three parameters. The use of CDA is acknowledged as more appropriate for research than clinical

practice, although clinicians may use CDA as a tool to validate clinical judgements (Snow et al., 2000). In addition, CDA has been used to guide the development of 20 items from the La Trobe Communication Questionnaire (LCQ), which is a measure of perceived communicative ability (Douglas et al., 2000; Douglas et al., 2007).

La Trobe Communication Questionnaire (LCQ)

The LCQ (Douglas et al., 2000; Douglas et al., 2007) is a self- and other report form for documenting the frequency of social communication behaviors in everyday conversational settings. Since it is primarily a personal rating of communication behavior, it was not included in the list of clinician rating scales above. Nevertheless, it has great applicability to this population and is frequently used by clinicians to obtain client and caregiver perceptions of communication skills (Frith et al., 2014), and its reliability and validity with the TBI population has been documented (Douglas et al., 2007). Scores range from 30 to 120, with higher scores indicating the respondent perceives a higher frequency of communication problems. Recent recommendations suggest the use of a video-recorded sample to assist with the rating process (Hoepner & Turkstra, 2013).

Box 10–4 references additional scales available for use by individuals with TBI to self-rate their communication; these may be completed by everyday communication partners.

Conversation Analysis

As outlined in Chapter 7, conversation analysis (CA) is an ethnomethodological approach to analyzing the different facets of conversational organization. Since this

> ### BOX 10–4. Tools for Self/ Communication Partner Rating of Conversational Skills
>
> - La Trobe Communication Questionnaire (LCQ; Douglas et al., 2000; Douglas et al., 2007)
> - Social Communication Skills Questionnaire–Adapted (SCSQ-A; Dahlberg et al., 2006)
> - Social Skills Questionnaire–Traumatic Brain Injury (SSQ-TBI; Francis et al., 2017)
> - Conversational rating scale from the "Protocole Montreal d'Evaluation de la Communication" (MEC; Joanette et al., 2004)
> - Communication Participation Item Bank (CPIB; Baylor et al., 2013)

analysis is an examination of data collected from naturally occurring collaborative conversation, it is especially conducive to examining conversational exchanges (Wilkinson, 2019). The focus of this analysis is not only on the deficits and difficulties that occur in conversation but also on strengths and skills. This primarily involves analyses of turn taking, topic management, and repair, and examines the collaborative contributions of all communication partners in the exchange. Conversational analysis has been extensively applied to aphasia (see Chapter 7). However, there have been some preliminary applications of CA to the conversations of individuals with TBI (Azios & Archer, 2018; Barnes, 2012; Body & Parker, 2005; Denman & Wilkinson, 2011; Friedland & Miller, 1998; Mann et al., 2015). Friedland and Miller (1998) found that CA methods allowed for a greater description of functional pragmatic difficulties than were cap-

tured on formal assessments. CA has been effective in supporting the systematic examination of how individuals with TBI use nonverbal communication (Denman & Wilkinson, 2011), topic bias and repetition (Body & Parker; 2005), questions (Mann et al., 2015), planning talk (Barnes, 2012), and singing behaviors (Azios & Archer, 2018).

Systemic Functional Linguistics

Systemic Functional Linguistics (SFL) is a theory that conceptualizes language or discourse as a social, meaning-based resource (Eggins & Slade, 1997; Halliday & Matthiessen, 2014). SFL focuses on three metafunctions: interpersonal (e.g., roles and relations), ideational (e.g., genre or topic focus), and textual (e.g., cohesive devices). SFL encompasses a variety of analytic tools that are useful for examining language use and conversational discourse after TBI.

Exchange Structure Analysis (ESA), for example, allows for an examination of the functions of the utterances used. Functions include giving information, offering goods and services, asking questions, or demanding goods and services. ESA has been used extensively to examine the discourse of individuals after TBI, as well as those interacting with them, as it allows for a thorough description of their contributions as relevant to the context of the interaction (Bogart et al., 2012; Guo & Togher, 2008; Jorgensen & Togher; 2009; Keegan et al., 2021; Rietdijk et al., 2019; Sim et al., 2013; Togher, 2000; Togher et al., 1996, 1997; Togher et al., 2006; Tu et al., 2011). The companion website provides a sample that includes an ESA analysis, and a manual that provides examples of utterance types and information on how to classify them is available on request.

Modality analysis involves examining conversation to identify expressions that convey probability (e.g., *would*), potential (e.g., *could*), usuality (e.g., *everyday*), inclination (e.g., *want*), and obligation (e.g., *must*). Several researchers have found utility in applying this approach to the investigation of language use in conversation after TBI (Keegan et al., 2021; Meulenbroek & Cherney, 2019; Meulenbroek & Turkstra, 2016; Togher & Hand, 1998). In addition, the potential of emphasizing modality (specifically politeness markers) to enhance conversational abilities in vocational settings has been recognized (Meulenbroek & Cherney, 2019).

Appraisal analysis reveals how a speaker uses graduation (qualification or intensification), engagement (linguistic tools to engage the listener), and evaluation (attitudes expressed to behavior, things, and feelings). Recently, appraisal analyses have facilitated the understanding of the linguistic and conversational strengths of individuals with TBI (Keegan & McAdam, 2016; Keegan et al., 2021). Transitivity analysis, an examination of the clause processes, has been used to provide insight into how individuals with TBI construe and present their experiences (Keegan & Müller, in press). It is expected that future research will continue to investigate this topic.

Goal Attainment Scaling

Goal Attainment Scaling (GAS) is a system of measuring progress toward goals by assimilating achievement in individual goals into a single aggregated score (Turner-Stokes, 2009). It therefore allows a client and clinician to collaboratively set individualized communication goals, as related to conversational communication, and develop a scale on which to measure progress toward these goals. Initially goals are scaled from −2 to +2; however, scales of 0 to 4 and 1 to 5 have been proposed and utilized with clients to avoid the distress of negative rating (Behn et al., 2019, Keegan et al., 2020; Malec, 1999). A sample scaled goal is presented in Box 10–5.

GAS has proven to be more responsive and sensitive to gains than many other standardized measures (Turner-Stokes, 2009), and the flexibility it allows is ideal for examining contextualized interaction. GAS provides a measurable, individualized, person-centered outcome based on concrete behaviors that are observed. It has been identified as an effective measure of functional progress in brain injury rehabilitation (Turner-Stokes, 2009).

BOX 10–5. Goal Attainment Scaling (GAS)

Goal: I will ask topic-relevant questions of my communication partner, without prompting, in*:	**GAS Level**	**Levels of Attainment**
0 out of 5 opportunities	−2	Much less than expected outcome
1 out of 5 opportunities	−1	Starting point
2 out of 5 opportunities	0	Expected outcome*
3 out of 5 opportunities	1	Somewhat more than expected outcome
4–5 out of 5 opportunities	2	Much more than expected outcome

Expected outcome to be achieved in four treatment sessions

GAS is also known for its excellent inter-rater reliability and good concurrent validity as compared to other outcome measures (Krasny-Pacini et al., 2016; Malec, 1999). However, Krasny-Pacini et al. (2016) caution that, to ensure reliability and validity, one must carefully construct and scale the goals. Grant and Ponsford's (2014) checklist for evaluating the scales was adapted here to provide a tool that minimizes the likelihood of poorly constructed goals (Box 10–6).

GAS scores can be converted to T-scores through the assignment of weights based on the importance and difficulty level of each goal (Turner-Stokes, 2009). Information on training and resources related to GAS and the use of T-scores can be found at the King's College website (https://www.kcl.ac.uk/cicelysaunders/resources/tools/gas). This method of assigning T-scores allows performance to be aggregated across multiple goals for comparison between participants that would otherwise be difficult to compare (Grant & Ponsford, 2014) and for communication goal setting (Finch et al.,

2017). However, caution should be used when aggregating such goals to parametric analyses. Thus, some researchers have used nonparametric approaches to examine GAS progress, including Friedman's test (Behn et al., 2019) and mixed multilevel analyses (Keegan et al., 2019).

This comprehensive outcome measurement system is gaining popularity as a tool that is used to examine communication after TBI (Behn et al., 2019; Doig et al., 2009; Keegan et al., 2020) as it is particularly responsive to changes in social communication (Behn et al., 2019; Braden et al., 2010; Dahlberg et al., 2007; Finch et al., 2019). Due to the way in which goals are collaboratively developed and measured, it allows for assessment of progress that is very sensitive to the individual's values and aspirations. Finally, it should be noted that Electronic Goal Attainment Scaling (eGAS) is currently being studied, and preliminary investigations of an electronic application show promise for aiding clinicians in goal setting and scaling (Kucheria et al., 2020).

BOX 10–6. Goal Attainment Scaling (GAS) Checklist for Conversations

- ☐ Individuals are involved in setting their own goals.
- ☐ Context and communication partners are considered/involved during goal setting.
- ☐ Videotaped conversations guide goal-setting discussions.
- ☐ Goals may target discrete communication skills and/or communication participation.
- ☐ Each goal targets a single communicative behavior (or variable).
- ☐ Each goal is specific, measurable, achievable, realistic, and time based (i.e., SMART).

- ☐ Each of the five outcome levels are carefully defined and continuous but differentiated, with an equal distance between each level.
- ☐ An independent team member reviews the scaled goal.
- ☐ Each goal is measured at follow-up.
- ☐ Multiple people involved in the intervention (e.g., person with ABI, therapist, communication partner) rate each goal.
- ☐ Other outcome measures are used to supplement GAS when tracking progress.

Future Directions

Assessment of conversations is an area that is well poised to improve in the coming years. First, the recent emphasis on examining participation in communicative and sociocultural context rather than solely communication impairment (MacDonald, 2017) has increased general appreciation for conversational samples that allow the clinician to obtain detailed information about how the individual with TBI communicates and socially participates in typical everyday interactions. Second, there are currently ongoing efforts to streamline the training procedures and improve the reliability data supporting the rating scales outlined in this chapter. Third, corpus data (e.g., TBIBank, see Chapter 17 of this book) is being compiled; as it grows, it will provide additional comparative data about communication strengths and difficulties of individuals with TBI. Finally, technology is continually improving, allowing for the use of automated measures and artificial intelligence in the collection, transcription, and analysis of conversational data (e.g., INT, outlined earlier in the chapter). Similarly, the rise of telehealth and telepractice services on online platforms engage individuals in their everyday environments with typical communication partners or as part of groups, and provide the clinician with insight into optimal contexts for assessment of conversations.

References

Azios, J. H., & Archer, B. (2018). Singing behavior in a client with traumatic brain injury: A conversation analysis investigation. *Aphasiology, 32*(8), 944–966. https://doi.org/10.1080/02687038.2018.1466106

Barnes, S. (2012). Planning talk and traumatic brain injury: An exploratory application of conversation analysis. *Journal of Interactional Research in Communication Disorders, 3*(2), 115–140. https://doi.org/10.1558/jircd.v3i2.115

Baylor, C., Yorkston, K., Eadie, T., Kim, J., Chung, H, & Amtmann, D. (2013). The Communicative Participation Item Bank (CPIB): Item bank calibration and development of a disorder-generic short form. *Journal of Speech, Language, and Hearing Research, 56*(4), 1190-1208. https://doi.org/10.1044/1092-4388 (2012/12-0140)

Bedrosian, J. L. (1985). An approach to developing conversational competence. In D. N. Ripich & F. M. Spinelli (Eds.), *Social discourse problems*. College Hill Press.

Bedrosian, J.L. (1993). Making minds meet: Assessment of conversational topic in adults with mild to moderate mental retardation. *Topics in Language Disorders, 13*, 36–46. https://psycnet.apa.org/doi/10.1097/0001 1363-199305000-00006

Behn, N., Francis, J., Togher, L., Hatch, E., Moss, B., & Hilari, K. (2021). Description and effectiveness of communication partner training in TBI: A systematic review. *Journal of Head Trauma Rehabilitation, 36*(1), 56–71. https://doi.org/10.1097/HTR.0000000000000580

Behn, N., Marshall, J., Togher, L., & Cruice, M. (2019a). Feasibility and initial efficacy of project-based treatment for people with ABI. *International Journal of Language and Communication Disorders, 54*(3), 465–478. https://doi.org/10.1111/1460-6984.12452

Behn, N., Marshall, J., Togher, L., & Cruice, M. (2019b). Setting and achieving individualized social communication goals for people with acquired brain injury (ABI) within a group treatment. *International Journal of Language and Communication Disorders, 54*(5), 828–840. https://doi.org/10.1111/1460-6984.12488

Behn, N., Togher, L., Power, E., & Heard, R. (2012). Evaluating communication training for paid carers of people with traumatic brain injury. *Brain Injury, 26*(13–14), 1702–1715. https://doi.org/10.3109/02699052.2012.722258

Body, R., & Parker, M. (2005). Topic repetitiveness after traumatic brain injury: An emergent, jointly managed behaviour. *Clinical Linguistics and Phonetics, 19*(5), 379–392. https://doi.org/10.1080/02699200400027189

Bogart, E., Togher, L., Power, E., & Docking, K. (2012). Casual conversations between individuals with traumatic brain injury and their friends. *Brain Injury, 26*(3), 221–233. https://doi.org/10.3109/02699052.2011.648711

Bond, F., & Godfrey, H. P. (1997). Conversation with traumatically brain injured individuals: A controlled study of behavioral changes and their impact. *Brain Injury, 11*(5), 319–330. https://doi.org/10.1080/026990597123476

Bouwens, S. F., Van Heugten, C. M., & Verhey, F. R. (2009). The practical use of goal attainment scaling for people with acquired brain injury who receive cognitive rehabilitation. *Clinical Rehabilitation, 23*(4), 310–320. https://doi.org/10.1177/0269215508101744

Braden, C., Hawley, L., Newman, J., Morey, C., Gerber, D., & Harrison-Felix, C. (2010). Social communication skills group treatment: A feasibility study for persons with traumatic brain injury and comorbid conditions. *Brain Injury, 24*(11), 1298–1310. https://doi.org/10.3109/02699052.2010.506859

Brassel, S., Kenny, B., Power, E., Elbourn, E., McDonald, S., Tate, R., . . . Togher, L. (2016). Conversational topics discussed by individuals with severe traumatic brain injury and their communication partners during subacute recovery. *Brain Injury, 30*(11), 1329–1342. https://doi.org/10.1080/02699052.2016.1187288

Cannizzaro, M., Allen, E. M., & Prelock, P. (2011). Perceptions of communicative competence after traumatic brain injury: Implications for ecologically driven intervention targets. *International Journal of Speech-Language Pathology, 13*(6), 549–559. https://doi.org/10.3109/17549507.2011.596571

Cherney, L. R., Shadden, B. B., & Coelho, C. A. (Eds.). (1998). *Analyzing discourse in communicatively impaired adults.* Aspen Publishers.

Cicchetti, D., & Sparrow, S. A. (1981). Developing criteria for establishing interrater reliability of specific items: Applications to assessment of adaptive behavior. *American Journal of Mental Deficiency, 86*, 127–137.

Coelho, C. A., Liles, B. Z., & Duffy, R. J. (1991). Analysis of conversational discourse in head-injured adults. *Journal of Head Trauma Rehabilitation, 6*(2), 92–98. https://doi.org/10.1097/00001199-199106000-00011

Coelho, C. A., Youse, K. M., & Le, K. N. (2002). Conversational discourse in closed-head-injured and non-brain-injured adults. *Aphasiology, 16*(4–6), 659–672. https://doi.org/10.1080/02687030244000275

Coulthard, M. (1984). Conversation analysis and social skills training. In P. Trower (Ed.), *Radical approaches to social skills training.* Croom Helm.

Dahlberg, C. A., Cusick, C. P., Hawley, L. A., Newman, J. K., Morey, C. E., Harrison-Felix, C. L., & Whiteneck, G. G. (2007). Treatment efficacy of social communication skills training after traumatic brain injury: A randomized treatment and deferred treatment controlled trial. *Archives of Physical Medicine and Rehabilitation, 88*(12), 1561–1573. https://doi.org/10.1016/j.apmr.2007.07.033

Dahlberg, C., Hawley, L., Morey, C., Newman, J., Cusick, C. P., & Harrison-Felix, C. (2006). Social communication skills in persons with postacute traumatic brain injury: Three perspectives. *Brain Injury, 20*(4), 425–435. https://doi.org/10.1080/02699050600664574

Denman, A., & Wilkinson, R. (2011). Applying conversation analysis to traumatic brain injury: Investigating touching another person in everyday social interaction. *Disability and Rehabilitation, 33*(3), 243–252. https://doi.org/10.3109/09638288.2010.511686

Doig, E., Fleming, J., Cornwell, P. L., & Kuipers, P. (2009). Qualitative exploration of a client centered, goal-directed approach to community-based occupational therapy for adults with traumatic brain injury. *American Journal of Occupational Therapy, 63*(5), 559–568. https://doi.org/10.5014/ajot.63.5.559

Douglas, J. M., Bracy, C. A., & Snow, P. C. (2007). Measuring perceived communicative ability after traumatic brain injury: Reliability and validity of the La Trobe Communication Questionnaire. *The Journal of Head Trauma*

Rehabilitation, 22(1), 31–38. https://doi.org/10.1097/00001199-200701000-00004

Douglas, J. M., O'Flaherty, C. A., & Snow, P. C. (2000). Measuring perception of communicative ability: The development and evaluation of the La Trobe Communication Questionnaire. *Aphasiology, 14*(3), 251–268. https://doi.org10.1080/026870300401469

Eggins, S., & Slade, D. (1997). *Analyzing casual conversation.* Equinox.

Ehrlich, J., & Barry, P. (1989). Rating communication behaviors in the head-injured adult. *Brain Injury, 3*, 193–198. https://doi.org/10.3109/02699058909004552

Ehrlich, J. S., & Sipes, A. L. (1985). Group treatment of communication skills for head trauma patients. *Cognitive Rehabilitation, 3*(1), 32–37.

Farrell, A. D., Rabinowitz, J. A., Wallander, J. L., & Curran, J. P. (1985). An evaluation of two formats for the intermediate-level assessment of social skills. *Behavioral Assessment, 7*, 155–171.

Finch, E., Copley, A., McLisky, M., Cornwell, P. L., Fleming, J. M., & Doig, E. (2019). Can goal attainment scaling (GAS) accurately identify changes in social communication impairments following TBI? *Speech, Language, and Hearing, 22*(3), 183–194. https://doi.org/10.1080/2050571X.2019.1611220

Finch, E., Cornwell, P., Copley, A., Doig, E., & Fleming, J. (2017). Remediation of social communication impairments following traumatic brain injury using metacognitive strategy intervention: A pilot study. *Brain Injury, 31*(13–14), 1830–1839. https://doi.org/10.1080/02699052.2017.1346284

Flanagan, S., McDonald, S., & Togher, L. (1995). Evaluating social skills following traumatic brain injury: The BRISS as a clinical tool. *Brain Injury, 9*(4), 321–338. https://doi.org/10.3109/02699059509005773

Francis, H. M., Osborne-Crowley, K., & McDonald, S. (2017). Validity and reliability of a questionnaire to assess social skills in traumatic brain injury: A preliminary study. *Brain Injury, 31*(3), 336–343. https://doi.org/10.1080/02699052.2016.1250954

Friedland, D., & Miller, N. (1998). Conversation analysis of communication breakdown after closed head injury. *Brain Injury, 12*(1), 1–14. https://doi.org/10.1080/026990598122818

Frith, M., Togher, L., Ferguson, A., Levick, W., & Docking, K. (2014). Assessment practices of speech-language pathologists for cognitive communication disorders following traumatic brain injury in adults: An international survey. *Brain Injury, 28*(13–14), 1657–1666. https://doi.org/10.3109/02699052.2014.947619

Grant, M., & Ponsford, J. (2014). Goal attainment scaling in brain injury rehabilitation: Strengths, limitations and recommendations for future applications. *Neuropsychological Rehabilitation, 24*(5), 661–677. https://doi.org/10.1080/09602011.2014.901228

Grice, H. P. (1975). Logic and conversation. In P. Cole & J. L. Morgan (Eds.), *Syntax and semantics: Speech acts* (Vol. 3). Academic Press.

Guo, Y. E., & Togher, L. (2008). The impact of dysarthria on everyday communication after traumatic brain injury: A pilot study. *Brain Injury, 22*(1), 83–98. https://doi.org/10.1080/02699050701824150

Halliday, M. A. K., & Matthiessen, C. M. I. M. (2014). *An introduction to functional grammar* (4th ed.). Arnold Publishing.

Hoepner, J. K., & Turkstra, L. S. (2013). Video-based administration of the La Trobe Communication Questionnaire for adults with traumatic brain injury and their communication partners. *Brain Injury, 27*(4), 464–472. https://doi.org/10.3109/02699052.2013.765600

Honan, C. A., McDonald, S., Tate, R., Ownsworth, T., Togher, L., Fleming, J., . . . Ponsford, J. (2019). Outcome instruments in moderate to severe adult traumatic brain injury: Recommendations for use in psychosocial research. *Neuropsychological Rehabilitation, 29*(6), 896–916. https://doi.org/10.1080/09602011.2017.1339616

Howell, S. (2018). *Measuring outcomes from a peer-led social communication skills intervention for adults following acquired brain injury* [Doctoral dissertation, University College London]. https://discovery.ucl.ac.uk/id/eprint/10059713

Howell, S., Beeke, S., Pring, T., & Varley, R. (2021). Measuring outcomes of a peer-led social communication skills intervention for adults with acquired brain injury: A pilot investigation. *Neuropsychological Rehabilitation*, *31*(7), 1069–1090. https://doi.org/10.10 80/09602011.2020.1760892

Howell, S., Varley, R., Sinnott, E. L., Pring, T., & Beeke, S. (2021). Measuring group social interactions following acquired brain injury: An interrater reliability evaluation. *Aphasiology*, *35*(11), 1505–1517. https://doi.org/10.10 80/02687038.2020.1836315

Iwashita, H., & Sohlberg, M. M. (2019). Measuring conversations after acquired brain injury in 30 minutes or less: A comparison of two pragmatic rating scales. *Brain Injury*, *33*(9), 1219–1233. https://doi.org/10.1080/0269905 2.2019.1631487

Joanette, Y., Ska, B., & Côté, H. (2004). *Protocole Montreál d'évaluation de la communication (*Montreal Communication Evaluation Protocol). Ortho Édition.

Jorgensen, M., & Togher, L. (2009). Narrative after traumatic brain injury: A comparison of monologic and jointly produced discourse. *Brain Injury*, *23*(9), 727–740. https://doi .org/10.1080/02699050903133954

Kagan, A., Winckel, J., Black, S., Felson Duchan, J., Simmons-Mackie, N., & Square, P. (2004). A set of observational measures for rating support and participation in conversation between adults with aphasia and their conversation partners. *Topics in Stroke Rehabilitation*, *11*(1), 67–83. https://doi.org/10.1310/ CL3V-A94A-DE5C-CVBE

Keegan, L. C., & McAdam, H. (2016). Swearing after traumatic brain injury: A linguistic analysis. *Journal of Interactional Research in Communication Disorders*, *7*(1), 101–122. https://doi.org/10.1558/jircd.v7i1.21570

Keegan, L. C., & Müller, N. (in press). The influence of context on identity construction after traumatic brain injury. *Journal of Interactional Research in Communication Disorders, Forthcoming Special Issue.*

Keegan, L. C., Murdock, M., Suger, C., & Togher, L., (2020). Improving social interaction: Group rehabilitation after traumatic brain injury. *Neuropsychological Rehabilitation*, *30*(8), 1497–1522. https://doi.org/10.1080/09 602011.2019.1591464

Keegan, L. C., Suger, C., & Togher, L. (2021). Discourse analysis of humor after traumatic brain injury. *American Journal of Speech-Language Pathology*, *30*(2S), 949–961. https://doi .org/10.1044/2020_AJSLP-20-00059

Keegan, L. C., Togher, L., Murdock, M., & Hendry, E. (2017). Expression of masculine identity in individuals with traumatic brain injury. *Brain Injury*, *31*(12), 1632–1641. https://doi .org/10.1080/02699052.2017.1332389

Krasny-Pacini, A., Evans, J., Sohlberg, M. M., & Chevignard, M. (2016). Proposed criteria for appraising goal attainment scales used as outcome measures in rehabilitation research. *Archives of Physical Medicine and Rehabilitation*, *97*(1), 157–170. https://doi .org/10.1016/j.apmr.2015.08.424

Kucheria, P., Sohlberg, M. M., Machalicek, W., Seeley, J., & DeGarmo, D. (2020). A single-case experimental design investigation of collaborative goal setting practices in hospital-based speech-language pathologists when provided supports to use motivational interviewing and goal attainment scaling. *Neuropsychological Rehabilitation*, *5*, 1–32. https:// doi.org/10.1080/09602011.2020.1838301

Linscott, R., Knight, R., & Godfrey, H. (1996). The Profile of Functional Impairment in Communication (PFIC): A measure of communication impairment for clinical use. *Brain Injury*, *10*(6), 397–412. https://doi.org/10.10 80/026990596124269

Linscott, R., Knight, R., & Godfrey, H. (2018). *Profile of Pragmatic Impairment in Communication (PPIC).* Authors. https://www.lulu .com/shop/richard-linscott-and-robert-knight-and-hamish-godfrey/profile-of-prag matic-impairment-in-communication/ebook/ product-23746385.html?page=1&pageSize=4

MacDonald, S. (2017). Introducing the model of cognitive-communication competence: A model to guide evidence-based communication interventions after brain injury. *Brain Injury*, *31*(13–14), 1760–1780. https://doi.org/ 10.1080/02699052.2017.1379613

MacLennan, D. L., Cornis-Pop, M., Picon-Nieto, L., & Sigford, B. (2002, March 7–10). *The prevalence of pragmatic communication impairments in traumatic brain injury* [Conference presentation]. National Brain Injury Association Conference, Minneapolis, MN. https://eatspeakthink.com/wp-content/uploads/2018/12/PRAGMATIC_EVAL2002.pdf

Malec, J. F. (1999). Goal attainment scaling in rehabilitation. *Neuropsychological Rehabilitation, 9*(3-4), 253–275. https://psycnet.apa.org/doi/10.1080/096020199389365

Mann, K., Power, E., Barnes, S., & Togher, L. (2015). Questioning in conversations before and after communication partner training for individuals with traumatic brain injury. *Aphasiology, 29*(9), 1082–1109. https://doi.org/10.1080/02687038.2015.1035226

Marsh, N. V., & Knight, R. G. (1991). Behavioral assessment of social competence following severe head injury. *Journal of Clinical and Experimental Neuropsychology, 13*(5), 729–740. https://doi.org/10.1080/01688639108401086

McDonald, S., & Flanagan, S. (2004). Social perception deficits after traumatic brain injury: The interaction between emotion recognition, mentalizing ability and social communication. *Neuropsychology, 18*, 572–579. https://doi.org/10.1037/0894-4105.18.3.572

McDonald, S., Tate, R., Togher, L., Bornhofen, C., Long, E., Gertler, P., & Bowen, R. (2008). Social skills treatment for people with severe, chronic acquired brain injuries: A multicenter trial. *Archives of Physical Medicine and Rehabilitation, 89*(9), 1648–1659. https://doi.org/10.1016/j.apmr.2008.02.029

Mentis, M., & Prutting, C. A. (1991). Analysis of topic as illustrated in a head-injured and normal adult. *Journal of Speech and Hearing Research, 34*, 583–595. https://doi.org/10.1044/jshr.3403.583

Meulenbroek, P., & Cherney, L. R. (2019). The voicemail elicitation task: Functional workplace language assessment for persons with traumatic brain injury. *Journal of Speech, Language, and Hearing Research, 62*(9), 3367–3380. https://doi.org/10.1044/2019_JSLHR-L-18-0466

Meulenbroek, P., & Turkstra, L. S. (2016). Job stability in skilled work and communication ability after moderate-severe traumatic brain injury. *Disability and Rehabilitation, 38*(5), 452–461. https://doi.org/10.3109/09638288.2015.1044621

Milton, S. B., Prutting, C. A., & Binder, G. M. (1984). *Appraisal of communicative competence in head-injured adults.* http://aphasiology.pitt.edu/802/1/14-14.pdf

Mortensen, L. (2005). Written discourse and acquired brain impairment: Evaluation of structural and semantic features of personal letters from a systemic functional linguistic perspective. *Clinical Linguistics and Phonetics, 19*(3), 227–247. https://doi.org/10.1080/02699200410001698652

Penn, C., & Cleary, J. (1988). Compensatory strategies in the language of closed head injured patients. *Brain Injury, 2*(1), 3–17. https://doi.org/10.3109/02699058809150928

Prutting, C. A, (1982). Pragmatics as social competence. *Journal of Speech and Hearing Disorders, 47*, 123–134. https://doi.org/10.1044/jshd.4702.123

Prutting, C. A., & Kirchner, D. M. (1983). Applied pragmatics. In T. M. Gallagher & C. A. Prutting (Eds.), *Pragmatic assessment and intervention issues in language* (pp. 29–64). College-Hill Press.

Prutting, C. A., & Kirchner, D. M. (1987). A clinical appraisal of the pragmatic aspects of language. *Journal of Speech and Hearing Disorders, 52*(2), 105–119. https://doi.org/10.1044/jshd.5202.105

Rietdijk, R., Power, E., Attard, M., Heard, R., & Togher, L. (2020). Improved conversation outcomes after social communication skills training for people with traumatic brain injury and their communication partners: A clinical trial investigating in-person and telehealth delivery. *Journal of Speech, Language, and Hearing Research, 63*(2), 615–632. https://doi.org/10.1080/09602011.2018.1554533

Rietdijk, R., Power, E., Brunner, M., & Togher, L. (2019). A single case experimental design study on improving social communication skills after traumatic brain injury using communication partner telehealth training. *Brain Injury, 33*(1), 94–104. https://doi.org/10.1080/02699052.2018.1531313

Scott, J. (2017). *Social network analysis* (4th ed.). SAGE Publications.

Searle, J.R. (1969). *Speech acts*. Cambridge University Press.

Sim, P., Power, E., & Togher, L. (2013). Describing conversations between individuals with traumatic brain injury (TBI) and communication partners following communication partner training: Using exchange structure analysis. *Brain Injury*, *27*(6), 717–742. https://doi.org/10.3109/02699052.2013.775485

Snow, P., & Douglas, J., (2000). Subject review: Conceptual and methodological challenges in discourse assessment with TBI speakers: Towards an understanding. *Brain Injury*, *14*(5), 397–415. https://doi.org/10.1080/026990500120510

Snow, P., Douglas, J., & Ponsford, J. (1997). Conversation assessment following traumatic brain injury: A comparison across two control groups. *Brain Injury*, *11*(6), 409–429. https://psycnet.apa.org/doi/10.1080/026990597123403

Snow, P., Douglas, J., & Ponsford, J. (1998). Conversational discourse abilities following severe traumatic brain injury: A follow up study. *Brain Injury*, *12*(11), 911–935. https://doi.org/10.1080/026990598121981

Sohlberg, M. M., MacDonald, S., Byom, L., Iwashita, H., Lemoncello, R., Meulenbroek, P., & O'Neil-Pirozzi, T. M. (2019). Social communication following traumatic brain injury, part I: State-of-the-art review of assessment tools. *International Journal of Speech-Language Pathology*, *21*(2), 115–127. https://doi.org/10.1080/17549507.2019.1583280

Steel, J., & Togher, L. (2019). Social communication assessment after traumatic brain injury: A narrative review of innovations in pragmatic and discourse assessment methods. *Brain Injury*, *33*(1), 48–61. https://doi.org/10.1080/02699052.2018.1531304

Togher, L. (2000). Giving information: The importance of context on communicative opportunity for people with traumatic brain injury. *Aphasiology*, *14*(4), 365–390. https://doi.org/10.1080/026870300401414

Togher, L., & Hand, L. (1998). Use of politeness markers with different communication partners: An investigation of five subjects with traumatic brain injury. *Aphasiology*,

12(7/8), 755–770. https://doi.org/10.1080/02687039808249571

Togher, L., Hand, L., & Code, C. (1996). A new perspective in the relationship between communication impairment and disempowerment following head injury in information exchanges. *Disability and Rehabilitation*, *18*(11), 559–566. https://doi.org/10.3109/09638289609166317

Togher, L., Hand, L., & Code, C. (1997). Analyzing discourse in the traumatic brain injury population: Telephone interactions with different communication partners. *Brain Injury*, *11*(3), 169–190. https://doi.org/10.1080/026990597123629

Togher, L., McDonald, S., Code, C., & Grant, S. (2004). Training communication partners of people with traumatic brain injury: A randomized controlled trial. *Aphasiology*, *18*(4), 313–335. https://doi.org/10.1080/02687030344000535

Togher, L., McDonald, S., Tate, R., Power, E., & Rietdijk, R. (2013). Training communication partners of people with severe traumatic brain injury improves everyday conversations: A multicenter single-blind clinical trial. *Journal of Rehabilitation Medicine*, *45*, 637–645. https://doi.org/10.2340/16501977-1173

Togher, L., Power, E., Tate, R., McDonald, S., & Rietdijk, R. (2010). Measuring the social interactions of people with traumatic brain injury and their communication partners: The adapted Kagan scales. *Aphasiology*, *24*(6–8), 914–927. https://doi.org/10.1080/02687030903422478

Togher, L. Taylor, C., Aird, V., & Grant, S. (2006). The impact of varied speaker role and communication partner on the communicative interactions of a person with traumatic brain injury: A single case study using systemic functional linguistics. *Brain Impairment*, *7*(3), 190–201. https://doi.org/10.1375/brim.7.3.190

Togher, L., Wiseman-Hakes, C., Douglas, J., Stergiou-Kita, M., Ponsford, J., Teasell, R., . . . Turkstra, L. S. (2014). INCOG Recommendations for management of cognition following traumatic brain injury, Part IV. *Journal of Head Trauma Rehabilitation*,

29(4), 353–368. https://doi.org/10.1097/HTR.0000000000000071

Tu, L. V., Togher, L., & Power, E. (2011). The impact of communication partner and discourse task on a person with traumatic brain injury: The use of multiple perspectives. *Brain Injury, 25*(6), 560–580. https://doi.org/10.3109/02699052.2011.571655

Turner-Stokes, L. (2009). Goal attainment scaling (GAS) in rehabilitation: A practical guide. *Clinical Rehabilitation, 23*(4), 362–370. https://doi.org/10.1177/0269215508101742

Wasserman, S., & Faust, K. (1994). *Social network analysis: Methods and applications.* Cambridge University Press.

Wilkinson, R. (2019). Atypical interaction: Conversation analysis and communicative impairments. *Research on Language and Social Interaction, 52*(3), 281–299. https://doi.org/10.1080/08351813.2019.1631045

Williamson, J., & Isaki, E. (2015). Facial affect recognition training through telepractice: Two case studies of individuals with chronic traumatic brain injury. *International Journal of Telerehabilitation, 7*(1), 13. https://doi.org/10.5195/IJT.2015.6167

Wiseman-Hakes, C., Stewart, M. L., Wasserman, R., & Schuller, R. (1998). Peer group training of pragmatic skills in adolescents with acquired brain injury. *Journal of Head Trauma Rehabilitation, 13*(6), 23–38. https://doi.org/10.1097/00001199-199812000-00005

11 Assessing Discourse in People With Right Hemisphere Disorders

Melissa D. Stockbridge, Jamila Minga, Alexandra Zezinka Durfee, and Melissa Johnson

Introduction

Examining discourse among individuals with right hemisphere brain damage (RHD) may not strike many readers as a necessary, obvious, or even interesting thing to do. Indeed, the RH's involvement in language and communication is often so eclipsed by the role of the left that, for many people, it can be tempting to simplify language as a wholly left-lateralized activity. However, as specialists in the clinical treatment of communication, we know this is not so. Communication is a whole-brain activity—one of the most challenging and uniquely human activities in which a person can engage. Adult speakers are so keenly aware of the nuanced performance of the specialized skill of discourse that even the mildest disruption or peculiarity registers as odd, even if it takes some time to build an evidentiary toolbox and clinical vocabulary with which to identify and describe those differences in a meaningful, objective, and reproducible way. Such is the circumstance of discourse following a RH lesion.

People with RHD often demonstrate some form of impaired communication (Benton & Bryan, 1996; Ferré et al., 2009; Ramsey & Blake, 2020). Discourse following RH damage has been referred to as "an impairment between sentences" (Brownell, 1988) that may demonstrate a paucity of specific detail or take on tangential, egocentric, or pragmatically inappropriate qualities (Blake, 2006; Brownell & Martino, 1998; Myers, 2001; Tompkins, 1995; Tompkins et al., 2012). This frequently occurs in the context of microlinguistic discourse features that are grossly intact (Marini, 2012), resulting in an impression that the language is fluent and intelligible. However, the ability to measure differences in discourse due to RHD has grown substantially since initial interest took hold in the 1960s.

It can be tempting to dismiss the macrolinguistic changes to communication as subclinical or too nuanced, especially when contrasted with the overt presentations of aphasia and agrammatism that can result from left hemisphere damage. Speech-language pathologists (SLPs) report feeling ill prepared to assess and diagnose impaired communication following RHD, yet are fairly confident in identifying the presence of a communication problem based primarily on observation and clinical judgment

(Ramsey & Blake, 2020). However, patients with RHD experience significant social consequences of their disability. They may have difficulty participating in social interactions to the extent that they can alienate listeners and face considerable social, vocational, and emotional consequences of their discourse and pragmatic impairments (Hewetson et al., 2021; Tompkins et al., 2012). Conversational partners may respond and adapt to their discourse behavior by providing unsupportive responses (e.g., minimal acknowledgments and explicit rejections), thereby ignoring or reinforcing, rather than repairing, the atypical patterns of their discourse (Barnes et al., 2020).

In this chapter, we begin with a brief theoretical orientation to RHD and the contribution of the RH to discourse-level language. Next, we discuss the key areas of discourse that have been identified as the most vulnerable to RHD. Finally, we provide guidance on how to capture these differences reliably in patients using descriptive, narrative, and conversational discourse tasks. In doing so, we discuss the ways in which research is contributing to the emerging foundation for interpreting discourse performance in RHD.

Throughout this discussion, a cautionary note pervades. Due to the eclipsing role of the left hemisphere in language at all structural levels of inquiry and limited knowledge of the RH's contributions to communication, individuals with RHD are not always evaluated for language or communication. Studies of communication and cognition in this population are notoriously small, contributing to a patchwork of empirical evidence, even for deficits such as emotional aprosodia, apragmatism, and visuospatial neglect that are considered core features of the population (Myers, 2001; Sheppard et al., 2022; Stockbridge, Sheppard, et al., 2021; Tompkins, 1995).

Right Hemisphere's Role in Discourse: Theoretical Perspectives

Although discourse assessment generally refers to a patient's ability to produce language, it is helpful to first introduce the theoretical foundations that underpin our understanding of how the RH contributes to discourse. Those foundations are laid in discourse comprehension. Adults with lesions in the "ineloquent" hemisphere have classically observed difficulties in discourse comprehension that bear heavily on their capacity and opportunities to participate in discourse. Discourse comprehension deficits are particularly salient when inferencing and integration are required (Blake, 2009; Brownell et al., 1992).

Two highly influential theories have shaped the investigation of discourse in RHD for the last 40 years: the coarse coding hypothesis and the suppression deficit hypothesis. Initially viewed as competing, these are now seen as complementary explanations of lesion-specific deficits that may be present in isolation or in concert within a given individual with RHD.

The first theoretical foundation for understanding discourse comprehension deficits is the Bilateral Activation, Inhibition, and Selection (BAIS) model (Jung-Beeman, 2005), an updated and expanded account based on the principles first introduced in the **coarse coding** hypothesis. By this account, the RH's role in lexical semantic encoding is one of coarse granularity resulting from diffuse activation in contrast to the left hemisphere's fine-grained representation (Beeman, 1998). In heathy adults, the complementary representation of coarse lexical semantic encoding facilitates novel, distant, and subordinate semantic relationships (Mashal et al., 2007). For example, when comprehending the word *bark*, the left hemisphere would support the mental representation of the "woof" itself, while the RH's broader encoding includes the concepts of *dog, sound*, and even *tree*. In some individuals with RHD, coarse diffuse representations are thought to be interrupted, leading to the hallmarks of RHD comprehension, namely, difficulties with inferencing and interpreting nonliteral language (Brownell et al., 1986; Tompkins et al., 2008). Functional imaging-based analyses have suggested that lesions specific to posterior parietal areas result in impairments best accounted for by poor coarse coding (Tompkins et al., 2008).

The second theoretical foundation for discourse comprehension deficits is the Structure Building Framework (Gernsbacher et al., 1990). In this view, a listener builds a hypothesis about the structure of information they are about to receive from a speaker, then new information is integrated into this hypothesis, elaborating upon and adapting it. If new information conflicts, the listener's working structure evolves to accommodate it. An important function necessary to this process is weight-based **suppression** of information that is less appropriate. Thus, one explanation for the comprehension deficits in RHD is that there is an inefficiency in suppressing this kind of information once it has been incorporated (Tompkins et al., 2000; Tompkins et al., 1997), leading to incorrect associations (Rehak et al., 1992) and flawed inferencing (Tompkins & Lehman, 1998). Lesions to the inferior frontal gyrus and associated basal ganglia result in impairments best accounted for by poor suppression (Yang et al., 2015).

From the perspective of clinical practice, a compelling dimension of this theoretical discussion is that it has given rise to concrete complementary lines of therapeutic

innovation. Contextual constraint treatment, in which patients receive context to constrain the intended interpretations of stimulus items, has been investigated in individuals with coarse coding deficits (Blake et al., 2015; Tompkins et al., 2012). Individuals with deficits due to suppression have been treated through the use of contextual cues to identify relevant versus irrelevant information and dismiss the inappropriate (Tompkins & Lehman, 1998). Difficulties suppressing prepotent responses to language that can convey multiple meanings may be best addressed by treating the ability to determine relevance of alternative meanings, rather than practicing generating the various meanings that could be present. As the associated deficits are not mutually exclusive, innovative treatment approaches have attempted to marry these complementary underlying processes to serve a broader range of individuals with RHD (Tompkins et al., 2011).

Identifying Right Hemisphere Discourse Skills

Main Concepts

Individuals with RHD include and exclude information inappropriately, resulting in an impression of wandering discourse. An important constellation of skills underlying effective communication is the ability to identify what information is central to a given topic or purpose and including that information in a logical sequence. For information that is not central, a speaker must decide what details are sufficiently relevant to include.

Consider Example 1 in Box 11–1. There is plenty of information conveyed, but the information is not central to the overall

> ### BOX 11–1. Example 1: Description of the Cookie Theft Picture by an Individual in the Chronic Phase of Recovery From RH Stroke
>
> There's a woman[1] in the picture who's cleaning up the dishes [GC4]. There are dishes and a curtain or a drape [GC2]. I don't know which[E]. There are cabinets on the bottom of the—of the counter [GC2]. This counter I'll call it[E] [GC1]. There's a light [GC2]. It's daytime [GC2]. There's a hanger hanging in the window [GC2]. It's daytime because it's light outside [GC1]. There are handles on the cabinets below the counter[D] [GC2]. There are also curtains on the window [GC2]. And I don't know if this a light or what [GC1]. But there are plates up on the counter also and two bowls and several plates [GC2], I can't count them[E] [GC1]. Certainly 4 or 5—3 or 4 and another couple bowls and a sink and a faucet over the sink and a water spray beside the faucet[D] [GC2]. And you can move it[2] from left to right—the arm of the faucet[2]—it seems[D] [GC1]. And there's a woman[1] who is now cleaning the plate [GC4]. She[1] actually looks like she's[1] smiling [GC3]. Maybe she[1] likes doing dishes[X] [GC3]. Now I see some more plates, maybe four more and more bowls[X] [GC1]. And on the floor, there's something [GC3]. I don't know, it looks like something spilled over from the—from the sink onto the floor [GC4].
>
> *Note:* [GC] = Global coherence rating. Utterance[D]: Divergent information, Utterance[E]: Egocentric information, Utterance[X]: Erroneous information. Superscript numbers track cohesion.

theme of the image. The statements with a subscript *D* demonstrate a clear divergence from what most would deem relevant to include. A listener could easily hear this description and never know that a portion of the image described depicts a mother who is daydreaming and not aware the sink is overflowing onto the floor.

Individuals with RHD tend to include less information than a healthy adult under similar circumstances, even if they speak a similar amount overall. This has been observed across a variety of elicitation tasks, including picture story sequences (Bloom et al., 1992; Joanette et al., 1986) and procedural descriptions (Cherney & Canter, 1993; Cummings, 2019). It may particularly impact inferred content versus explicit content (Mackisack et al., 1987).

Coherence

In addition to the inclusion and exclusion of the appropriate level of relevant detail, individuals with RHD also tend to more frequently fail to suppress tangential, irrelevant information (Blake, 2006; Ferré et al., 2011). This has led some to suggest that the difficulties associated with structure building in comprehension may be mirrored in production (Marini, 2012; Marini et al., 2005; Stemmer & Joanette, 1998). However, the ability to inhibit inappropriate information has been associated with right frontal lesions (Mar, 2004).

Coherence refers to the semantic relationships between distant utterances within a given discourse and captures the inclusion of information that is tangential or conceptually incongruous. Measuring coherence is an effective way of operationalizing the tangential and often egocentric quality in RHD discourse. Measures of coherence can be divided into local and global aspects. Local coherence is the extent to which each utterance builds meaning from the utterance before it. One way that global coherence can be operationalized is as a surrogate for topic maintenance. This can be assessed using a 4-point scale ranging from a completely unrelated, egocentric, and/or off-topic utterance (score of 1) to a completely on-topic utterance directly related to the topic at hand (score of 4; Wright et al., 2013). Scores of 2 and 3 are assigned when utterances are indirectly related to the stimulus or contain nonessential information. Self-referential remarks can be seen in Example 1 in Box 11–1 (statements with a subscript *E*) and suggest an apragmatic lack of awareness that the picture description task is occurring in the context of language assessment.

Cohesion

Another way in which discourse differences between the sentences has been understood is through cohesion. Cohesion is defined as the reference to content across sentences within discourse (see Chapter 1). This skill relies heavily both on tracking referents and accounting for the listener's knowledge over time. It is correlated with measures of executive function (Mozeiko et al., 2011), word finding (Coelho et al., 2005), and theory of mind (Balaban et al., 2016).

Differences in cohesion have been observed following RH damage (Davis et al., 1997; Stockbridge, Berube, et al., 2021), using speech elicited from single-picture and picture sequence description

tasks. The most common differences that have been observed are inappropriate use of pronouns and lexical coreference, in which the speaker is expected to use the word *the* (versus *a*) to signal that a noun already has been introduced (Barker et al., 2017; Davis et al., 1997). Individuals with RHD may use these inappropriately, as though something has been introduced previously when it has not, or ambiguously. For example, in "The cat and dog ran inside. *It* jumped on the sofa," *it* could refer either to the dog or the cat. Incidents of ambiguous or erroneous reference ties make it difficult to follow the speaker's train of thought and can contribute to exponentially increasing communication breakdown and frustration if they are not repaired and, instead, aggregate over the course of a conversation.

Another type of cohesion is lexical, in which subjects are renamed but refer to the same target. Adults with RHD tend to rename referential targets. For example, "The woman is cleaning. The lady has a dress. The mom isn't paying attention," all having the same referent rather than being consistent with the same subject label (Stockbridge, Berube, et al., 2021). This can result in an atypical quality to their discourse, even when their use of personal pronouns is intact.

Story Grammar

Story grammar captures the set of rules underlying the serialization and hierarchy of information provided during narrative discourse. It dictates the structure of necessary and sufficient information needed to describe a series of events in a logically causal or consequential way. It introduces agents, including the events leading up to some central conflict or theme, then describes that peak and the resolution that follows. In this way, story grammar adheres to a canonical anticipated syntax, not just across sentences, but also across events. Although difficulties sequencing have been observed in this population (Delis et al., 1983), more recent work suggests frontal damage is most associated with difficulties organizing information to produce stories with an anticipated structure and flow (Kaczmarek, 1984; Mar, 2004).

Conversation

Conversation is another circumstance in which information utilization is made increasingly complex by adding an overarching structure of expected behaviors. Individuals with RHD may experience difficulties in conversation that impact all levels of the experience. There is evidence that individuals with RHD have difficulty adequately maintaining an exchange of information (Blake, 2006; Hird & Kirsner, 2003). They may not adhere to turn-taking norms (Barnes et al., 2019) or maintain and initiate topics poorly (Brady et al., 2003; Kennedy, 2000). They also may produce discourse that diverges from the listener's expected organization. The discourse may be incomplete and omit vital information (Bartels-Tobin & Hinckley, 2005; Brady et al., 2003; Sherratt & Bryan, 2012, 2019).

Complementary to including appropriate information is the ability to identify when central information has not been provided by the listener in the conversation and then form and produce relevant, appropriate questions. Once the question is answered, one must integrate the newly provided information in a way that resolves the missingness. Questions also may be used to initiate and maintain conversation. Those with RHD also may demonstrate differences

making requests (Brownell & Stringfellow, 1999), though it is not clear why. It is possible that this is due to a specific deficit in recognizing that information is missing or in formulating questions needed to address missing information or other discourse goals, or it may relate to contrived task demands associated with assessing requests. Regardless, individuals with RHD may produce fewer questions overall (Minga et al., in press; Minga et al., 2020), and yes/no or polar questions have been associated with difficulty.

Selecting and Interpreting Right Hemisphere Tasks

Having reviewed the differences one can see in discourse following RHD, we will now pivot to examining the tasks best suited to reliably capturing these differences in a clinical or research setting. Importantly, some of the qualities of discourse highlighted in the profile of RHD exist on a spectrum in which variability has been noted due to normal aging. As reviewed in Chapters 2 to 4, nearly 1 in 5 older adults also includes anomalous, irrelevant, and self-referential content in discourse, which can reduce coherence. Thus, it is important for the SLP to determine whether the differences seen in patients with RHD are present over and above age-related discourse changes and whether those differences are *clinically* relevant deficits.

Due to the nuanced nature of many of these difficulties, task selection becomes perhaps the most important part of reliably observing change (Marini et al., 2005; Ska & Joanette, 1996). Individuals with RHD often perform well on skills most often captured on assessments of aphasia (Côté et al., 2004). Discourse tasks used in the assessment of individuals with RHD should be more complex, cognitive-linguistically integrated, and ecologically valid than those used in the appraisal of aphasia if SLPs wish to avoid ceiling performance when attempting to gauge capacity (Marini et al., 2005; Tompkins et al., 2000).

There are three commonly used elicitation techniques, each with its own strengths and weaknesses: single-picture or picture series description tasks, storytelling tasks, and spontaneous and conversation samples (Figure 11–1). Elicitation procedures used in research typically have included pictures or picture sequences rather than auditory-oral retellings, conversation, or spontaneous elicitations (see also Chapter 3). However, discourse assessments should rely on more than one task. This allows the SLP to parse those deficits that are discourse specific versus those that are reverberations of other domain general cognitive skills observed in the context of discourse. More recently, new tasks have been developed with an eye toward resolving some of the common weaknesses in these approaches, such as thinking-out-loud tasks.

Description of the Boston Diagnostic Aphasia Examination (BDAE) Cookie Theft picture (Goodglass et al., 2001) has been the primary basis upon which *clinical relevance* of discourse differences has been examined. Reduced use of appropriate information, reduced mention of inferential concepts, and inefficient inclusion of appropriate information have been noted as clinically relevant changes associated with RHD (Hillis Trupe & Hillis, 1985; Myers, 2005; Tompkins et al., 1993). Recently, a more complex Cookie Theft image has been developed. It is colorized and includes richer content that may enhance SLPs' ability to capture clinically relevant discourse differences in this population (Berube et al., 2019), although psychometric properties

of this stimulus are still being established as of this writing. For both versions, main ideas and concepts (content units), as well as inferred content, have been identified through norming samples of age-matched healthy adults; these may be used as a basis for interpreting performance. A key drawback of picture-description tasks is that they often elicit simple agent-action constructions (e.g., "The girl is playing," "The man is swimming") to the exclusion of more complex sentences, though this is less common when a picture is designed to have inferential content (e.g., the Cookie Theft picture). Picture description tasks require sustained visual attention and may be less appropriate for evaluating discourse in those with significant visual neglect.

Storytelling and retelling tasks, such as the *Cinderella* retelling, have increased ecological validity in contrast to single-picture description tasks. They may or may not rely on an initially presented picture, picture series, or movie, each of which presents increasing demands on memory and organization of information for the speaker. Story telling tasks can be useful and efficient cognitive-linguistic litmus tests, even in populations with relatively mild impairments (Kazhuro & Fischer-Baum, 2021; Stockbridge & Newman, 2019). Story grammars with content units have been developed and normed for the *Cinderella* task (Stark, 2010) and the *Pigeon: Impossible* wordless short film (Stockbridge & Newman, 2019), among other stimuli. Speakers receive credit for each proposition (generally defined by a core verb and the surrounding phrase).

In certain tasks, such as picture descriptions and story retelling, individuals with RHD occasionally adopt a strategy of listing simple sentences, either joined by a conjunction or not, grossly impacting cohesion (e.g., "She's reaching. He is standing and he

Figure 11–1. Characteristics of RH discourse analysis targets.

Greater basis for interpretation →

Greater ecological validity →

	Key targets & Examples	Strengths	Weaknesses
Picture & picture series description	• Information & Inference Mackisack et al., 1987 • Cohesion Stockbridge, Berube, et al., 2021 Marini, 2012 • Coherence Marini, 2012	• Strong basis for interpreting performance • Strong basis for determining clinical relevance • Brief & easy	• May be too easy for some patients • Vulnerable to visual neglect • Responders may list picture contents
Storytelling & retelling	• Information & Inference Frederiksen & Stemmer, 1993 • Cohesion Uryase, Duffy, & Liles, 1991 • Coherence Davis et al., 1997 • **Story grammar**	• Greater complexity than single pictures • Unfamiliar story retelling can detect differences due to mild impairments	• Places demands on memory and organization • May take longer than more structured measures
Spontaneous & conversational sampling	• Information & Inference Joanette et al., 1986 Brady et al., 2006 • Cohesion • Coherence • **Topic maintenance** • **Question asking** Minga et al., in press	• Many examples of topic-structured or topic-directed approaches • High ecological validity	• May take longer than more structured measures • Impacted by cultural and interpersonal dynamics • Vulnerable to pragmatic deficits

Bolded targets are considered unique to the task.

is reaching and he is getting a cookie and he is going to fall."). This can be informative, but SLPs may wish to supplement tasks that are performed in this way with additional discourse contexts that encourage more varied and complex language.

Spontaneous samples and conversational samples are a common, highly ecologically valid means of eliciting discourse (see Chapters 4, 7, and 10). Topic-structured or topic-directed procedures for eliciting conversational samples have been developed (Brady et al., 2006; Ripich & Terrell, 1988), in which a target topic is introduced at the onset using an open-ended question or request for information (e.g., "Tell me about your health"). The weakness of conversational tasks is that the language an SLP has to analyze is limited to what the patient produces. For example, if the patient responds to "Tell me about your health" by saying "It's fine," then there is little the SLP may use to assess the patient. In the other extreme, individuals may take the prompt as an invitation to begin a personal narrative, rather than a conversation with a greater degree of turn taking. This contrasts with the strength of picture-description and story retelling tasks, which can be expected to elicit similar specific content in most people, leading to a straightforward basis for interpretation. Contrived or legitimate first encounter conversations may also circumvent patients' tendency to simply produce monologues (Kennedy et al., 1994). Eliciting conversational discourse offers an avenue to examine turn taking and question asking—two important facets for constructing order and meaning in discourse. SLPs may want to examine conversation using the Discourse Contribution Measure (Minga et al., in press), which specifically addresses the need for a simple, reproducible measure of turn taking in conversation (see companion website).

Given the burden associated with extensive conversation transcription and analysis, it is useful to discuss the issue of how much discourse constitutes an analyzable discourse sample. Samples should have at least 50 utterances, but more than 100 is not necessarily beneficial (Miller et al., 2016; Paul & Norbury, 2012). This amounts to 10 to 15 minutes of conversational elicitation (for an extensive discussion of this issue, see Guo and Eisenberg (2015). However, shorter samples have been used, particularly if they sample the middle of a longer interaction; for example, the middle 8 minutes of a 10-minute conversation (Kennedy, 2000).

As mentioned before, there are innovations in discourse assessment that have sought to minimize the contributions of other nondiscourse skills that can mask or exacerbate a patient's discourse performance. Thinking-out-loud tasks may provide complementary information to that which is gained from picture descriptions and story retellings without diminishing the structure to the extent of conversation. Thinking out loud refers to verbalizing thoughts while completing a task, such as a puzzle. Memory and other cognitive demands can be diminished further by using a written modality (Olson et al., 2018). Substantial differences in inclusion of tangential and egocentric information have been observed between those with RHD and healthy older adults in thinking-out-loud tasks (Blake, 2006).

It can be helpful to see just how much task selection skews the lens with which deficits may or may not be appreciated. Consider how performance on the Cookie Theft task differs from performance in a first encounter conversation for a single patient (Example 2 in Box 11–2). As above, this patient produces a cohesive description, though it does seem to have some atypical inferences marked with a subscript X (e.g.,

---

BOX 11–2. Example 2: Contrast of Cookie Theft Description and First Encounter Conversation With an Individual in the Chronic Phase of Recovery From RH

Patient: Mommy, Mommy[1] is washing dishes and wiping up the floor$_X$ [GC2] because she[1] has turned the pipe off$_X$ [GC1]. "Oh boy!" Here is John[2] trying to get in the cookie jar [GC4]. He's[2] gonna break his[2] leg anyway because stool is gonna fall from underneath him[2] [GC4] and his[2] sister's[3] asking him[2] for one of the cookies not paying attention$_X$ [GC4]. He's[2] not looking even looking at her [GC3]. [3] His[2] sister is gonna fall off the stool [GC3]. <u>He's[2] still enjoying the cookie</u>$_X$ not even looking at his[2] sister asking him[2] for more [GC3] and he's[2] gonna break his[2] leg by falling off the stool [GC3]. Mommy,[1] Mommy[1] not even paying attention that her[1] shoes is getting wet [GC4]. All her[1] interested is just what? [GC2] Drying the dishes$_X$ [GC3]. The dish she[1] has in her[1] hand [GC2].

Assistant: So just tell me about anything that you would like to. So maybe what you've been up to this week or today or anything exciting.

Patient: Well, uh uh as a matter of fact I tell you what I did over the weekend is I I watched golf—Quicken Loans Golf Championship. [GC4]

Assistant: Perfect. Mhm.

Patient: Are you interested in golf? [GC4]

Assistant: Oh yeah, a little bit. I watch it every once in a while.

Patient: You watch it every once in ... Do you understand the game? [GC4]

Assistant: I wouldn't say I totally understand it, but I enjoy watching it though.

Patient: So ...

Assistant: So tell me a little bit about it.

Patient: So a question for ... I had a question for you. [GC4]

You say you watch it, so I was just about to ask you a question. When they say "It's a hole in one," what does that mean? [GC4]

Assistant: That means you hit the ball one time and then it goes in, right?

Patient: Huh, no, you're supposed to tell me. [GC4]

Note: [GC] = Global coherence rating. Utterance$_D$: Divergent information, Utterance$_E$: Egocentric information, Utterance$_X$: Erroneous information. Superscript numbers track cohesion.

---

the boy is facing the girl, but the patient says the boy does not see her; the mother is daydreaming while looking out the window as the sink spills over) and at least one pronoun error (underlined; the girl is the person eating a cookie in the image). However, the patient's conversation with the student

about the golf tournament he watched does not.

Based on these findings and what is known about the contribution of the RH to discourse, a gold-standard approach to discourse assessment in this population should adapt to the patient's comprehensive medical and cognitive profile and overall level of functioning. The approach may include picture description to target information and inferencing, story retelling to target coherence and story grammar, and brief conversational sampling to target all four key discourse targets in a more generalizable context (Table 11–1). Additional tasks may be included to parse out the contribution of domain general cognitive and executive capacities, such as neglect and other relevant comorbidities (Sheppard et al., 2022).

These tasks overlap with guidelines outlined in the protocol for the banking of discourse samples via the RHDBank (see Chapter 17). The RHDBank protocol includes scripts and tasks that pair with a growing bank of available data from other patients with similarly lateralized lesions (N = 34 patients as of 2021). Additionally, task parameters include suggested time limits, which can facilitate time management in the clinic and standardized administra-

tions from visit to visit. The RHDBank can be used to provide additional insights into a patient's performance over and above their recovery from their own initial baseline, as compared to controls (N = 43) or to individuals with left-lateralized lesions (N in the 1000s). Choosing to bank patient data supports the expanded utility of the RHD-Bank for future analyses and understanding of discourse after RHD, as further discussed in Chapter 17.

Many tasks used to assess discourse production following RHD, including those in the RHDBank, likely overlap with activities SLPs are inclined to do anyway. For example, most clinical interactions begin with a short, informal first encounter conversation. First encounter conversations are a useful source of information about discourse (Barnes et al., 2019; Kennedy, 2000; Minga et al., 2022; Minga et al., 2020) included in the RHDBank protocol. Adding minimal artificial structure to this encounter (e.g.,

Table 11–1. Gold-Standard Approach to Discourse Assessment in RHD

	RHDBank	*Time*
Picture description	Cookie Theft (Goodglass et al., 2001)	3 min
	Cat rescue (Nicholas & Brookshire, 1993)	3 min
Narrative retelling	Cinderella	5 min
Conversation	First Encounter (Kennedy, Strand, Burton, & Peterson, 1994)	5 min
	Open conversation	10 min
	Additional Assessments	*Time*
Procedural discourse	Peanut butter and jelly sandwich	1–2 min
Question generation	Unfamiliar object task	10 min
General cognition	Cognitive Linguistic Quick Test (Helm-Estabrooks, 2001)	15–30 min
Hemispatial neglect	Apples Test (Bickerton, Samson, Williamson, & Humphreys, 2011)	5 min
	Indented Paragraph Test (Caplan, 1987)	1–2 min

prompting the patient that you would like to get to know one another, asking if you can place a recording device on the table) can be the difference between using this exchange purely to build rapport and establish medical history and using it to those ends in addition to growing our understanding of the patient's communication needs. Automated transcription software options are increasingly available to facilitate the process of dictation and analysis.

As a final thought, it is important for SLPs and other related clinicians to appreciate that our understanding of the role of the RH is in its relative infancy. However, we urge clinicians and clinical researchers to adopt an inquisitive, curious approach regarding patients with RH lesions and their discourse. It is important to counsel patients and their families about nuanced changes they may notice about discourse and pragmatics more generally (Davidson & Wallace, 2021), even if structured language evaluation has not elucidated the overt differences that we are most inclined to anticipate under the broad category of "discourse deficits." Clinicians should guide patients and their families toward an understanding that changes in discourse and pragmatics following a RH lesion are no less important than visuospatial neglect. Numerous resources are available to support clinicians, patients, families, and caregivers throughout this process, including the American Speech-Language-Hearing Association (ASHA) practice portal (www.asha.org/practice-portal/clinical-topics/right-hemisphere-damage/) and RightHemisphere.org.

References

Balaban, N., Friedmann, N., & Ariel, M. (2016). The effect of theory of mind impairment on language: Referring after right-hemisphere damage. *Aphasiology, 30*(12), 1424–1460. https://doi.org/10.1080/02687038.2015.1137274

Barker, M. S., Young, B., & Robinson, G. A. (2017). Cohesive and coherent connected speech deficits in mild stroke. *Brain and Language, 168*, 23–36. https://doi.org/10.1016/j.bandl.2017.01.004

Barnes, S., Beeke, S., & Bloch, S. (2020). How is right hemisphere communication disorder disabling? Evidence from response mobilizing actions in conversation. *Disability and Rehabilitation*, 1–14. https://doi.org/10.1080/09638288.2020.1766123

Barnes, S., Toocaram, S., Nickels, L., Beeke, S., Best, W., & Bloch, S. (2019). Everyday conversation after right hemisphere damage: A methodological demonstration and some preliminary findings. *Journal of Neurolinguistics, 52*(100850). https://doi.org/10.1016/j.jneuroling.2019.100850

Bartels-Tobin, L. R., & Hinckley, J. J. (2005). Cognition and discourse production in right hemisphere disorder. *Journal of Neurolinguistics, 18*(6), 461–477. https://doi.org/10.1016/j.jneuroling.2005.04.001

Beeman, M. (1998). Coarse semantic coding and discourse comprehension. In M. Beeman & C. Chiarello (Eds.), *Right hemisphere language comprehension: Perspectives from cognitive neuroscience* (pp. 255–284). Lawrence Erlbaum.

Benton, E., & Bryan, K. (1996). Right cerebral hemisphere damage: incidence of language problems. *International journal of rehabilitation research. Internationale Zeitschrift fur Rehabilitationsforschung. Revue internationale de recherches de readaptation, 19*(1), 47–54. http://europepmc.org/abstract/MED/8730543

Berube, S., Nonnemacher, J., Demsky, C., Glenn, S., Saxena, S., Wright, A., . . . Hillis, A. E. (2019). Stealing cookies in the twenty-first century: Measures of spoken narrative in healthy versus speakers with aphasia. *American Journal of Speech-Language Pathology, 28*(1S), 321–329. https://doi.org/10.1044/2018_AJSLP-17-0131

Bickerton, W. L., Samson, D., Williamson, J., & Humphreys, G. W. (2011). Separating forms of neglect using the Apples Test: Validation and functional prediction in chronic and acute stroke. *Neuropsychology, 25*(5), 567. https://doi.org/10.1037/a0023501

Blake, M. L. (2006). Clinical relevance of discourse characteristics after right hemisphere brain damage. *American Journal of Speech-Language Pathology, 13*(3), 255–267. https://doi.org/10.1044/1058-0360(2006/024)

Blake, M. L. (2009). Inferencing processes after right hemisphere brain damage: Effects of contextual bias. *Journal of Speech, Language, and Hearing Research, 52*(2), 373–384. https://doi.org/10.1044/1092-4388(2009/07-0172)

Blake, M. L., Tompkins, C. A., Scharp, V. L., Meigh, K. M., & Wambaugh, J. (2015). Contextual constraint treatment for coarse coding deficit in adults with right hemisphere brain damage: Generalisation to narrative discourse comprehension. *Neuropsychological Rehabilitation, 25*(1), 15–52. https://doi.org/10.1080/09602011.2014.932290

Bloom, R. L., Borod, J. C., Obler, L. K., & Gerstman, L. J. (1992). Impact of emotional content on discourse production in patients with unilateral brain damage. *Brain and Language, 42*(2), 153–164. https://doi.org/10.1016/0093-934X(92)90122-U

Brady, M., Armstrong, L., & Mackenzie, C. (2006). An examination over time of language and discourse production abilities following right hemisphere brain damage. *Journal of Neurolinguistics, 19*(4), 291–310. https://doi.org/10.1016/j.jneuroling.2005.12.001

Brady, M., Mackenzie, C., & Armstrong, L. (2003). Topic use following right hemisphere brain damage during three semi-structured conversational discourse samples. *Aphasiology, 17*(9), 881–904. https://doi.org/10.1080/02687030344000292

Brownell, H. H. (1988). Appreciation of metaphoric and connotative word meaning by brain-damaged patients. In C. Chiarello (Ed.), *Right hemisphere contributions to lexical semantics* (pp. 19–31). Springer Berlin Heidelberg. https://doi.org/10.1007/978-3-642-73674-2_2

Brownell, H. H., Carroll, J. J., Rehak, A., & Wingfield, A. (1992). The use of pronoun anaphora and speaker mood in the interpretation of conversational utterances by right hemisphere brain-damaged patients. *Brain and Language, 43*(1), 121–147. https://doi.org/10.1016/0093-934X(92)90025-A

Brownell, H. H., & Martino, G. (1998). Deficits in inference and social cognition: The effects of right hemisphere brain damage. In M. Beeman & C. Chiarello (Eds.), *Right hemisphere language comprehension: Perspectives from cognitive neuroscience* (pp. 309–328). Lawrence Earlbaum.

Brownell, H. H., Potter, H. H., Bihrle, A. M., & Gardner, H. (1986). Inference deficits in right brain-damaged patients. *Brain and Language, 27*(2), 310–321. https://doi.org/10.1016/0093-934X(86)90022-2

Brownell, H. H., & Stringfellow, A. (1999). Making requests: Illustrations of how right-hemisphere brain damage can affect discourse production. *Brain and Language, 68*(3), 442–465. https://doi.org/10.1006/brln.1999.2122

Caplan, B. (1987). Assessment of unilateral neglect: A new reading test. *Journal of Clinical and Experimental Neuropsychology, 9*(4), 359–364. https://doi.org/10.1080/01688638708405056

Cherney, L. R., & Canter, G. J. (1993). Informational content in the discourse of patients with probable Alzheimer's disease and patients with right brain damage. In M. Lemme (Ed.), *Clinical aphasiology* (Vol. 21, pp. 123–134). Pro-Ed.

Coelho, C. A., Grela, B., Corso, M., Gamble, A., & Feinn, R. (2005). Microlinguistic deficits in the narrative discourse of adults with traumatic brain injury. *Brain Injury, 19*(13), 1139–1145. https://doi.org/10.1080/02699050500110678

Côté, H., Moix, V., & Giroux, F. (2004). Évaluation des troubles de la communication des cérébrolésés droits. *Rééducation orthophonique, 42*(219), 107–122.

Cummings, L. (2019). On making a sandwich: Procedural discourse in adults with right-hemisphere damage. In A. Capone, M. Carapezza, & F. Lo Piparo (Eds.), *Further advances in pragmatics and philosophy: Part 2, theories and applications* (Vol. 20, pp. 331–355). Springer. https://doi.org/10.1007/978-3-030-00973-1

Davidson, C. S., & Wallace, S. E. (2021). Information needs for carers following a family member's right hemisphere stroke. *Aphasiology*, 1–26. https://doi.org/10.1080/02687038.2021.1873906

Davis, G. A., O'Neil-Pirozzi, T. M., & Coon, M. (1997). Referential cohesion and logical coherence of narration after right hemisphere stroke. *Brain and Language*, 56(2), 183–210. https://doi.org/10.1006/brln.1997.1741

Delis, D. C., Wapner, W., Gardner, H., & Moses, J. A. (1983). The contribution of the right hemisphere to the organization of paragraphs. *Cortex*, 19(1), 43–50. https://doi.org/10.1016/S0010-9452(83)80049-5

Ferré, P., Clermont, M. F., Lajoie, C., Côté, H., Ferreres, A., Abusamra, V., . . . Joanette, Y. (2009). Identification de profils communicationnels parmi les individus cérébrolésés droits: Profils transculturels. *Revista neuropsicologia latinoamericana*, 1(1), 32–40.

Ferré, P., Ska, B., Lajoie, C., Bleau, A., & Joanette, Y. (2011). Clinical focus on prosodic, discursive and pragmatic treatment for right hemisphere damaged adults: What's right? *Rehabilitation Research and Practice, 2011*. https://doi.org/10.1155/2011/131820

Frederiksen, C. H., & Stemmer, B. (1993). Conceptual processing of discourse by a right hemisphere brain-damaged patient. In H. Brownell & Y. Joanette (Eds.), *Narrative discourse in neurologically impaired and normal aging adults* (pp. 239–278). Singular Publishing.

Gernsbacher, M. A., Varner, K. R., & Faust, M. E. (1990). Investigating differences in general comprehension skill. *Journal of Experimental Psychology: Learning, Memory, and Cognition*, 16(3), 430–445. https://doi.org/10.1037/0278-7393.16.3.430

Goodglass, H., Kaplan, E., & Weintraub, S. (2001). *BDAE: The Boston Diagnostic Aphasia Examination*. Lippincott Williams & Wilkins.

Guo, L.-Y., & Eisenberg, S. (2015). Sample length affects the reliability of language sample measures in 3-year-olds: Evidence from parent-elicited conversational samples.

Language, Speech, and Hearing Services in Schools, 46(2), 141–153. https://doi.org/10.1044/2015_LSHSS-14-0052

Helm-Estabrooks, N. (2001). *Cognitive Linguistic Quick Test: CLQT*. Psychological Corporation.

Hewetson, R., Cornwell, P., & Shum, D. H. (2021). Relationship and social network change in people with impaired social cognition post right hemisphere stroke. *American Journal of Speech-Language Pathology*, 30(2S), 962–973. https://doi.org/10.1044/2020_AJSLP-20-00047

Hillis Trupe, E., & Hillis, A. (1985). *Paucity vs. verbosity: Another analysis of right hemisphere communication deficits*. Clinical aphasiology: Proceedings of the Conference,

Hird, K., & Kirsner, K. (2003). The effect of right cerebral hemisphere damage on collaborative planning in conversation: An analysis of intentional structure. *Clinical Linguistics and Phonetics*, 17(4-5), 309–315. https://doi.org/10.1080/0269920031000080037

Joanette, Y., Goulet, P., Ska, B., & Nespoulous, J.-L. (1986). Informative content of narrative discourse in right-brain-damaged right-handers. *Brain and Language*, 29(1), 81–105. https://doi.org/10.1016/0093-934X(86)90035-0

Jung-Beeman, M. (2005). Bilateral brain processes for comprehending natural language. *Trends in Cognitive Sciences*, 9(11), 512–518. https://doi.org/10.1016/j.tics.2005.09.009

Kaczmarek, B. L. (1984). Neurolinguistic analysis of verbal utterances in patients with focal lesions of frontal lobes. *Brain and Language*, 21(1), 52–58. https://doi.org/10.1016/0093-934X(84)90035-X

Kazhuro, K., & Fischer-Baum, S. (2021). *Unfamiliar storytelling as a measure of language and cognition after a stroke*. Academy of Aphasia [Online]. https://easychair.org/publications/preprint/WZ4R

Kennedy, M. R. (2000). Topic scenes in conversations with adults with right-hemisphere brain damage. *American Journal of Speech-Language Pathology*, 9(1), 72–86. https://doi.org/10.1044/1058-0360.0901.72

Kennedy, M. R., Strand, E. A., Burton, W., & Peterson, C. (1994). Analysis of first-encounter conversations of right-hemisphere-damaged adults. *Clinical aphasiology.* http://aphasiology.pitt.edu/id/eprint/159

Mackisack, E. L., Myers, P. S., & Duffy, J. R. (1987). Verbosity and labeling behavior: The performance of right hemisphere and non-brain-damaged adults on an inferential picture description task. *Clinical aphasiology.* http://aphasiology.pitt.edu/id/eprint/928

Mar, R. A. (2004). The neuropsychology of narrative: Story comprehension, story production and their interrelation. *Neuropsychologia, 42*(10), 1414–1434. https://doi.org/10.1016/j.neuropsychologia.2003.12.016

Marini, A. (2012). Characteristics of narrative discourse processing after damage to the right hemisphere. *Seminars in Speech and Language, 33*(01), 68–78. https://doi.org/10.1055/s-0031-1301164

Marini, A., Carlomagno, S., Caltagirone, C., & Nocentini, U. (2005). The role played by the right hemisphere in the organization of complex textual structures. *Brain and Language, 93*(1), 46–54. https://doi.org/10.1016/j.bandl.2004.08.002

Mashal, N., Faust, M., Hendler, T., & Jung-Beeman, M. (2007). An fMRI investigation of the neural correlates underlying the processing of novel metaphoric expressions. *Brain and Language, 100*(2), 115–126. https://doi.org/10.1016/j.bandl.2005.10.005

Miller, J. F., Andriacchi, K., Nockerts, A., Westerveld, M., & Gillon, G. (2016). *Assessing language production using SALT software: A clinician's guide to language sample analysis.* SALT Software, LLC

Minga, J., Fromm, D., Jacks, A., Stockbridge, M. D., Nelthropp, J., & MacWhinney, B. (2022). The effect of right hemisphere brain damage on question asking during conversation. *Journal of Speech, Language, and Hearing Research, 65*(2), 727–737. doi: 10.1044/2021_JSLHR-21-00309

Minga, J., Fromm, D., Williams-DeVane, C., & MacWhinney, B. (2020). Question use in adults with right-hemisphere brain damage. *Journal of Speech, Language, and Hearing Research, 63*(3), 738–748. https://doi.org/10.1044/2019_JSLHR-19-00063

Mozeiko, J., Le, K., Coelho, C. A., Krueger, F., & Grafman, J. (2011). The relationship of story grammar and executive function following TBI. *Aphasiology, 25*(6-7), 826–835. https://doi.org/10.1080/02687038.2010.543983

Myers, P. S. (2005). CAC Classics Profiles of communication deficits in patients with right cerebral hemisphere damage: Implications for diagnosis and treatment. *Aphasiology, 19*(12), 1147–1160. doi: 10.1080/02687030500331585

Myers, P. S. (2001). Toward a definition of RHD syndrome. *Aphasiology, 15*(10-11), 913–918. https://doi.org/10.1080/02687040143000285

Nicholas, L. E., & Brookshire, R. H. (1993). A system for quantifying the informativeness and efficiency of the connected speech of adults with aphasia. *Journal of Speech, Language, and Hearing Research, 36*(2), 338–350. https://doi.org/10.1044/jshr.3602.338

Olson, G. M., Duffy, S. A., & Mack, R. L. (2018). Thinking-out-loud as a method for studying real-time comprehension processes. In D. E. Kieras & M. A. Just (Eds.), *New methods in reading comprehension research* (pp. 253–286). Routledge.

Paul, R., & Norbury, C. (2012). *Language disorders from infancy through adolescence—E-Book: Listening, speaking, reading, writing, and communicating.* Elsevier Health Sciences.

Ramsey, A., & Blake, M. L. (2020). Speech-language pathology practices for adults with right hemisphere stroke: What are we missing? *American Journal of Speech-Language Pathology, 29*(2), 741–759. https://doi.org/10.1044/2020_AJSLP-19-00082

Rehak, A., Kaplan, J. A., Weylman, S. T., Kelly, B., Brownell, H. H., & Gardner, H. (1992). Story processing in right-hemisphere brain-damaged patients. *Brain and Language, 42*(3), 320–336. https://doi.org/10.1016/0093-934X(92)90104-M

Ripich, D. N., & Terrell, B. Y. (1988). Patterns of discourse cohesion and coherence in Alzheimer's disease. *Journal of Speech and Hearing Disorders, 53*(1), 8–15. https://doi.org/10.1044/jshd.5301.08

Sheppard, S. M., Stockbridge, M. D., Keator, L. M., Murray, L. L., Blake, L. M., & Right Hemisphere Damage working group, Evidence-Based Clinical Research Committee, Academy of Neurological Communication Disorders and Sciences. (2022). The company prosodic deficits keep following right hemisphere stroke: A systematic review. *Journal of the International Neuropsychological Society, 6*, 1–16. doi: 10.1017/S1355617721001302

Sherratt, S., & Bryan, K. (2012). Discourse production after right brain damage: Gaining a comprehensive picture using a multi-level processing model. *Journal of Neurolinguistics, 25*(4), 213–239. https://doi.org/10.1016/j.jneuroling.2012.01.001

Sherratt, S., & Bryan, K. (2019). Textual cohesion in oral narrative and procedural discourse: the effects of ageing and cognitive skills. *International Journal of Language and Communication Disorders, 54*(1), 95–109. https://doi.org/10.1111/1460-6984.12434

Ska, B., & Joanette, Y. (1996). Discourse in older adults: Influence of text, task, and participant characteristics. *Canadian Journal of Speech Language Pathology and Audiology, 20*, 101–108. https://cjslpa.ca/files/1996_JSLPA_Vol_20/No_02_85-168/Ska_Joanette_JSLPA_1996.pdf

Stark, J. A. (2010). Content analysis of the fairy tale Cinderella–A longitudinal single-case study of narrative production: "From rags to riches." *Aphasiology, 24*(6-8), 709–724. https://doi.org/10.1080/02687030903524729

Stemmer, B., & Joanette, Y. (1998). The interpretation of narrative discourse of brain damaged individuals within the framework of a multilevel discourse model. In M. Beeman & C. Chiarello (Eds.), *Right hemisphere language comprehension: Perspectives from cognitive neuroscience* (pp. 329–348). Erlbaum.

Stockbridge, M. D., Berube, S., Goldberg, E., Suarez, A., Mace, R., Ubellacker, D., & Hillis, A. E. (2021). Differences in linguistic cohesion within the first year following right- and left-hemisphere lesions. *Aphasiology, 35*(3), 357–371. https://doi.org/10.1080/02687038.2019.1693026

Stockbridge, M. D., & Newman, R. (2019). Enduring cognitive and linguistic deficits in individuals with a history of concussion. *American Journal of Speech-Language Pathology, 28*(4), 1554–1570. https://doi.org/10.1044/2019_AJSLP-18-0196

Stockbridge, M. D., Sheppard, S. M., Keator, L. M., Murray, L. L., Blake, M. L., & Right Hemisphere Disorders Evidence-Based Clinical Research Committee. (2021). Aprosodia subsequent to right hemisphere brain damage: A systematic review and meta-analysis. *Journal of the International Neuropsychological Society*, 1–27. https://doi.org/10.1017/S1355617721000825

Tompkins, C. A. (1995). *Right hemisphere communication disorders: Theory and management*. Singular Publishing.

Tompkins, C. A., Baumgaertner, A., Lehman, M. T., & Fassbinder, W. (2000). Mechanisms of discourse comprehension impairment after right hemisphere brain damage: Suppression in lexical ambiguity resolution. *Journal of Speech, Language, and Hearing Research, 43*(1), 62–78. https://doi.org/10.1044/jslhr.4301.62

Tompkins, C. A., Baumgaertner, A., Lehman, M. T., & Fossett, T. R. D. (1997). Suppression and discourse comprehension in right brain-damaged adults: A preliminary report. *Aphasiology, 11*(4-5), 505–519. https://doi.org/10.1080/02687039708248487

Tompkins, C. A., Blake, M. T., Wambaugh, J., & Meigh, K. (2011). A novel, implicit treatment for language comprehension processes in right hemisphere brain damage: Phase I data. *Aphasiology, 25*(6-7), 789–799. https://doi.org/10.1080/02687038.2010.539784

Tompkins, C. A., Boada, R., McGarry, K., Jones, J., Rahn, A. E., & Ranier, S. (1993). Connected speech characteristics of right-hemisphere-damaged adults: A re-examination. *Clinical Aphasiology: Proceedings of the Conference.* http://aphasiology.pitt.edu/id/eprint/1442

Tompkins, C. A., & Lehman, M. T. (1998). Interpreting intended meanings after right hemisphere brain damage: An analysis of evidence, potential accounts, and clinical implications. *Topics in Stroke Rehabilitation, 5*(1), 29–47. https://doi.org/10.1310/2NTF-GTQU-MXN0-L3U7

Tompkins, C. A., Scharp, V. L., Meigh, K. M., & Fassbinder, W. (2008). Coarse coding and discourse comprehension in adults with right hemisphere brain damage. *Aphasiology, 22*(2), 204–223. https://doi.org/10.1080/0268 7030601125019

Tompkins, C. A., Scharp, V. L., Meigh, K. M., Lehman Blake, M., & Wambaugh, J. (2012). Generalisation of a novel implicit treatment for coarse coding deficit in right hemisphere brain damage: A single-participant experiment. *Aphasiology, 26*(5), 689–708. https://doi.org/10.1080/02687038.2012.676869

Uryase, S. D., Duffy, R. J., & Liles, B. Z. (1991). Analysis and description of narrative discourse in right-hemisphere-damaged adults: A comparison with neurologically normal and left-hemisphere-damaged aphasic adults. In T. E. Prescott (Ed.), *Clinical aphasiology* (Vol. 19, pp. 125–138). Pro-Ed.

Wright, H. H., Capilouto, G. J., & Koutsoftas, A. (2013). Evaluating measures of global coherence ability in stories in adults. *International Journal of Language and Communication Disorders, 48*(3), 249–256. https://doi .org/10.1111/1460-6984.12000

Yang, Y., Tompkins, C. A., Meigh, K. M., & Prat, C. S. (2015). Voxel-based lesion symptom mapping of coarse coding and suppression deficits in patients with right hemisphere damage. *American Journal of Speech-Language Pathology, 24*(4), S939–S952. https://doi.org/ 10.1044/2015_AJSLP-14-0149

12 Using Technology and Telepractice to Evaluate Discourse After Traumatic Brain Injury

Rachael Rietdijk and Peter Meulenbroek

Introduction

Technology plays an increasing role in everyday communication. People regularly use technology in their daily lives for a range of spoken discourse tasks, including monologic discourse (e.g., leaving a voicemail for a coworker) and conversational discourse (e.g., joining a video call with your extended family). Written discourse is also commonly supported through technology as part of text messaging, email, and communication on social media. In addition to the increasing use of technology for communication in daily life, technology is also employed in the clinical assessment of discourse impairments after a traumatic brain injury (TBI).

During the COVID-19 pandemic, clinicians embraced technology in serving people with TBI as traditional in-person clinical services presented hazards. The rapid adoption of telepractice, including the use of telephone and video conferencing, emerged as a result (Malec et al., 2021). Even prior to the pandemic, clinicians and researchers were interested in the use of telepractice for discourse assessment of TBI, with the first research in this field being conducted more than 15 years ago (Brennan et al., 2004).

Technology can also provide the means to collect data about discourse in different contexts, including phone conversations with different communication partners (Togher et al., 1997), video conferencing to capture conversations in the home environment (Rietdijk et al., 2018), or virtual reality to evaluate discourse in a range of real-life situations, all without leaving the clinical setting (Vaezipour et al., 2021). In addition, technology can be used to support the clinical assessment process through automation of analysis processes or through the application of new methods to generate insights about the nature of discourse after TBI. This chapter provides an overview of the use of telepractice in discourse assessment, implementation of technology to support the analysis of discourse, and future directions in evaluating discourse via the application of new and emerging technologies.

Using Telepractice for Evaluation of Discourse

Telepractice has been defined as "the application of telecommunications technology to the delivery of speech-language pathology and audiology professional services at a distance by linking clinician to client or clinician to clinician for assessment, intervention, and/or consultation" (American Speech-Language-Hearing Association, n.d.). Interest in the use of telepractice to evaluate discourse was originally motivated by the aim of increasing access to services for people with TBI in rural and remote areas (Brennan et al., 2004). In more recent years, the broader benefits of telepractice services have been identified from the perspectives of people with TBI and their communication partners, including the convenience of scheduling appointments around other commitments and preservation of personal boundaries (Rietdijk et al., 2022). While telepractice may not be suitable for all clients or in all situations, there is evidence to support that service delivery enabled by technology can be acceptable to people with TBI (Vaezipour et al., 2019).

Considerations for Telepractice Assessment of Discourse

There are many considerations relating to the implementation of telepractice for assessment of discourse of people with TBI. These issues have been identified in telepractice policy and practice documentation from speech-language pathology and rehabilitation organizations (e.g., American Speech-Language-Hearing Association, n.d.; Brain Rehab Program and Mobility Innovations Centre, 2020; Speech Pathology Australia, 2014). Considerations relevant to the use of telepractice in discourse assessment encompass the organizational context, the technology, and the individual. While there may be some issues specific to local contexts, the checklist in Box 12–1 may serve as a guide for clinicians in conducting discourse assessment via telepractice.

The implementation of telepractice within a clinical service will be influenced by a range of policies, such as security and privacy protocols, licensure regulations, and reimbursement schemes. It is recommended that clinicians undertaking assessment become familiar with their local regulatory requirements related to telepractice and ensure the planned assessment is compliant with these requirements. Regarding the assessment of discourse via telepractice, clinicians should be particularly cognizant of the privacy and security of systems used to store or transfer audio or video recordings of discourse samples.

Planning to use telepractice to deliver a discourse assessment should be addressed through a task analysis that maps the clinical task to the technology. For example, a clinician conducting an assessment including collection of a video sample of conversation with a communication partner who does not live with the person with TBI may identify the clinical tasks required as (a) engage with both the client and communication partner across two different remote locations, (b) document consent for video recording of a conversation, (c) provide client and communication partner with instructions on how to complete the conversation task, (d) turn off camera and mute microphone during conversation task to minimize distractions, and (e) record and securely store the conversation sample.

After identifying these clinical tasks, a clinician may then identify the technology features required as follows: (a) secure group video conferencing that meets local regulatory requirements, (b) recording functionality to capture verbal consent of both participants and the conversation sample itself, (c) functionality for screen sharing prepared slides with task instructions, (d) functionality for the clinician to turn off his or her own camera and microphone during the conver-

---

BOX 12–1

Before the Telepractice Assessment

☐ Familiarize yourself with the regulatory requirements relevant to conducting an assessment via telepractice in your local context.

☐ Itemize the tasks required for conducting the assessment and prepare resources (e.g., slides, videos, scripts) to support the assessment.

☐ Conduct a task analysis to map the assessment tasks to the required features of the technology (see online companion resource for further detail).

☐ Evaluate suitability of the client for a telepractice assessment. Considerations may include cognitive status, technical ability, or presence of a support person.

☐ Conduct a risk assessment and identify a plan for how to address any technical or clinical concerns: What will you do if the technology fails? What will you do if you are concerned during a telepractice assessment about the health or well-being of the client?

☐ Obtain consent for telepractice assessment from the client (and communication partner, if participating), including consent for audio or video recording if this will occur.

☐ Ensure the quality of the connection is adequate to proceed with the assessment.

☐ Optimize the physical environment and your computer setup for the session.

During the Telepractice Assessment

☐ Consider potential impact of the mode of telepractice on the discourse sample (e.g., distractions in the home environment, stress if unfamiliar with using the technology).

☐ If a familiar communication partner is present, ask for feedback about whether performance is representative of usual ability.

After the Telepractice Assessment

☐ Ensure relevant policies are followed regarding storage and retention of any video or audio files captured during the discourse assessment.

☐ Engage in ongoing evaluation of the telepractice service, with consideration of service quality, client satisfaction, and updates to practice to reflect changes in regulation.

---

sation recording, and (e) access to a secure cloud-based platform for long-term storage of the recorded sample. The clinician can then review specific platforms to determine appropriateness for clinical use based on whether these features are supported. More broadly, a high-speed and stable connection is important for both administering assessments successfully and obtaining a good-quality audio or video sample of the client's discourse. Additional considerations for administering a discourse assessment via telepractice are included in the companion website.

Finally, clinicians must consider the suitability of telepractice for the individual client. The planning process needs to account for the client's cognitive and communication status, availability of technology to connect to the session, comfort and proficiency with using technology, need for and availability of support persons, and need for an interpreter. Additionally, the technology type and operating system on the client's end should be compatible with the clinician's, and the necessary protections on audio and video recordings need to allow for recordings and transfer. Clinicians may need to provide clients with support or training to access technology successfully for the purposes of telepractice. Clients must provide consent for the telepractice assessment before proceeding, including being informed of the benefits, risks, and availability of alternative service delivery options.

Validated Telepractice Measures

There is evidence for the feasibility of using telepractice with the TBI population (Ownsworth et al., 2018) and, more specifically, evidence for the validity of using telepractice for the administration of established assessment methods of discourse of people with TBI. The earliest study in this field (Brennan et al., 2004) analyzed discourse samples of speakers with a stroke or TBI, based on information units as per the Story Retell Procedure (Doyle et al., 1998) with comparison between in-person and video conferencing assessment modes. No significant differences were detected between the discourse samples collected during the two separate assessments. Similarly, for discourse samples from speakers with TBI collected with tasks from the Aphasia Bank protocol (MacWhinney et al., 2011),

a comparison of productivity measures (i.e., number of words, number of C-units) and quality measures (i.e., type-token ratio, number of mazes) found no significant differences for in-person and video conferencing assessments (Turkstra et al., 2012).

The Adapted Kagan Scales (Togher et al., 2010) and Global Impression Scales (Bond & Godfrey, 1997), described in Chapter 10 and the companion website, have been tested for video conferencing application to conversations between a person with TBI and a usual communication partner (Rietdijk et al., 2018). There were no significant differences in ratings between samples recorded in-person and samples recorded via video conferencing. The La Trobe Communication Questionnaire (LCQ) (Douglas et al., 2007) provides an alternative method to evaluate conversational discourse through administration of a questionnaire via interview with the person with TBI and/or a close other. The LCQ has also been validated for use via telepractice, with no significant difference in scores between telepractice and in-person administration (Rietdijk et al., 2017). Enhancement of LCQ administration has also been studied where 20-minute recordings of conversation between persons with TBI and a usual communication partner are reviewed as a reference to completing the LCQ to aid with memory impairments (Hoepner & Turkstra, 2013). The findings across these research studies demonstrate that video conferencing assessment of discourse after TBI can produce similar data to in-person assessment.

Using Technology to Collect and Analyze Discourse Data

Technology may also be applied to methods of collection and analysis of discourse data. The use of technology as part of a discourse assessment may serve multiple purposes. These purposes include providing information about an individual's ability to complete everyday communication tasks requiring use of technology, broadening the communication contexts that are sampled beyond what is possible in the in-person context, and increasing efficiency of discourse analysis. A number of studies have reported applications of technology to the evaluation of discourse after TBI that have potential for future clinical implementation.

The Voicemail Elicitation Task (VET)

The voicemail elicitation task (VET) is an example of using technology to evaluate discourse specific to a functional communication (Meulenbroek & Cherney, 2019). The VET involves a computer program that provides instructions for various scenarios, such as leaving a voicemail for a coworker, and records the spoken discourse sample produced for each scenario. The voicemail scenarios relate to different levels of status of the communication partner (superior, subordinate, or colleague) and different levels of familiarity (friends versus new coworkers). In subsequent research (Meulenbroek & Cherney, 2021), the VET has been integrated with software that enables automated transcription of the discourse sample and detection of politeness markers frequently used in workplace communication. The studies used a phone-handset speaker and microphone that plays the audio recording of an outgoing message. The screen provides the voicemail scenarios randomly one at a time. An example of a VET scenario is shown in Box 12–2.

Analysis of the use of politeness markers is central to the VET. Politeness markers include words that are of mainly modal verbs and adjuncts (Halliday & Matthies-

> **BOX 12–2. Example of Voicemail Scenario**
>
> Your car just broke down and will be in the shop for the rest of the week. Now you need a ride to work. You recently got to know a coworker named Stanley because you are working on a project together. Stanley mentioned he drives by your house on his way to work. Call your coworker Stanley on his office phone. Tell him about your car and ask him for some help getting to and from work for the next week.

sen, 2004). Examples of politeness markers include: *just, possibly, would, could, probably,* and so on. Politeness markers can also appear as phrases such as those in Box 12–3. The purpose of politeness markers is to denote ambiguity and provide *options* for the conversation partner, making it easier to avoid committing to things they might not want to do. Persons with TBI produce fewer politeness markers in conversation (Togher & Hand, 1998), possibly because of the cognitive challenges associated with this class of words. Without this category of words, speech can be curt or direct, and can be interpreted as rude or disrespectful. Beyond the impressions that omitting politeness markers provide, the speaker needs to consider the power of the speaker relative to the listener, social distance and familiarity between the speaker and the listener, and the amount of imposition being placed on the listener by the speaker (Brown & Levinson, 1987). Examples of politeness markers are included in Box 12–3.

Studies have shown that the VET is sensitive to discriminating people with TBI who are stably employed versus unstably employed (Meulenbroek & Cherney, 2019) and sensitive to change as a result

---

BOX 12–3. *Examples of Politeness Markers and Politeness Strategies*

Politeness Markers	Examples
Finite modal verbs	*will, would, could, should, may, might, wish*
Modal adjuncts	*probably, possibly, maybe, just, a bit, really*
Comment adjuncts	*please, frankly, unfortunately, hopefully*

Politeness Strategies	Examples
Examples provided for the act of requesting	*May I ask you a favor . . . could you pass the salt?*
	I hate to bother you . . . but could you pass the salt?
	If it's no bother . . . could you pass the salt?

---

of intervention (Meulenbroek & Cherney, 2021). Clinically, this platform could provide clinicians with the means to both evaluate this specific type of discourse and to efficiently track progress over time. Example analyses of three transcribed recordings are provided in Appendix 12–1. The recordings include a person with severe TBI who is unemployed, a second person with severe TBI who is employed stably after injury, and a third from a control. All samples were collected from persons who were employed in similar-level jobs before their injuries.

The unemployed individual with TBI who left the voicemail was a 43-year-old white male from the American Midwest. He experienced a severe TBI from a motor vehicle crash. The recording was made 14 years postinjury when he was still unable to manage his business or maintain stable employment. The recording from the employed person with TBI was from a 61-year-old white male also from the American Midwest. After experiencing a severe TBI due to a skiing accident at the age of 34, he was hospitalized for 6 months and had 6 years of vocational rehabilitation, where he served in many jobs and volunteer positions. At the time of the recording, he had been working for 3 years as an office manager in a small company with a more limited role. The control participant was an African American male from an urban location in the American Midwest employed as a custodial manager in a large office building.

The recording from the chronically unemployed person with TBI indicates the use of one politeness marker. Although he successfully conveys his message to the voicemail recipient, he does so with a prolonged sarcastic joke. By comparison, the recording of the employed person with TBI shows the use of 16 politeness markers in a minute-long voicemail message. Although his use of politeness markers is appropriate and he demonstrates some politeness strategies, the content of his voicemail message is disorganized. The voicemail message from the control participant reveals the use of eight politeness markers in a much shorter 39-second voicemail. The relative economy of words and time in this voicemail indicates that the control participant's rate of politeness marker use is slightly more efficient than the employed person with TBI.

Evaluating Emotion Perception and Theory of Mind

Another technology-supported approach to the collection of discourse involves an interaction with a virtual human that has previously been used in aphasia to evaluate discourse in situational scripts (Kalinyak-Fliszar et al., 2015). More recently, this technique was used to evaluate discourse in relation to theory of mind and emotion perception after TBI (Moreau et al., 2022). This study involved people with TBI using a platform similar to a video conferencing call, with the virtual human presenting different conversational situations. Tasks included scenarios where the virtual human used sarcasm during discussion of a plan to see a movie or expressed surprise in reaction to a suggestion of a gift to buy for a friend. The virtual human's conversational responses were delivered by the examiner manually selecting the best option out of a bank of prerecorded responses, depending on what the participant said.

The discourse samples generated from these interactions were evaluated to determine whether the speaker with TBI was able to identify the other speaker's emotional state and modify their verbal response appropriately. This initial experimental study found that these tasks discriminated effectively between the discourse of speakers with and without a TBI. Future implementation of this technology within clinical settings could provide a structured approach to evaluate deficits in emotion perception and theory of mind. Impairments in these domains after a TBI have a subtle, but important impact on conver-

sation discourse with family and friends. However, they are challenging to detect in naturalistic conversation samples.

Broadening Contexts of Assessment

Alongside structured contexts for discourse sampling such as those described above, it is also important to evaluate discourse with familiar communication partners in typical daily conversations. Technology can play a role in enabling collection of these discourse samples from communication partners who may not be available to attend in-person sessions. Even well-established technology, such as the telephone, can be useful for sampling conversational discourse with different communication partners (Togher et al., 1997). Video conferencing technology can also be used to evaluate conversation with usual communication partners within the client's home while the clinician is in a different location (Rietdijk et al., 2018). The application of video conferencing technology to discourse assessment could provide opportunities to evaluate an even broader range of conversations, such as a meeting with a workmate or a social catch-up with a friend. The functionality of group video conferencing may also offer a means to evaluate conversational discourse within a group conversation, given that the feasibility of group video conferencing involving people with TBI has been demonstrated (Tsaousides et al., 2017).

Evaluating Prosody

Another aspect of measurement of discourse is intonation—the pitch and intensity variations of voice during conversation.

TBI-related dysarthrias often affect respiratory, phonatory, articulatory, and/or resonatory systems, resulting in an accompanied aprosodia, or flat affect (Theodoros et al., 1995). Also present in the speech patterns of some individuals with TBI is an altered speaking rate that is generally slower in rate but can be faster (Wang et al., 2004). Research has previously applied specialized acoustic analysis software for the analysis of prosody and rate after TBI (Wang et al., 2005). Consumer-grade technology (i.e., technology intended for personal or household use) such as the PowerPoint Presenter Coach (Microsoft, n.d.) is now available, that provides a user with data on speech rate and pitch variation while delivering a presentation. This technology may increase the clinical feasibility of collecting this type of data. Use of this technology in clinical practice with people with TBI is a potential direction for future research.

Evaluating Written Discourse

Despite the frequency of use of technology-supported written communication in daily life, there has been little attention to evaluating the written discourse produced by people with TBI in their text messages, emails, or social media posts. People with TBI may find it challenging to use these types of written discourse, given impairments in cognitive-communication skills (Brunner et al., 2019). For clinical purposes, it may be useful to evaluate written discourse by applying consumer-grade technologies such as embedded spelling and grammar checks in word-processing software that can provide measures of productivity such as number of words and can automatically detect errors in spelling or sentence structure.

Recently developed technology goes beyond the analysis of spelling and grammar to automatically detect emotional tone

and degree of formality in written discourse (e.g., Grammarly, 2021; IBM, n.d.). These software applications provide feedback about emotional tone based on analyzing a sample of written text (e.g., email example) or a transcript of a spoken discourse sample. Given that people with TBI use technology such as social media and email for written communication at rates similar to people without TBI (Flynn et al., 2019), further investigations into the use of these communication platforms is an important consideration for research.

The frequency of use of technology to support communication also means that some individuals with TBI will have access to a repository of preinjury discourse samples such as recorded presentations, text messages, emails, and social media posts. With the individual's consent, these preinjury samples could be used as comparative data for evaluation of change in discourse patterns postinjury. For example, accessing a sample of preinjury social media posts has been recommended as an initial step to support people with TBI with social media use postinjury (Brunner et al., 2021; Morrow et al., 2021). This process, when carried out in partnership with the client and their close contacts, can inform the clinician about the individual's preinjury communication style, common patterns of communication via a particular online platform and, more specifically, the socially accepted communication practices within that individual's circle of contacts.

An important consideration for evaluating discourse in the context of technology-supported communication is the impact of the mode itself on the discourse. The social expectations of online communication differ from in-person communication, and even individual online platforms differ in how discourse is used. A helpful framework for understanding the expectations of online communication is generic structure potential analysis (Ventola, 1979). Examples of common genres in online communication include emailing a request, texting a birthday message, or posting a question on Twitter. Each of these genres contains a specific set of structural elements that may be used, depending on the field (topic or activity) and tenor (relationship between the communicators). For example, the obligatory structural elements in an email request to a stranger would include a greeting, introduction, request, and a close. In contrast, a post on Twitter to ask for information has fewer obligatory elements; it may contain only the request for information with optional additional elements such as tagging other Twitter users, inclusion of hashtags, use of emojis, and attachment of images. As online platforms for communication continue to evolve, and communities of users develop their own patterns of communication, clinicians may need to evaluate discourse in technological contexts that are not familiar to them. Observation of the discourse of other users of the platform can be clinically helpful as a comparison when evaluating how a person with TBI communicates on that platform.

Using Technology to Monitor Change in Discourse

Technology enables the clinician, client, and communication partner to capture and retain samples of discourse for later review that can assist in reflecting on communication skill and tracking change over time. Playback and review of discourse samples together with the client and the communication partner has been shown to facilitate involvement in the evaluation process and thus support collaborative identification of goals (Hoepner & Turkstra, 2013). The use of video recording to analyze interpersonal dynamics was standardized early in the psychology literature with the advent of Interpersonal Process Recall (Kagan et al., 1969). This established approach uses video playback and review with a clinician serving as a coach and has been found effective for persons with brain injury in the acute phase (Helffenstein & Wechsler, 1982). When recorded and saved in a manner compliant with confidentiality laws, the use of video playback may be a helpful tool in the inpatient phase when patient buy-in has been achieved.

Another example of using technology for ongoing evaluations comes from a related product to the VET, the Work-Related Communication (WoRC) program. This program is an online intervention that also completes automated speech to text, then automatically scores the text for politeness markers (Meulenbroek & Cherney, 2021). Whereas the VET collects a monologic discourse sample (voicemail), the WoRC program supports a two-person dialogue with one side of the dialogue being standardized. The software collects spoken performance while the clinician encourages review of conversational performance and aids with shaping speech to be more professional. This cyclical use of recording, review, self-assessment, clinician feedback, and rerecording is consistent with the use of role play to model social behavior that has been in use for decades (Meulenbroek et al., 2019).

Identifying Meaningful Data Points Within Discourse Data

The online companion website outlines evaluation tools discussed in this chapter that may be applicable to discourse after TBI and provides an illustrative case study of an assessment protocol with planning of relevant data sampling and measures.

Technology can provide clinicians with access to much more data than previously available through traditional evaluation approaches. To make the best clinical use of this information, the selection of key data points and interpretation of data must be based on what is known about key communication deficits after TBI and about typical discourse of people without a TBI. Data points that may be collected have already been mentioned, including mean length of utterance, politeness markers, aspects of vocal affect, or conversational tone from word choice as obtained using tone analyzer software (e.g., IBM, n.d.).

Other factors to consider are the types of turns that people make in discourse. For instance, turns can be taken to provide new information; examining the relative contribution of informational moves taken in conversation might uncover who is leading the conversation and who is not (Halliday & Matthiessen, 2004). Persons with TBI utilize fewer turns to inform than controls (Togher et al., 1997). Counting mental state terms as data points may also be a promising direction for identifying theory of mind or metacognitive deficits in persons with TBI (Byom & Turkstra, 2012). Clinical applications and future innovation in the use of technology for discourse assessment should be driven by knowledge about the core discourse deficits after TBI, as well as client-identified priorities regarding meaningful data.

Future Directions in Technology and Discourse Analysis

Technology Supporting the Analysis of Discourse Samples

A key reason why a clinician may not evaluate discourse after TBI is the time required for analysis (Maddy et al., 2015). An emerging technology in discourse assessment is the use of automated transcription and analysis that may address this barrier. The use of automated speech-to-text transcription has been applied to recordings of sentences produced by speakers with aphasia following a stroke (Jacks et al., 2019). While accuracy of automated transcription was lower than human transcription, there was excellent agreement between the two methods. Automated transcription may serve to supplement human transcription, with the automated process providing an initial transcript, which is then reviewed by a human rater. It is also important to note that individuals with dysarthric speech present more difficulty with reliability of speech-to-text transcription software applications, and so human transcription may still be required. In these cases, video of the speaker is preferable to audio-only recordings as it provides more contextual information to assist with transcription. There are currently efforts to improve accuracy of automated speech recognition of individuals with nontypical speech, such as Project Euphonia (Google AI, n.d.). Work in this field may be relevant to clinical discourse evaluation in the future.

A currently available tool to support manual transcription of discourse is the Computerized Language Analysis (CLAN) program, which is described in Chapter 17. This tool has been applied to automated analysis of discourse samples of people with aphasia (Fromm et al., 2020) and TBI (Byom & Turkstra, 2012). The CLAN program supports transcript preparation through time-linking utterances between a transcription file and audio or video file. The transcript can then be subjected to the automated measurement tools available through CLAN. CLAN commands can be used for automated calculation of generic discourse measures such as number of utterances, number of words, mean length of utterance, and type-token ratio. It is also possible to analyze samples collected using the AphasiaBank protocol for presence of words from the core lexicon lists for the discourse tasks. After the initial time for transcript preparation, the automated analyses run quickly and provide reliable quantitative data regarding discourse.

An alternative approach to transcription is the use of annotation software to count instances of a behavior while observing a discourse sample in real time. This has been applied to conversations of people with aphasia following a stroke to count occurrences of closed-ended questions, open-ended questions, yes/no questions, and long pauses, with point-by-point agreement of 81 to 99% (Croteau et al., 2018). If a specific target behavior of interest relevant to an individual's goals can be reliably identified, this approach can serve as a useful way to evaluate a conversation as well as monitor change over time.

One example of a novel implementation of analyzing communication behaviors is to examine the number of types of moves made in a conversational exchange, which has been applied in the field of aphasia (Armstrong et al., 2013; Husak, 2018). In this research, the Speech Function Network (Eggins & Slade, 2004) was used to categorize speech behaviors as openings, sustaining moves, reactions, rejoinders, and confronts. Each of these have submoves and, once learned, they can be used to complete online coding of conversation exchange.

There is also a growing field of research in the application of automated analyses to video samples of conversation. For example, the application EQclinic can automatically report data such as the amount of time each person speaks during a video conference and duration of nonverbal features such as nodding (Liu et al., 2016). Similarly, the software Affectiva (iMotions, n.d.) may be used for automated detection of facial expression from a video sample. The use of these applications in analyzing the discourse of TBI speakers has been investigated in two unpublished dissertations. EQclinic was used to analyze interactions between simulated patients with TBI and different communication partners (Naoum, 2019) and Affectiva was used to investigate differences in facial expression between speakers with a TBI and speakers without a TBI (Yiew, 2021). These preliminary studies have identified potential for future clinical application for assessment of communication after TBI

Use of Chatbots or Digital Conversation Agents

Conversation agents (CAs), or chatbots, are automatic, computerized systems that use decision logic to create an interactive spoken or written dialogue between a human and a computer. This technology is an emerging field within healthcare (Laranjo et al., 2018). However, there is currently little evidence specific to the field of TBI (Hocking et al., 2021). One reported application of this technology for people with TBI is the development of a prototype chatbot for the purpose of motivational interviewing and goal setting after TBI (Hocking & Maeder, 2021). Using artificial intelligence approaches, an algorithm could be developed based on a collection of language samples for a specific scenario (e.g., interviews, providing information) that the chatbot follows to evaluate natural language use in the patient with TBI. An example of this approach for assessment is seen in unpublished dissertation work by Musaji (2020). Application of this technology may be suitable for assessment of skill in participating in dialogue after a TBI. By programming the algorithm to introduce harder conversational situations (e.g., indicating anger, which requires recognition of emotion or stating information in a purposefully complex manner that demands verbal working memory), chatbots can be tailored to operate at a conversation level that is individualized for the client. They can also be designed to evaluate specific problems with conversational dialogue such as emotion recognition or memory deficits.

Assessment Using Virtual Reality

Clinicians have been limited to assessing discourse in the settings and with the communication partners that are available within their real-world environment or setting up role-play scenarios to observe a client's discourse in hypothetical communication situations. Virtual reality (VR) may further increase the range of possible communication contexts and the ecological validity for discourse assessment by placing the person with TBI into a realistic simulated environment. The clinical utility of VR for people with TBI has been noted by speech-language pathologists who trialed a VR system (Vaezipour et al., 2021). Perceived benefits included the ability to detect functional communication deficits in everyday scenarios for individuals who perform well on impairment-focused assessment and the capacity to manipulate task and environment complexity for each individual. However, a lack of research on the use of VR for discourse assessment was identified in a recent systematic review of VR in brain injury rehabilitation (Brassel et al., 2021).

Conclusions

As technology changes the ways people communicate, the ways that we evaluate discourse after a TBI must also evolve. Technology may create new opportunities to evaluate discourse beyond the traditional clinical setting and may deliver new efficiencies in analysis processes. Technology also introduces new questions to be considered as part of a discourse evaluation. These considerations include the privacy and safety of data storage, the interpretation of new types of data, and the social rules of communication within online spaces. This chapter has provided an overview of current practices in the application of technology and telepractice for discourse assessment after TBI and has mapped potential future directions in this field for both research and clinical applications.

References

American Speech-Language-Hearing Association. (n.d.). *Telepractice* [Practice portal]. http://www.asha.org/Practice-Portal/Profes sional-Issues/Telepractice/

Armstrong, E., Fox, S., & Wilkinson, R. (2013). Mild aphasia: Is this the place for an argument? *American Journal of Speech-Language Pathology, 22*(2), S268–S278. https://doi.org/ 10.1044/1058-0360(2012/12-0084)

Bond, F., & Godfrey, H. P. (1997). Conversation with traumatically brain injured individuals: A controlled study of behavioral changes and their impact. *Brain Injury, 11*(5), 319–330. https://doi.org/10.1080/026990597123476

Brain Rehab Program and Mobility Innovations Centre. (2020). *The Toronto rehab telerehabilitation toolkit for outpatient rehabilitation programs.* Toronto Rehabilitation Institute.

Brassel, S., Power, E., Campbell, A., Brunner, M., & Togher, L. (2021). Recommendations for the design and implementation of virtual reality for acquired brain injury rehabilitation: Systematic review. *Journal of Medical Internet Research, 23*(7), e26344. https://doi .org/10.2196/26344

Brennan, D. M., Georgeadis, A. C., Baron, C. R., & Barker, L. M. (2004). The effect of videoconference-based telerehabilitation on story retelling performance by brain-injured subjects and its implications for remote speech-language therapy. *Telemedicine Journal and e-Health, 10*(2), 147–154. https://doi .org/10.1089/tmj.2004.10.147

Brown, P., & Levinson, S. C. (1987). *Politeness: Some universals in language usage.* Cambridge University Press.

Brunner, M., Hemsley, B., Togher, L., Dann, S., & Palmer, S. (2021). Social media and people with traumatic brain injury: A metasynthesis of research informing a framework for rehabilitation clinical practice, policy, and training. *American Journal of Speech-Language Pathology, 30*(1), 19–33. https://doi.org/10 .1044/2020_AJSLP-20-00211

Brunner, M., Palmer, S., Togher, L., & Hemsley, B. (2019). "I kind of figured it out": The views and experiences of people with traumatic brain injury (TBI) in using social media—self-determination for participation and inclusion online. *International Journal of Language and Communication Disorders, 54*(2), 221–233. https://doi.org/10.1111/1460-6984.12405

Byom, L. J., & Turkstra, L. (2012). Effects of social cognitive demand on theory of mind in conversations of adults with traumatic brain injury. *International Journal of Language and Communication Disorders, 47*(3), 310–321. https://doi.org/10.1111/j.1460-6984 .2011.00102.x

Croteau, C., McMahon-Morin, P., Le Dorze, G., Power, E., Fortier-Blanc, J., & Davis, G. A. (2018). Exploration of a quantitative method for measuring behaviors in conversation. *Aphasiology, 32*(3), 247–263. https://doi.org/ 10.1080/02687038.2017.1350629

Douglas, J. M., Bracy, C. A., & Snow, P. C. (2007). Measuring perceived communicative ability after traumatic brain injury: Reliability and validity of the La Trobe Communication Questionnaire. *Journal of Head Trauma Rehabilitation, 22*(1), 31–38. https://doi.org/ 10.1097/00001199-200701000-00004

Doyle, P., McNeil, M., Spencer, K., Goda, A., Cotrell, K., & Lustig, A. (1998). The effects of concurrent picture presentation on retelling of orally presented stories by adults with

aphasia. *Aphasiology, 12,* 561–574. https:// doi.org/10.1080/02687039808249558

Eggins, S., & Slade, D. (1997). *Analyzing casual conversation.* Cassell.

Flynn, M. A., Rigon, A., Kornfield, R., Mutlu, B., Duff, M. C., & Turkstra, L. S. (2019). Characterizing computer-mediated communication, friendship, and social participation in adults with traumatic brain injury. *Brain Injury, 33*(8), 1097–1104. https://doi.org/10.1080/02 699052.2019.1616112

Fromm, D., Forbes, M., Holland, A., & MacWhinney, B. (2020). Using AphasiaBank for discourse assessment. *Seminars in Speech and Language, 41*(1), 10–19. https://doi.org/10.10 55/s-0039-3399499

Google AI. (n.d.). https://sites.research.google/ euphonia/about/

Grammarly. (2021). https://www.grammarly .com/

Halliday, G. M., & Matthiessen, C. M. I. M. (2004). *An introduction to functional grammar.* Hodder Arnold.

Helffenstein, D. A., & Wechsler, F. S. (1982). The use of interpersonal process recall (IPR) in the remediation of interpersonal and communication skill deficits in the newly brain injured. *Clinical Neuropsychology, 4*(3), 139–142.

Hocking, J., & Maeder, A. (2021). Motivational embodied conversational agent for brain injury rehabilitation. In A. J. Maeder, C. Higa, M. E. L. van den Berg, & C. Gough (Eds.), *Telehealth innovations in remote healthcare services delivery* (pp. 37–46). IOS Press. https://doi.org/10.3233/shti210026

Hocking, J., Oster, C., & Maeder, A. (2021). Use of conversational agents in rehabilitation following brain injury, disease, or stroke: A scoping review protocol. *JBI Evidence Synthesis, 19*(6), 1369–1381. https://doi.org/ 10.11124/JBIES-20-00225

Hoepner, J. K., & Turkstra, L. S. (2013). Video-based administration of the La Trobe Communication Questionnaire for adults with traumatic brain injury and their communication partners. *Brain Injury, 27*(4), 464–472. https://doi.org/10.3109/02699052.2013.765 600

Husak, R. S. (2018). *Joint decision-making in married couples affected by aphasia* [Doctoral dissertation, University of Kentucky]. https://doi.org/10.13023/ETD.2018.164

IBM. (n.d.). *Watson tone analyzer.* https://tone-analyzer-demo.ng.bluemix.net/

iMotions. (n.d.). *Affectiva—emotion AI.* https://imotions.com/affectiva

Jacks, A., Haley, K. L., Bishop, G., & Harmon, T. G. (2019). Automated speech recognition in adult stroke survivors: Comparing human and computer transcriptions. *Folia Phoniatrica et Logopaedica, 71*(5–6), 286–296. https://doi.org/10.1159/000499156

Kagan, N., Schauble, P., Resnikoff, A., Danish, S. J., & Krathwohl, D. R. (1969). Interpersonal process recall. *The Journal of Nervous and Mental Disease, 148*(4), 365–374. https://doi.org/10.1097/00005053-196904000-00004

Kalinyak-Fliszar, M., Martin, N., Keshner, E., Rudnicky, A., Shi, J., & Teodoro, G. (2015). Using virtual technology to promote functional communication in aphasia: Preliminary evidence from interactive dialogues with human and virtual clinicians. *American Journal of Speech-Language Pathology, 24*(4), S974–S989. https://doi.org/10.1044/2015_AJSLP-14-0160

Laranjo, L., Dunn, A. G., Tong, H. L., Kocaballi, A. B., Chen, J., Bashir, R., . . . Coiera, E. (2018). Conversational agents in healthcare: A systematic review. *Journal of the American Medical Informatics Association, 25*(9), 1248–1258. https://doi.org/10.1093/jamia/ocy072

Liu, C., Lim, R. L., McCabe, K. L., Taylor, S., & Calvo, R. A. (2016). A web-based telehealth training platform incorporating automated nonverbal behavior feedback for teaching communication skills to medical students: A randomized crossover study. *Journal of Medical Internet Research, 18*(9), e246. https://doi.org/10.2196/jmir.6299

MacWhinney, B., Fromm, D., Forbes, M., & Holland, A. (2011). Aphasia bank: Methods for studying discourse. *Aphasiology, 25*, 1286–1307. https://doi.org/10.1080/02687038.2011.589893

Maddy, K. M., Howell, D. M., & Capilouto, G. J. (2015). Current practices regarding discourse analysis and treatment following nonaphasic brain injury: A qualitative study. *Journal of Interactional Research in Communication Disorders, 6*(2), 211–236. https://doi.org/10.1558/jircd.v7i1.25519

Malec, J. F., Salisbury, D. B., Anders, D., Dennis, L., Groff, A. R., Johnson, M., . . . Smith, G. T. (2021). Response to the COVID-19 pandemic among posthospital brain injury rehabilitation providers. *Archives of Physical Medicine and Rehabilitation, 102*(3), 549–555. https://doi.org/10.1016/j.apmr.2020.10.137

Meulenbroek, P., & Cherney, L. R. (2019). The voicemail elicitation task: Functional workplace language assessment for persons with traumatic brain injury. *Journal of Speech, Language, and Hearing Research, 62*, 3367–3380. https://doi.org/10.1044/2019_JSLHR-L-18-0466

Meulenbroek, P., & Cherney, L. R. (2021). Computer-based workplace communication training in persons with traumatic brain injury: The work-related communication program. *Journal of Communication Disorders, 91*, 106104. https://doi.org/10.1016/j.jcomdis.2021.106104

Meulenbroek, P., Ness, B., Lemoncello, R., Byom, L., MacDonald, S., O'Neil-Pirozzi, T. M., & Moore Sohlberg, M. (2019). Social communication following traumatic brain injury part 2: Identifying effective treatment ingredients. *International Journal of Speech-Language Pathology, 21*(2), 128–142. https://doi.org/10.1080/17549507.2019.1583281

Microsoft. (n.d.). *Rehearse your slide show with Presenter Coach.* https://support.microsoft.com/en-us/office/rehearse-your-slide-show-with-presenter-coach-cd7fc941-5c3b-498c-a225-83ef3f64f07b

Moreau, N., Taché, E., & Champagne-Lavau, M. (2022). Speaking with virtual humans: Assessing social cognition in traumatic brain injury with a second-person perspective task. *Journal of Neuropsychology, 16*(1), 75–96. https://doi.org/10.1111/jnp.12257

Morrow, E. L., Zhao, F., Turkstra, L., Toma, C., Mutlu, B., & Duff, M. C. (2021). Computer-mediated communication in adults with and without moderate to severe traumatic brain injury: Survey of social media use. *JMIR Rehabilitation and Assistive Technologies*, *8*(3), e26586. https://doi.org/10.2196/26586

Musaji, I. Y. (2020). *Developing a chatbot-based screening tool for rapid assessment of computer-mediated communication impairment* [Doctoral dissertation, Wichita State University]. https://soar.wichita.edu/handle/10057/18814

Naoum, D. (2019). *Automated analysis of conversation after traumatic brain injury: Student and experienced speech pathologists' interactions with simulated patients* [Unpublished honors thesis, University of Sydney].

Ownsworth, T., Arnautovska, U., Beadle, E., Shum, D. H., & Moyle, W. (2018). Efficacy of telerehabilitation for adults with traumatic brain injury: A systematic review. *Journal of Head Trauma Rehabilitation*, *33*(4), E33–E46. https://doi.org/10.1097/HTR.0000000000000350

Rietdijk, R., Power, E., Attard, M., & Togher, L. (2022). Acceptability of telehealth-delivered rehabilitation: Experiences and perspectives of people with traumatic brain injury and their carers. *Journal of Telemedicine and Telecare*, *28*(2), 122–134. https://doi.org/10.1177%2F1357633X20923824

Rietdijk, R., Power, E., Brunner, M., & Togher, L. (2017). Reliability of videoconferencing administration of a communication questionnaire to people with traumatic brain injury and their close others. *Journal of Head Trauma Rehabilitation*, *32*(6), E38–E44. https://doi.org/10.1097/HTR.0000000000000282

Rietdijk, R., Power, E., Brunner, M., & Togher, L. (2018). The reliability of evaluating conversations between people with traumatic brain injury and their communication partners via videoconferencing. *Neuropsychological Rehabilitation*, *30*, 1074–1091. https://doi.org/10.1080/09602011.2018.1554533

Speech Pathology Australia. (2014). *Telepractice in speech pathology* [Position statement]. The Speech Pathology Association of Australia.

Theodoros, D. G., Murdoch, B. E., & Stokes, P. D. (1995). Variability in the perceptual and physiological features of dysarthria following severe closed head injury: An examina-tion of five cases. *Brain Injury*, *9*(7), 671–696. https://doi.org/10.3109/02699059509008225

Togher, L., & Hand, L. (1998). Use of politeness markers with different communication partners: An investigation of five subjects with traumatic brain injury. *Aphasiology*, *12*(7–8), 755–770. https://doi.org/10.1080/02687039808249571

Togher, L., Hand, L., & Code, C. (1997). Analyzing discourse in the traumatic brain injury population: Telephone interactions with different communication partners. *Brain Injury*, *11*(3), 169–190. https://doi.org/10.1080/026990597123629

Togher, L., Power, E., Tate, R., McDonald, S., & Rietdijk, R. (2010). Measuring the social interactions of people with traumatic brain injury and their communication partners: The adapted Kagan scales. *Aphasiology*, *24*(6–8), 914–927. https://doi.org/10.1080/02687030903422478

Tsaousides, T., Spielman, L., Kajankova, M., Guetta, G., Gordon, W., & Dams-O'Connor, K. (2017). Improving emotion regulation following web-based group intervention for individuals with traumatic brain injury. *Journal of Head Trauma Rehabilitation*, *32*(5), 354–365. https://doi.org/10.1097/HTR.0000000000000345

Turkstra, L. S., Quinn-Padron, M., Johnson, J. E., Workinger, M. S., & Antoniotti, N. (2012). In-person versus telehealth assessment of discourse ability in adults with traumatic brain injury. *Journal of Head Trauma Rehabilitation*, *27*(6), 424–432. https://doi.org/10.1097/HTR.0b013e31823346fc

Vaezipour, A., Whelan, B. M., Wall, K., & Theodoros, D. (2019). Acceptance of rehabilitation technology in adults with moderate to severe traumatic brain injury, their caregivers, and healthcare professionals: A systematic review. *Journal of Head Trauma Rehabilitation*, *34*(4), E67–E82. https://doi.org/10.1097/HTR.0000000000000462

Vaezipour, A., Aldridge, D., Koenig, S., Theodoros, D., & Russell, T. (2021). "It's really exciting to think where it could go": A mixed-method investigation of clinician acceptance, barriers, and enablers of virtual reality technology in communication rehabilitation. *Disability and Rehabilitation* [Online]. https://doi.org/10.1080/09638288.2021.1895333

Ventola, E. (1979). The structure of casual conversation in English. *Journal of Pragmatics*, *3*, 267–298. https://doi.org/10.1016/0378-2166(79)90034-1

Wang, Y.-T., Kent, R. D., Duffy, J. R., Thomas, J. E., & Weismer, G. (2004). Alternating motion rate as an index of speech motor disorder in traumatic brain injury. *Clinical Linguistic and Phonetics*, *18*, 57–84. https://doi.org/10.1080/02699200310001596160

Wang, Y.-T., Kent, R. D., Duffy, J. R., & Thomas, J. E. (2005). Dysarthria associated with traumatic brain injury: Speaking rate and emphatic stress. *Journal of Communication Disorders*, *38*(3), 231–260. https://doi.org/10.1016/j.jcomdis.2004.12.001

Yiew, K. (2021). *Differentiating use of facial expression between individuals with and without traumatic brain injury using Affectiva software: A pilot study* [Unpublished honors thesis, University of Sydney].

APPENDIX 12–1

Voicemail Elicitation Task (VET) Transcripts

Scenario

William reports to you for a project at work you are in charge of. You notice that he has not been following the dress code recently. The weather outside has warmed up and he started wearing shorts every other day. Call your assistant William on his office phone. Remind him of the rule that shorts are not allowed in the workplace and ask him to follow the dress code rules.

Transcription of Person with TBI—Unemployed

Hello William. Uh, do we need to relocate the office to the beach so you can, uh wear appropriate clothing every day? If so, tell me and we'll relocate it down there and you can dress in your shorts. Well, get back to me. Have a *great* day. Bye.

Transcription of Person with TBI—Employed

Hey, hi William this is (First and Last Name). Say, first of all I want to let you know I *really appreciate* the work you're doing on this project that we—that we're working on together. Uh, you're doing a *nice* job *thank you so very much*. Uh, the second thing that I wanted to let—let you know, though is—and I figured you'd rather hear this from me than somebody else and that is that, um, I've noticed that the, you're, because it's got-

ten warmer out you're *not really* following the dress code. You're wearing shorts, which, which, well, which I'm sure you're *probably* aware of is *not really* allowed in the office. There's a couple reasons for that. One of which is, um, well you never know in the course of a day who I might be, who you *might* be meeting with. Um, it *could* be someone important from another company and I think *just* the other thing is— the other reason for the policy is that, um, you know, having a dress code means that people dress in a, uh, certain manner. So, if you have any questions, by all means, uh, let me know. I'm *sure you know* I'm sure *happy* to talk with you about it. Uh, again, *thank you* for the work you're doing.

Transcription of Healthy Control—Employed

Hi William. Um, this is (First name). Um, I'm calling in reference to your recent, um, dress code at work. Uh, I *do understand* that the weather has warmed up, but we are not allowed to wear shorts in the office. Not at the workplace. Uh, *we do have* a strict dress code and *if you need any* reference to that *we do have* the policy here and *you can* review it. Uh, give me a call to let me know that you did, in fact, receive this message and *if you have* any other further questions regarding this you can give me a call. Uh, xxx-xxx-xxxx. *Thank you, have a good day*. (See Table A12–1 on following page.)

Table A12–1. Summary Scores			
Person	*Politeness Markers*	*Minutes*	*Politeness Markers per Minute*
TBI—Unemployed	1	0.43	2.32
TBI—Employed	16	1.18	13.56
Healthy Control	8	0.65	12.31

SECTION IV
Discourse of People Living With Neurodegenerative Disorders

J. B. Orange, Topic Chair

Introduction

The term *neurodegenerative disorders* represents multidimensional progressive conditions in which there are declines involving one or both of the peripheral and central nervous systems, often eventually leading to organ and musculoskeletal system failures. Documentation from ancient times shows awareness of and fascination with those whose mental, psychological, behavioral, communicative, musculoskeletal, or neurological functions declined over time. Religious, spiritual, philosophical, cultural, and even political leaders debated for centuries the underlying basis of neurodegenerative disorders. They postulated Satanic and demonic possession, absence of a soul, inferior genetics, heredity, and environmental influences, among among other origins. (Jennekens, 2014).

The seminal scientific writings of giants in neurodegenerative disorders, including Alois Alzheimer (1907), James Parkinson (1817), and Friedrich Lewy (1912), described behavioral, neuropathological, psychological, and musculoskeletal features of their unique patients. Some of their noteworthy scientific documenta-

tions also included descriptions of their patients' speech production, language, and communication.

Today, neuropathology researchers typically use the term *diseases* within the context of neurodegeneration based on autopsy-confirmed neuropathological findings linked to clinical behaviors and biomarkers, where available. They reserve the word *disorders* for clinical, nonautopsy-based cases. The terms diseases and disorders often are used interchangeably in the literature of language and communication sciences, so both terms are used by authors within this topic section.

Scientific leaders in the field of language and communication sciences and those in multiple disciplines such as neuropsychology, sociolinguistics, cognitive neurology, and geriatrics have explored in greater depth and detail the language, communication, discourse productions, and neural underpinnings of persons living with neurodegenerative conditions (e.g., Asp & de Villiers, 2010; Bayles et al., 2020; Davis, 2005; Guendouzi & Muller, 2006; Hickey & Bourgeois, 2011; Theodoros & Ramig, 2011). As noted by Coelho and colleagues in Chapter 1, it is important to address both the spoken and written discourse in those with a neurodegenerative disorder. To date, the majority of discourse studies have focused on spoken output, although there are recent published efforts documenting the written discourse performances of persons with neurodegenerative disorders such as amyotrophic lateral sclerosis (ALS) and mild cognitive impairment (e.g., Ichikawa et al., 2010; Ichikawa et al., 2011; Kim et al., 2021). There also are analyses of recorded spoken and written discourse samples of public figures such as U.S. President Ronald Reagan (Berisha et al., 2015) and prominent U.K. novelists Iris Murdoch and Agatha Christie (Le et al., 2011), who likely suffered from dementia years before diagnosis. There now are myriad other empirical, experimentally driven studies that reinforce the importance and value of analyzing spoken and written discourse performances to mark the onset and the progression of neurodegenerative disorders such as dementia (Orange & Kertesz, 2000).

Importantly, some investigators sought to uncover unique differences and profiles of traditional neurodegenerative diagnostic groups, including their discourse differences. Mesulam's (1982) groundbreaking documentation of what he referred to at that time as "slowly progressive aphasia" is an example of a current trailblazer who revolutionized how we conceptualize subgroups within the diagnostic category of frontotemporal dementia. His efforts led to others (e.g., Gorno-Tempini et al., 2011; Harciarek & Kertesz, 2011) documenting even greater details of subgroups within the overall grouping of what is now referred to as *primary progressive aphasia* (see Chapter 13). Others have looked for commonalities in behavioral, language, and discourse performances, seeking evidence for shared discourse and neural processing features (Farhan et al., 2017; Ingram et al., 2020; Murley et al., 2020; Sajjadi et al., 2012). Currently,

we are at a nexus where researchers use sophisticated and innovative tools for data collection and analysis to identify and to predict group assignments and shared features of discourse performances (e.g., Fraser et al., 2019; Le et al., 2011). The development of DementiaBank (https://dementia.talkbank.org/access/) within the larger TalkBank data set (see Chapter 17) marks the advancement of and access by researchers and clinicians to a collection of useful comparative discourse performances.

The Chapters in This Section

The four chapters gathered in this topic section capture, as representative samples, the breadth and depth of current thinking of the multidimensional, shared, and distinct discourse performances of persons living with primary progressive aphasia (PPA), Alzheimer's dementia, Parkinson's disease, and amyotrophic lateral sclerosis (ALS). These representative chapters build on and expand from the foundational work of discourse analysis contained in the well-known "green book" of Cherney, Shadden, and Coelho (1998).

Dalton, Hubbard, and Richardson (Chapter 13) open with a description of the conceptual foundation of PPA situated within the current category of frontotemporal dementia. They document the distinctive and important roles that speech-language pathologists (SLPs) play in conducting early and ongoing language and discourse assessments and treatments of persons living with PPA. Using several case examples, Dalton and colleagues make compelling arguments for using the "clinically friendly" microstructural Core Lexicon analysis (CoreLex) and the hybrid micro- and macrostructural levels measure Main Content Analysis (MCA) to identify performance differences among the currently accepted variants of PPA and to track progressive changes over time. They present coded transcripts and interpretations of findings from their cases, along with support from the extant literature, that demonstrate the usefulness of discourse measures, including CoreLex and MCA. They conclude with caveats related to discourse assessments in clinical practice.

In Chapter 14, Guendouzi offers an appraisal of the value of using conversational data for discourse analyses framed within "the lens of psycholinguistic theories" for persons living with dementia. Guendouzi includes a brief overview of common communication and discourse performances of persons living with dementia of the Alzheimer's type (DAT). She acknowledges the limitations of well-known stroke aphasia-based assessment tools and linguistic-communication measures standardized on persons with DAT to measure conversational interactions. Guendouzi devotes the majority of her chapter to providing a strong rationale for the value of measuring features of given information in conversations with persons living with DAT. She uses case scenarios and extracts from conversations she held with "Flo," an 82-year-old neighbor with whom she has held an extended relationship. Persons living with DAT progressively lose access to, retrieval from, and ultimately the representative content of their reservoir of shared knowledges. Such losses mean conversation partners must make greater efforts to facilitate rewarding and fulfilling conversations. The value of using scripts and schemas to help scaffold interactions in conversations is illustrated in the conversational extracts between Guendouzi and Flo, making clear the clinical utility of such measures in the assessment of and conversation-based

treatment options for persons living with DAT.

Aveni and Roberts (Chapter 15) present an overview of the value of undertaking a multilevel analysis of the discourse of persons living with Parkinson's disease (PD). Aveni and Roberts offer a summary of key motor and cognitive impairments in persons living with PD, highlighting the crucial, and sometimes neglected, importance of how cognitive impairment manifests in persons living with PD and how it affects their language and discourse performances. The majority of their chapter, however, is devoted to systematic coverage of the multilevel micro-, macro-, and superstructural changes in the discourse of persons living with PD. The authors include clinically doable processes for conducting their multilevel discourse analyses. The multilevel discourse analysis protocol is grounded in current models of discourse processing, and offers a clear, logical, and clinically sound pathway for researchers and clinicians alike to assess and to monitor treatment outcomes that are discourse based for persons living with PD.

Finally, in Chapter 16, Ash and Shellikeri offer a comprehensive discussion of the interplay among discourse, language, motor, and executive function in persons living with ALS. ALS is now recognized as a multisystem neurodegenerative disorder rather than only as a motor disorder. As a result, cognitive impairments in persons living with ALS have recently received attention. Ash and Shellikeri summarize the language and discourse performance of persons living with ALS. Their findings show that the wide range of expressive discourse problems of persons living with ALS is influenced, in large part, by executive dysfunction and its highly heterogenous manifestations. Chapter 16 illustrates how traditional discourse assessment tasks (e.g., single picture description, narrative story retelling) and classic discourse measures (e.g., speaking rate, MLU, T-units, number of words, content measures) can help advance our clinical understanding of the complex discourse performance of persons living with ALS. Critical work with neuroimaging to identify the connections between motor, cognitive, and discourse performance and underlying neural structures is also illustrated on the companion website.

Conclusions

Neurodegenerative disorders, often associated with aging and older adults, represent a rapidly growing proportion of our clinical caseloads. The disorders also continue to garner high-impact research attention. Each neurodegenerative condition can be viewed as a distinct entity with reasonably well-delineated clinical and neuropathological profiles. However, recent research findings, especially from studies of discourse, show a network of multiple interconnected and overlapping commonalities across conditions.

The contributing authors to the chapters in this topic section provide comprehensive, thought-provoking, and clinically meaningful discussions of discourse assessment considerations and recommendations from their representative areas of expertise. They offer markers for valid and distinguishing discourse performance features across four representative neurodegenerative disorders while giving pause for readers to consider the commonalities within disorder subgroups and across disorders.

Serving clients living with neurodegenerative disorders requires expert, interprofessional support because of multisystem involvement including cognitive, neural, musculoskeletal, speech production, language, and discourse domains. The contributions of the authors acknowledge the heterogenous presentations even within a single diagnostic category. They highlight the need for multiple discourse tasks and analyses cross-referenced with measures of cognition (e.g., executive function), speech production (e.g., motor control, speaking rate), and language (e.g., grammaticality). Such comprehensives assessments are necessary to capture the diverse array of performance that will inform the development of future novel, well-planned, discourse-based communication therapies.

References

Alzheimer, A. (1907). Über eine eigenartige Erkrankung der Hirnrinde [On an Unusual Illness of the Cerebral Cortex]. *Allgemeine Zeitschrift fur Psychiatrie under Psychisch-Gerichtliche Medizin, 64*, 146–148. http://info-centre.jenage.de/assets/pdfs/library/stelzmann_et_al_alzheimer_CLIN_ANAT_1995.pdf

Asp, E. D., & de Villiers, J. (2010). *When language breaks down: Analyzing discourse in clinical contexts*. Cambridge University Press. https://doi.org/10.1017/CBO9780511845352

Bayles, K. A., McCullough, K., & Tomoeda, C. (2020). *Cognitive-communication disorders of MCI and dementia—Definition, assessment, and clinical management* (3rd ed.). Plural Publishing.

Berisha, V., Wang, S., LaCross, A., & Liss, J. (2015). Tracking discourse complexity preceding Alzheimer's disease diagnosis: A case study comparing the press conferences of presidents Ronald Reagan and George Herbert Walker Bush. *Journal of Alzheimer's Disease, 45*(3), 959–963. https://doi.org/10.3233/JAD-142763

Cherney, L. R., Shadden, B. B., & Coelho, C. A. (Eds.). (1998). *Analyzing discourse in communicatively impaired adults*. Aspen Publishers.

Davis, B. (Ed.). (2005). *Alzheimer talk, text and context: Enhancing communication*. Springer. https://doi.org/10.1057/9780230502024

Farhan, S. M., Bartha, R., Black, S. E., Corbett, D., Finger, E., Freedman, M., . . . Strong, M. J. (2017). The Ontario Neurodegenerative Disease Research Initiative (ONDRI). *Canadian Journal of Neurological Sciences, 44*(2), 196–202. https://doi.org/10.1017/cjn.2016.415

Fraser, K. C., Linz, N., Li, B., Fors, K. L., Rudzicz, F., König, A., . . . Kokkinakis, D. (2019, June 2–7). Multilingual prediction of Alzheimer's disease through domain adaptation and concept-based language modelling [Conference presentation]. ACL Conference Proceedings, Minneapolis. *ACL Anthology, I.* https://acl anthology.org/N19-1367/

Gorno-Tempini, M. L., Hillis, A. E., Weintraub, S., Kertesz, A., Mendez, M., Cappa, S. F., . . . Grossman, M. (2011). Classification of primary progressive aphasia and its variants. *Neurology, 76*(11), 1006–1014. https://doi .org/10.1212/WNL.0b013e31821103e6

Guendouzi, J. A., & Muller, N. (2006). *Approaches to discourse in dementia.* Psychology Press.

Harciarek, M., & Kertesz, A. (2011). Primary progressive aphasias and their contribution to the contemporary knowledge about the brain-language relationship. *Neuropsychology Review, 21*(3), 271–287. https://doi.org/ 10.1007/s11065-011-9175-9

Hickey, E., & Bourgeois, M. S. (Eds.). (2011). *Dementia: From diagnosis to management— A functional approach.* Taylor & Francis.

Ichikawa, H., Hieda, S., Ohno, H., Ohnaka, Y., Shimizu, Y., Nakajima, M., & Kawamura, M. (2010). Kana versus kanji in amyotrophic lateral sclerosis: A clinicoradiological study of writing errors. *European Neurology, 64*(3), 148–155. https://doi.org/10.1159/000317011

Ichikawa, H., Ohno, H., Murakami, H., Ohnaka, Y., & Kawamura, M. (2011). Writing error may be a predictive sign for impending brain atrophy progression in amyotrophic lateral sclerosis: A preliminary study using X-ray computed tomography. *European Neurology, 65*(6), 346–351. https://doi.org/10.1159/ 000328216

Ingram, R. U., Halai, A. D., Pobric, G., Sajjadi, S., Patterson, K., & Lambon Ralph, M. A. (2020). Graded, multidimensional intra- and intergroup variations in primary progres-sive aphasia and poststroke aphasia. *Brain, 143*(10), 3121–3135. https://doi.org/10.1093/ brain/awaa245

Jennekens, F. G. I. (2014). A short history of the notion of neurodegenerative disease. *Journal of the History of the Neurosciences, 23*(1), 85–94. https://doi.org/10.1080/09647 04X.2013.809297

Kim, H., Walker, A., Shea, J., & Hillis, A. E. (2021). Written discourse task helps to identify progression from mild cognitive impairment to dementia. *Dementia and Geriatric Cognitive Disorders. 50*(5), 446–453. https:// doi.org/10.1159/000519884

Le, X., Lancashire, I., Hirst, G., & Jokel, R. (2011). Longitudinal detection of dementia through lexical and syntactic changes in writing: A case study of three British novelists. *Literary and Linguistic Computing, 26*(4), 435–461. https://doi.org/10.1093/llc/fqr013

Lewy, F. H. (1912). Paralysis agitans. 1. Pathologische anatomie. In M. Lewandowsky (Ed.), *Handbuch der Neurologie, Dritter Band, Spezielle Neurologie I* (pp. 920–933). Springer.

Mesulam, M. M. (1982). Slowly progressive aphasia without generalized dementia. *Annals of Neurology, 11*(6), 592–598. https://doi .org/10.1002/ana.410110607

Murley, A. G., Coyle-Gilchrist, I., Rouse, M. A., Jones, P. S., Li, W., Wiggins, J., . . . Rowe, J. B. (2020). Redefining the multidimensional clinical phenotypes of frontotemporal lobar degeneration syndromes. *Brain, 143*(5), 1555–1571. https://doi.org/10.1093/brain/awaa097

Orange, J. B., & Kertesz, A. (2000). Discourse analyses and dementia. *Brain and Language, 71*(1), 172–174. https://doi.org/10.1006/brln .1999.2243

Parkinson, J. (1817). *An essay on the shaking palsy.* Whittingham and Rowland for Sherwood, Neely, and Jones.

Sajjadi, S. A., Patterson, K., Arnold, R. J., Watson, P. C., & Nestor, P. J. (2012). Primary progressive aphasia: A tale of two syndromes and the rest. *Neurology, 78*(21), 1670–1677. https:// doi.org/10.1212/WNL.0b013e3182574f79

Theodoros, D., & Ramig, L. (Eds.). (2011). *Communication and swallowing in Parkinson's disease.* Plural Publishing.

13 Clinical Implications of Discourse Analysis for Individuals With Primary Progressive Aphasia

Sarah Grace Dalton, H. Isabel Hubbard, and Jessica D. Richardson

Overview of Primary Progressive Aphasia

Primary progressive aphasia (PPA) refers to a unified group of neurodegenerative conditions caused by underlying protein pathologies, such as tau, TDP-43, and beta amyloid (Bergeron et al., 2018; Grossman, 2010). Unlike more commonly occurring dementias, PPA is characterized by an initial and primary impairment of language, rather than by other cognitive skills (e.g., memory) or motor control. This reflects the primarily left hemisphere perisylvian locus of neurodegeneration, at least in the early clinical stages of the disease. As the underlying pathology progresses, individuals with PPA experience worsening language impairment as cognitive deficits also begin to emerge and progress. International consensus for PPA diagnosis states that language impairment must be the initial and primary concern in the early clinical stages of the syndrome and that language impairment is the cause of impaired activities of daily living (Gorno-Tempini et al., 2011). Additionally, the language impairment is not better explained by other stable neurological, medical, or psychiatric concerns and there are no initial difficulties with visual or episodic memory, visuoperceptual skills, or behavioral impairments. There are additional diagnostic criteria for three PPA variants—semantic, nonfluent/agrammatic, and logopenic (Gorno-Tempini et al., 2011).

The international criteria provide a conceptually sound framework for discussing this condition and its variants, common symptomatology, and progression. However, in clinical practice, individuals do not always present with the clear, distinct patterns of speech and/or language strengths and weaknesses described in the criteria. Most often, unless the speech-language pathologist (SLP) is located in a specialized care center for individuals with dementia (such as a memory and aging center or a specialty neurology clinic), they are likely to encounter individuals later in the syndrome progression who present with both language and cognitive deficits. SLPs are a critical but underutilized and underrecognized component of an interprofessional team-based approach to PPA care, possessing the education, skills, and training necessary to recognize mild deficits early in progression, aid in PPA and variant diagnosis, and ameliorate the impact of language impairment on everyday life (Henry et al., 2018; Henry et al., 2019; Ruggero et al., 2020).

The Role of the SLP in Identification of PPA

While other professionals are frequently consulted when exploring a diagnosis of PPA, the complementary depth of experience and knowledge of language provided by an SLP are necessary to identify subtle language impairments and attribute them to the appropriate causes. SLPs in acute inpatient settings may play an important role in identifying PPA in individuals admitted for nonneurological medical concerns, but who complain of language changes. One such case is expertly demonstrated in the literature by Chandregowda (2020). Here we present the case of Mrs. Hernandez, who experienced a 5-year delay in diagnosis while presenting language difficulties that were attributed to a psychological foundation. Eventually, a diagnosis of PPA was confirmed with behavioral testing and clinical neuroimaging.

The Case of Mrs. Hernandez

History and Chart Review: Mrs. Hernandez reported a slow onset of communication difficulties that began approximately 4 years prior to the date of our evaluation. She stated, *"I couldn't get my words out"* and her mother noticed that she was having trouble conversing. She went to the hospital and was quickly discharged without a diagnosis or follow-up plan. Her husband stated that these difficulties coincided with significant life stressors—getting married, moving, etc. He commented that *"She had*

trouble expressing herself . . . she couldn't hear or understand."

In the ensuing years, she sought several additional medical evaluations. At one time, an MRI showed *"a small area of hyperintensity involving the posterior left periatrial region"* and *"minimal diffuse cortical volume loss."* Although these evaluations identified reduced cognitive and linguistic abilities, the team ruled out core speech and language problems as a primary concern. They indicated a speech and language disturbance, specifically PPA, was not present, stating that the constellation of symptoms and her history (including recent stressors) seemed most consistent with conversion disorder.

Results and Recommendations: Four years after her initial hospital visit, Mrs. Hernandez sought an extensive speech-language and cognitive evaluation at our clinic. Word-finding difficulties in conversation, accompanied by compensatory gestures, were immediately observed by the evaluating team. She also demonstrated impaired naming and significant phonological impairment: deficits in repeating sentences, phonological errors in naming and spontaneous language production (often self-corrected), and inability to complete a phonological assessment. While she did demonstrate low or below-average performance on several cognitive assessments, many of these were linguistically loaded (e.g., California Verbal Learning Test). She performed within normal limits for spatial perception, face perception, and emotion naming, but slightly below average for design fluency.

Mrs. Hernandez's performance on naming was only mildly impaired, producing 53/60 items on the Boston Naming Test. However, when asked to describe the Broken Window picture sequence she said:

"Okay. So, so there's a, he kicked his the ball . . . And c— c— crack . . . well it

*looks like it go uh crashed . . . and then
and then (laughs) he was um . . . the dad
. . . um . . . I don't know, and then . . .
I don't know, I don't know what there the
last thing is I don't know."*

Her discourse was inefficient (this low-content sample was produced in 45 seconds) and sparse. She did not produce many of the vocabulary items specific to the stimulus, and a listener unfamiliar with the stimulus would not understand the gist of the story depicted in the stimulus. Mrs. Hernandez's performance was consistent with a clinical diagnosis of logopenic variant PPA (lvPPA). Our report advised meeting with a neurologist to review our findings and do additional testing, including neuroimaging, to determine if lvPPA was the appropriate diagnosis. Five years after Mrs. Hernandez first noticed her deficits, she received an imaging and clinically supported diagnosis of lvPPA from two independent neurologists who specialized in neurodegenerative diseases.

This case highlights the importance of in-depth language assessment, including discourse analysis, by the qualified SLP to ensure appropriate diagnosis and treatment management, particularly when a degenerative process is suspected. It is critical that SLPs advocate for their role in the diagnosis and management of these individuals to ensure timely services are provided.

Discourse Measurements for PPA—Core Lexicon Analysis and Main Concept Analysis

There are more than 500 discourse measures available in the published literature (Bryant et al., 2016), and many studies that examine discourse in PPA report numerous measures across language domains (e.g., phonology, morphology, semantics, syntax). To date, microlinguistic measures that investigate a specific domain of language have been the primary means of describing discourse production in PPA variants. In this chapter, we focus on two clinically friendly measures with well-developed checklists, freely available training materials, and normative data to highlight behaviors of interest throughout the cases. Core Lexicon analysis (CoreLex) is a microlinguistic measure, while Main Concept Analysis (MCA) is a hybrid measure that provides some information about both microlinguistic and macrolinguistic performance. We also present efficiency measures (e.g., the number of CoreLex items produced per minute; the number of accurate and complete main concepts produced per minute) to demonstrate differences within variants and over time. We previously reported on the utility of these measures in PPA (Dalton, Hubbard, et al., 2020).

CoreLex is a measurement of the typicality of words produced during a discourse sample. CoreLex checklists have been developed for the AphasiaBank tasks (picture sequence, picture scene, procedure, story retell) (see Chapter 17) and novel storytelling from wordless picture books (Dalton, Kim, et al., 2020). CoreLex is scored by comparing an individual's productions to the associated checklist (see Dalton, Kim, et al., 2020, or the "Discourse Analysis" topic on the AphasiaBank website for lists and detailed scoring rules). One point is scored for each CoreLex item produced, regardless of inflection or part of speech. Using previously published norms, SLPs can then compare client performance to healthy controls.

MCA measures how well an individual can communicate the gist or essential elements of a story (Kong, 2009; Nicholas & Brookshire, 1995; Richardson & Dalton, 2016). MCA checklists have been developed for the AphasiaBank tasks described above (see Richardson & Dalton, 2016, or the "Discourse Analysis" topic on the AphasiaBank website for complete main concept lists and detailed scoring rules). Main concepts consist of multiple essential elements; the discourse samples are scored for the accuracy and completeness of these essential elements. If all essential elements in a main concept are present and accurate, it is scored as "accurate/complete." If there are missing or inaccurate essential elements in the production, the main concept can be scored as "accurate/incomplete," "inaccurate/complete," or "inaccurate/incomplete." If the client does not produce a statement related to the main concept, it is coded as "absent." These codes can be converted to numerical scores, which are summed to yield a main concept composite score.

MCA for the *Cinderella* task recently has been extended to include sequencing and story grammar scoring (Greenslade et al., 2020). This new measure, Main Concept, Sequencing, and Story Grammar (MSSG), characterizes superstructural abilities that also are known to impact the comprehensibility of otherwise linguistically well-formed utterances. The MSSG analyses may be particularly useful for identifying the impact of cognitive deficits on communication, as sequencing and story grammar rely on both linguistic and general cognitive processes (Richardson et al., 2021). Combined with CoreLex, MSSG may be an efficient way to measure discourse across microlinguistic, macrolinguistic, and superstructural levels of performance.

International Consensus Variants of PPA

In our discussion of each variant, we present cases to illustrate the discourse changes that occur in this progressive condition. While we focus on the PPA variants with broad international consensus, various groups have presented alternative or additional variants, which are listed on the companion website.

Semantic Variant PPA

The diagnostic criteria for semantic variant PPA (svPPA) are described in Box 13–1.

> ### BOX 13–1. Diagnostic Criteria for Semantic Variant PPA (svPPA)
>
> Diagnosis of svPPA requires two core features: impaired confrontation naming and impaired single-word comprehension (Gorno-Tempini et al., 2011). At least two supporting features are also required, which could include impaired object knowledge (especially for low-frequency or low-familiarity objects), surface dyslexia and/or dysgraphia, intact repetition, and intact motoric and grammatical speech production (Gorno-Tempini et al., 2011).

Individuals with svPPA typically present with profound naming impairment seen during confrontation naming and spontaneous spoken or written language tasks. Naming impairments can be present in all word classes, but nouns are most prominently impacted (Riello et al., 2018). Generally, less-frequent words tend to be affected earlier (Lambon Ralph et al., 2011). The loss of semantic information for a given word or concept is gradual, usually initially presenting as difficulty retrieving the label in naming or discourse, but still recognized as the correct label when supplied. Over time, further degradation of semantic information is associated with other deficits in object recognition (e.g., recognizing label, describing function) and spelling (Lambon Ralph et al., 2011; Neophytou et al., 2019). Progression is marked by the degradation of semantic concepts and increasing degradation of multimodal representation of those concepts. Language impairments may progress to include an increasing number of phonological paraphasias and neologisms (Dalton et al., 2018) as well as other cognitive and/or behavioral symptoms (e.g., rigidity, apathy, disinhibition, compulsivity, prosopagnosia, and loss of empathy) that reflect the progression of atrophy (Pressman & Miller, 2014). The case below illustrates some of the language and behavioral symptoms that may be observed in individuals with svPPA.

The Case of Mr. Damien

History and Chart Review: Mr. Damien's family noticed a slow onset of communication difficulties approximately 2 years prior to our assessment. Approximately 6 months before our assessment, he was seen by the neurologist, who ordered an MRI and referred him for a cognitive-linguistic evaluation. When the SLP asked Mr. Damien why he had an MRI of his brain, he reported that it was for general screening purposes since he is in his mid-50s. This lack of insight into the reported difficulties (as also reported by his wife) is not uncommon for individuals with svPPA, especially in the earliest stages.

Mr. Damien was accompanied to the evaluation by his wife. During the preassessment interview, Mrs. Damien reported that her husband has difficulty *"remembering basic words."* She also reported difficulty with short-term memory and recounted a conversation where she asked Mr. Damien to fix a casserole for dinner. He went to make a note in his notepad and asked, *"What did you say you wanted me to do?"* Finally, Mrs. Damien reported that her husband uses the word *component* frequently when he cannot access the word he wants. When Mr. Damien was asked by the SLP if he had any trouble communicating, his response was, *"Well it depends on who you're talking to. Everyone has different expectations for everything . . ."*

Following extensive cognitive-linguistic testing, findings showed that Mr. Damien's test results and reported history were most consistent with a diagnosis of semantic variant PPA (svPPA). He presented with a severe spoken naming impairment, particularly when compared to relative sparing of other language domains. He demonstrated impaired single-word comprehension, object knowledge, surface alexia and agraphia, and spared repetition and motor speech abilities.

Mr. Damien completed several discourse tasks. Outlined below is his Broken Window picture sequence description. The Broken Window stimulus has eight main concepts and 24 CoreLex items, including 11 content (noun, verb, adjective, adverb) and 13 function words (e.g., auxiliary verb, preposition, conjunction). When asked to tell the Broken Window story, he said (MC, **CoreLex**):

> *"**He** looks like he's kidding, **kicking the** thing but I don't see other team members around there so I think he's doing **it** solo **out** on the middle of **a** meadow or something. That **looks** like maybe it went **through** the **window into** the house. **And** that looks like maybe his father or his brother is catching it there. Look like it **broke** through the window. And that's coincidental because that's what [name] did."*

Mr. Damien attempted 4/8 main concepts (MCs). Three concepts were accurate/complete, where all essential elements were produced correctly. The first concept was accurate/incomplete—"the thing" was too vague to receive credit for a production of "the ball." He produced 14/24 CoreLex items. While his sample included a high proportion of functors and light verbs, Mr. Damien produced some nouns and verbs specific to this task (e.g., *kick, broke, father, window*).

During the discourse tasks and in conversation, Mr. Damien displayed many of the characteristics of an individual with svPPA. He used (and was overreliant on) vague vocabulary. For example, despite the question or topic, he frequently used the terms *party people, the basics, components,* and *technology.* He demonstrated impaired word finding, particularly for nouns, as evidenced by CoreLex for the task above (consistent with his picture-naming performance). These features highlight the decline in semantic knowledge and subsequent reliance on more familiar and high-frequency vocabulary. Generally, Mr. Damien spoke in complete, grammatically well-formed sentences despite the lack of content. He often produced off-topic statements or asides, which may again reflect his overreliance on vague, high-frequency vocabulary and/or problems with working memory or sustained attention. Finally, Mr. Damien demonstrated a lack of insight into his communication difficulties; for example, failing to connect his neuroimaging results to communication partners' complaints and equivocating about whether he experienced communication difficulties.

Nonfluent/Agrammatic Variant PPA

The diagnostic criteria for nonfluent/agrammatic variant PPA (nfvPPA) are described in Box 13–2. Future research and clinical observation will shed light on the classification of PPA involving agrammatism, apraxia of speech (AOS), and/or dysarthria.

Here we use international consensus criteria, in which nfvPPA is a single condition with varying presentations.

> ### BOX 13–2. Diagnostic Criteria for Nonfluent/Agrammatic Variant PPA (nfvPPA)
>
> Diagnosis of nfvPPA requires at least one core feature: inconsistent speech sound errors and/or agrammatism in spoken language production. At least two supporting features are required, which could include impaired comprehension of grammatically complex sentences, spared single-word comprehension, and spared object knowledge (Gorno-Tempini et al., 2011). Since only one core feature (plus two supporting features) is required, initial presentation and progression of nfvPPA varies widely. Further, some clinicians and researchers consider cases that present with only one core feature as separate conditions.

Features of agrammatism include syntactic difficulties in production and comprehension, which are critical for adequate discourse superstructure. Agrammatism can impact completeness and/or accuracy of discourse (e.g., omission of verbs or copulas, omission/accuracy of pronouns, omission of a negative marker) as well as production of typical vocabulary, especially for closed-class words. When motor speech involvement is present, features of AOS are common, including distortions, irregular prosody, segmentation or increasing errors in multisyllabic words, substitutions, ommissions, and additions. AOS may negatively impact efficiency of discourse production (e.g., slowed speaking rate, increased pause length, multiple attempts at self-correction), but may not impact accuracy and completeness.

Dysarthric symptoms are less frequently observed in nfvPPA and are characterized by more consistent errors (unless there is significant spasticity). Breathiness or harsh vocal quality, poor air maintenance during speech production, and imprecise articulation can be seen, consistent with spastic, hypokinetic, or mixed dysarthria (Duffy et al., 2014). Yes/no confusion and Parkinsonism are also common difficulties that can develop alongside nfvPPA symptoms.

Two Presentations of nfvPPA

Discourse measures in nfvPPA can be affected both from a linguistic (aphasia, agrammatism) and/or motoric (AOS, dysarthria) impairment. The cases of Mrs. Jackson and Mr. Michael elucidate this variability.

The Case of Mrs. Jackson

At the time of her referral, Mrs. Jackson had been diagnosed with nfvPPA by her treating neurologist. Her speech production was slow, deliberate, aprosodic, and segmented, especially for multisyllabic words. Her sentences were complete and grammatical. Three years later, however, her speech pro-

duction was more significantly impacted, resulting in an increased number and duration of pauses, aprosodia, and further reduction in speaking rate and intelligibility. Despite these speech production difficulties, she still conveyed her narrative in complete sentences, but with simplified and nonvarying syntax.

The Case of Mr. Michael

Mr. Michael first noticed difficulty keeping time with faster-paced songs in his choir. Two years after these initial observations, Mr. Michael sought a comprehensive evaluation from our team. At this time, he presented with a markedly reduced speaking rate, agrammatism in spoken and written productions (e.g., missing functor and plural markings, switching verb tenses), and speech-sound errors consistent with moderate AOS (e.g., slow, effortful speech with inconsistent errors).

Comparison

While the linguistic content of Mrs. Jackson's message did not change drastically over time, her efficiency declined substantially, consistent with a significant increase in apraxia severity and relatively preserved language (Table 13–1). In contrast, while

Table 13–1. Mrs. Jackson and Mr. Michael's CoreLex and MCA Performance on the Broken Window Task

Broken Window	Jackson (nfvPPA— AOS only)		Michael (nfvPPA— agrammatism + AOS)
	Year 1	Year 3	Year 1
MC Composite (max = 24)	12	15	8
MC Attempts (max = 8)	4	5	3
MCA AC/min	10	3.8	3.8
CoreLex Score (max = 24)	18	19	9
CoreLex/min	45	14.6	16.9

Mr. Michael's efficiency at his initial visit was comparable to Mrs. Jackson's efficiency at her third visit, Mr. Michael was also less informative (as measured by MCA and CoreLex). This observation coincided with his agrammatism, which Mrs. Jackson did not demonstrate. MCA and CoreLex may be more vulnerable to changes in grammatical ability because of their inclusion of grammatical morphemes (CoreLex) and focus on the verb and its constituent arguments (MCA).

Logopenic Variant PPA

The diagnostic criteria for logopenic variant PPA (lvPPA) are described in Box 13–3.

BOX 13–3. Diagnostic Criteria for Logopenic Variant PPA (lvPPA)

Diagnosis of lvPPA requires both core features: impaired single-word lexical retrieval in confrontation naming or spontaneous spoken language; and impaired repetition of phrases and sentences (Gorno-Tempini et al., 2011). At least three supporting features are required, which could include phonological errors in naming and/or spontaneous spoken language, intact motor speech abilities, intact grammatical abilities, and intact single-word comprehension and object knowledge.

The primary underlying difficulty associated with lvPPA is impaired phonological processing in speaking (e.g., phonological paraphasias) or writing (e.g., spelling difficulty), as well as phonological loop or verbal working memory impairment (e.g., difficulty repeating phrases and sentences) (Gorno-Tempini et al., 2011). As these difficulties progress, lexical retrieval becomes increasingly difficult, especially in time-bound contexts (i.e., discourse) and with increasing disruption to confrontation naming. Additionally, the capacity for remembering and/or manipulating phonological information decreases, resulting in repetition impairment in shorter phrases or even difficulty repeating multisyllabic words. This diminishing capacity for processing phonological information can eventually lead to comprehension difficulties, especially for longer or more complex sentences (e.g., passive or object cleft sentences) (Gorno-Tempini et al., 2008).

During periods of lexical search, speakers with lvPPA may use a number of strategies to help them grasp the threads of their intended message. Over time, strategies such as circumlocution may become less effective in retrieving the intended word because speakers may get lost in their own attempts at self-cueing, resulting in unrelated comments or abandoned utterances. Fluency may vary, with some speakers displaying frequent word finding that reduces fluency and others exhibiting almost hyperfluent productions (e.g., logorrhea) due to circumlocution (Faroqi-Shah et al., 2020; Wilson et al., 2010).

The Case of Mr. Park

History and Chart Review: Mr. Park first noticed word-finding difficulty in conversation. Two years after he first noticed these difficulties, he sought out a neurological examination. The neurologist noted cerebral atrophy, ischemic demyelination, generalized volume loss with gliosis and encephalomalacia in left parietal and frontal lobes, and evidence of iron deposits in the same regions extending posteriorly. During behavioral tasks, the neurologist noted primary difficulties with language and referred Mr. Park to us for evaluation.

Results and Recommendations: Our initial evaluation 6 months after the neurologist's visit confirmed the reported difficulties and revealed additional concerns. Mr. Park demonstrated impaired phoneme blending and replacement; repetition of long, nonmeaningful sentences; and reading of nonwords. Compared to performance on language tasks, cognitive tasks were relatively intact. His pattern of strengths and weaknesses best aligned with a diagnosis of lvPPA.

Longitudinal Tracking: Over the next several years, Mr. Park participated in research assessments every 6 to 12 months, all of which included discourse sampling. We use Broken Window picture sequence description to highlight patterns in discourse performance over time. Figures 13–1A and 13–1B show his scores and percentile ranks at each assessment.

At the time of diagnosis, Mr. Park's spoken discourse was relatively intact (MCs, **CoreLex**):

> *"Okay so **a boy is he** is **out** uh **kicking** a um **soccer ball**. **And** that soccer ball **goes** right **through** somebody's **window** and **it** comes **in** into this guy's **window**. **Looks** like he's **sitting** down and um **the** the ball not only comes in, but knocks **over** a lamp. And he was probably sitting there watching television or something like that. Then he picks **up** the ball and he looks out the window to see who throw that ball through his window."*

Eight months later, Mr. Park's performance had deteriorated substantially. More than half of the omitted CoreLex items were content words, reflecting the typical word-finding deficits observed in individuals with lvPPA. For most of the 8 months between

diagnosis and this assessment, Mr. Park participated in a phonological treatment focused on improving spelling, which was causing significant disruptions to everyday life. While he showed a marked therapy response and reported finding it useful, this therapy did not result in discourse maintenance or improvement.

Approximately 1.5 years after diagnosis, Mr. Park's performance stayed relatively stable. More than half of the omitted CoreLex items were content words. In the months before this assessment, Mr. Park participated in phonological components analysis therapy in a group setting with other individuals with PPA. Mr. Park showed good response to the intervention, which was reflected in his picture naming and maintenance of discourse performance. At this time, he produced the following:

> *"Okay. Alright so this **boy is kicking** a soccer barl ball. **And** uh **he** kicks **it** through the neighbor's **window**. **Goes** right **in** there. And then it comes in and here's the guy. I don't know maybe that's his father. Could be someone else, whatever. But anyway it has come through. And he sees it okay. And then he sees the big hole and he's standing **up**. And he's got the ball. And you don't know what he's going **to** do with it. I don't xxx."*

Two years after diagnosis, Mr. Park's performance was maintained or improved compared to 8 months after diagnosis. Prior to this assessment, Mr. Park participated in group script-training therapy where participants developed and practiced personally relevant, meaningful scripts (Hubbard et al., 2020). The VISTA hierarchy (Henry et al., 2018) was adapted for use in a group setting because it includes activities intended to facilitate generalization to conversation. Mr. Park showed good response

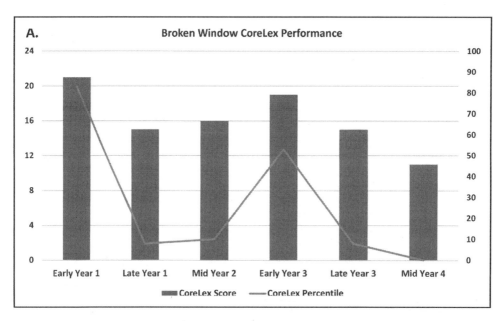

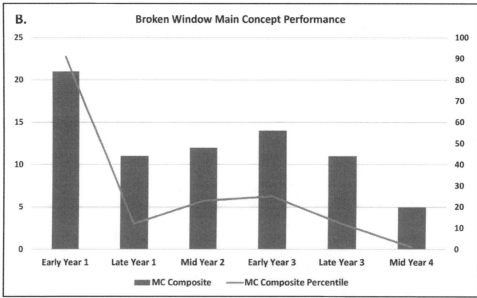

Figure 13–1. Mr. Park's discourse performance on the Broken Window task is tracked over time for (A) CoreLex score and percentile rank and (B) MC composite score and percentile rank.

to the intervention, reflected in his performance on script-related measures and discourse performance. In contrast to previous assessments, more CoreLex function words than content words were omitted, perhaps reflecting treatment gains.

Two and a half years after diagnosis, Mr. Park's performance once again declined, not unexpectedly given the progressive neurodegenerative nature of PPA. While his numerical performance was similar to performance 8 months after diagnosis, he omitted far more content words than function words, including words that are critical for communicating the idea of the story. Although still attending group script training, rapid decline across domains was observed, including significant impairments in procedural memory (no longer consistently recognizing eating utensils and consuming nonfood/nonedible items on multiple occasions) and significant weight loss (secondary to increased falls, insomnia, and gastrointestinal issues). At this time, he also became unable to engage in important recreational activities due to safety concerns. However, executive function and general orientation remained relatively intact.

At the final assessment 3 years after diagnosis, Mr. Park's performance continued to decline, although he remained capable of consenting to and enthusiastic about participating in clinical research. He continued to omit most content words and demonstrated increased difficulty producing function words. In response to the Broken Window stimulus, he said:

> "Okay. So here's _here's this_ **boy**. Okay. **And** right there _he was_ **kicked** this thing. Alright. I can't get exactly what _it_ says there but that's what it is okay. Alright so **the** next thing because he had _he had kicked this thing alright_. And it **went** down there. Okay. And that was that was . . . Well _this person here you know is living_ **in** _the next place alright_. The the that thing came right here into it. Alright it went there. Okay and he saw the c— it it went right **through** there. Okay. Alright so that's the end **of** it."

In summary, Mr. Park showed significant deterioration in discourse, moderated by speech-language therapy, until neurodegeneration and behavioral symptoms became widespread. While Mr. Park demonstrated improvements in trained behaviors following therapy, only those designed to improve verbal production corresponded to discourse maintenance or improvement. Both MCA and CoreLex tracked Mr. Park's language performance. There was a general tendency for higher scores on MC composite than CoreLex. MCA allows for greater variation in production since the goal is to measure how well the gist of the story is produced. In contrast, CoreLex measures the typicality of vocabulary use, and only the specific CoreLex items are correct. CoreLex may better track the primary lexical retrieval deficits experienced by individuals with lvPPA.

Clinical Implication of Discourse Analysis in PPA

Differential Diagnosis

Discourse analysis is a beneficial addition to diagnosis of PPA since individuals often report initial problems with discourse, sometimes years before seeking an evaluation. Discourse may also prove useful for differential diagnosis of PPA variants (e.g., Faroqi-Shah et al., 2020). However, at present, there is insufficient data to draw direct relationships between discourse performance and PPA variant. Indeed, some discourse findings may not align with the international consensus diagnostic criteria. For example, individuals with svPPA may produce phonological paraphasias at higher-than-reported rates during discourse production (see Dalton et al., 2018). This was observed in Mr. Damien's case (produced _kidding_ for _kicking_).

Diagnosis of PPA variants is most challenging in the initial and end clinical stages of the syndrome. In the initial clinical stage, the unique language impairments of each variant may only be observed during challenging, highly decontextualized language tasks (e.g., diadochokinetic rate, complex syntax comprehension, phoneme manipulation). Individuals with initial clinical stage PPA show variable performance on discourse measures, and the subtle changes observed may not be sufficient to differentially diagnose variants in isolation; additional assessments may be required. However, it is important to note that even if discourse is not obviously impaired, performance may represent a significant change from the individual's baseline, and monitoring discourse performance during this period may prove useful. Relatedly, in late clinical stages, language impairments are severe and co-occur with substantial cognitive impairments, making standardized discourse and classic language assessments challenging. In later clinical stages, discourse assessment may not provide actionable information for treatment planning.

Clinicians should expect reduced word finding at semi-spontaneous language and conversational levels of discourse (Ash et al., 2019; Dalton, Hubbard, et al., 2020). Generally, nfvPPA may be more distinguishable from lvPPA and svPPA due to reduced fluency and syntactic impairments (Faroqi-Shah et al., 2020). However, nfvPPA with a motor presentation may be harder to distinguish from lvPPA as they share overt behavioral features (e.g., phonological/phonemic errors) that arise from different underlying damage (e.g., phonological impairment versus motor planning/execution impairment). Individuals with nfvPPA may be relatively protected from loss of informativeness, especially when presenting with primary motor speech impairment, though efficiency may be more impacted (e.g., Mrs. Jackson). This contrasts with individuals with svPPA, who are more likely to demonstrate impaired content with spared function-word production (e.g., Mr. Damien).

Monitoring Change Over Time

Given the heterogeneity of clinical presentations, especially in the middle clinical stages of progression, it is not surprising that there is little published evidence documenting the gradual decline of discourse performance in PPA. Most investigators instead seek to establish the features of discourse impairments within each variant or to differentiate among variants, to aid in differential diagnosis. As a result, few studies document the longitudinal changes exhibited in discourse within each variant.

Thompson and colleagues (1997) are perhaps the first to report this type of longitudinal data in a small cohort of individuals with nfvPPA (note that this was prior to consensus diagnostic criteria; some of the individual descriptions more closely resemble present-day lvPPA than nfvPPA). Similarly, Hilger and colleagues (2014) reported a longitudinal case study of an individual with lvPPA over the course of 2 years. Most recently, changes in connected spoken-language performance in all three variants were evaluated (Ash et al., 2019). While these studies investigated speech and language performance in discourse, all measures used were microlinguistic in nature, spanning phonology (e.g., number of uncorrected sound errors), morphology (e.g., verb morphology index), semantics (e.g., semantic paraphasias), and syntax (e.g., percentage grammatically complete sentences produced).

While the microlinguistic measures reported in these studies were sensitive to changes over time, the use of only microlinguistic measures limits our understanding of how changes contribute to the overall quality or functionality of the discourse.

Microlinguistic measures cannot speak to issues such as essential content, organization, and coherence, which impact successful communication of a message and are more reliant on cognitive abilities. Further research is desperately needed to examine macrolinguistic and superstructural discourse measures such as cohesion, local and/or global coherence, MCA, MSSG, story grammar, and sequencing that may better relate to functional communication. However, we recognize that applying macrolinguistic and superstructural measures in clinical settings can be challenging. We focused on CoreLex and MCA in this chapter in part because these measures are designed to be clinically feasible. They are checklist based, have published norms and freely available training materials, and have web-based apps for scoring that are in the final stages of development (Cavanaugh, Dalton, et al., 2021; Cavanaugh, Richardson, et al. 2021). However, we encourage the use of multidimensional discourse analysis using the most appropriate measures for a given individual. As discourse continues to emerge as a critical dimension with which to measure communication abilities and treatment outcomes, we expect future studies will present detailed data on longitudinal discourse abilities at microlinguistic, macrolinguistic, and superstructural levels in all variants.

Assessing Treatment Response

Most PPA treatment research has focused on single-word retrieval, with generally positive outcomes and some generalization and/or maintenance of gains (e.g., Croot, 2018). Studies investigating augmentative alternative communication (Mooney et al., 2018), reading (Henry et al., 2013; Rogalski & Edmonds, 2007), script training (Henry et al., 2018; Hubbard et al., 2020), spelling

(Tsapkini & Hillis, 2013), and verb retrieval in sentences (Schneider et al., 1996) have been reported. Direct treatment of discourse in PPA has only been investigated using NARNIA, a metalinguistic treatment that trains a framework for narrative discourse (Whitworth et al., 2018). Discourse has been investigated as a direct outcome of treatment in only a few studies (e.g., Dalton, Hubbard, et al., 2020; Kim, 2017), although there is an increasing trend to include discourse outcomes. Mr. Park's case highlights the potential benefits of measuring discourse in addition to more direct treatment outcomes since effective therapy response was realized even as Mr. Park's discourse continued to decline.

Planning Ahead

Despite the broad clinical presentations that are possible among PPA variants, there is unfortunately a commonality in the progression of each case. Ultimately, each variant leads to mutism and global cognitive impairment as demonstrated by Mr. Park. Therefore, no discussion of PPA can conclude before discussing how best to plan for future decline. Maintaining functional communication for as long as possible is the ultimate clinical goal and has the largest potential impact on quality of life. With planning, steps can be taken to help foster functional communication as long as possible. Initial planning may include narrative treatment approaches (e.g., Whitworth et al., 2018), script training (e.g., Henry et al., 2018), alternative augmentative communication strategies (e.g., Beukelman et al., 2007; Cadório et al., 2021; Cress & King, 1999; King et al., 2007; Mooney et al., 2018; Rogers et al., 2000), and voice banking. These techniques may be especially beneficial in the early to middle clinical stages when it is possible to capitalize on preserved function and work on maintenance of narrative skills.

However, it can be difficult to gain clients' buy-in for voice banking or alternative augmentative communication (AAC) when they are still able to communicate verbally. As a result, this topic must be broached sensitively with supporting client and caregiver education. The timing of such discussions may need to wait until the client and their family have reached some degree of acceptance of the diagnosis, which may differ dramatically across individuals. But, with no disease-altering medical treatments available at present for the underlying neuropathological processes, it is critical that we prepare our clients and their families to be successful in communication. AAC, story banking, and voice banking may allow individuals with PPA to speak with their own voice and to tell stories in their own words, even when they are no longer able to do so independently.

Challenges and Barriers to Clinical Implementation of Discourse Assessment in PPA

We recognize that for many clinicians, discourse analysis may be difficult to implement in practice. The barriers clinicians experience are well described in the stroke-induced aphasia literature and include the time needed to transcribe and analyze discourse, lack of training resources for implementing specific measures, the huge number of measures published in the literature, and the lack of adequate psychometric data (Bryant et al., 2017; Pritchard et al., 2018; see also Chapters 5 and 6). In addition to these challenges, clinicians working with individuals with PPA may experience unique

barriers, such as difficulty interpreting and applying results given limited research, the variability in presenting characteristics of discourse impairments across individuals, effects of treatment on performance, and lack of research into how discourse measures are related to quality of life, among several other important considerations. These challenges are further magnified by the importance of getting it right the first time for individuals with a progressive neurodegenerative disease.

Summary

The growing work of recognizing, diagnosing, and treating PPA has led to an explosion of research articles and an emerging understanding of its variants. Just as in stroke-induced aphasia, the increasing emphasis on discourse analysis as a reliable, informative tool and target for treatment is critical for providing care that meets the desires of individuals with PPA and their loved ones. As measures improve and task demands are reduced through faster transcription methods or transcriptionless analysis, discourse assessment and analysis are becoming more clinically feasible. Further research is warranted, especially focusing on macrolinguistic and superstructural aspects of discourse that may better reflect functional communication abilities and identifying longitudinal patterns of change in relation to participation and function among persons living with PPA.

References

Ash, S., Nevler, N., Phillips, J., Irwin, D. J., McMillan, C. T., Rascovsky, K., & Grossman, M.

(2019). A longitudinal study of speech production in primary progressive aphasia and behavioral variant frontotemporal dementia. *Brain and Language, 194*(4), 46–57. https://doi.org/10.1016/j.bandl.2019.04.006

Bergeron, D., Gorno-Tempini, M. L., Rabinovici, G. D., Santos-Santos, M. A., Seeley, W., Miller, B. L., . . . Ossenkoppele, R. (2018). Prevalence of amyloid-β pathology in distinct variants of primary progressive aphasia. *Annals of Neurology, 84*(5), 729–740. https://doi.org/10.1002/ana.25333

Beukelman, D. R., Fager, S., Ball, L., & Dietz, A. (2007). AAC for adults with acquired neurological conditions: A review. *Augmentative and Alternative Communication, 23*(3), 230–242. https://doi.org/10.1080/07434610701553668

Bryant, L., Ferguson, A., & Spencer, E. (2016). Linguistic analysis of discourse in aphasia: A review of the literature. *Clinical Linguistics and Phonetics, 30*(7), 489–518. https://doi.org/10.3109/02699206.2016.1145740

Bryant, L., Spencer, E., & Ferguson, A. (2017). Clinical use of linguistic discourse analysis for the assessment of language in aphasia. *Aphasiology, 31*(10), 1105–1126. https://doi.org/10.1080/02687038.2016.1239013

Cadório, I., Figueiredo, D., Martins, P., Cardoso, R., Santos, J., & Lousada, M. (2021). Combined restorative and compensatory treatment for primary progressive aphasia: A case report. *Aphasiology, 35*(2), 222–239. https://doi.org/10.1080/02687038.2019.1687842

Cavanaugh, R., Dalton, S. G., & Richardson, J. (2021). *CoreLexicon: An open-source web app for scoring core lexicon analysis.* R package version 0.0.1.0000. https://github.com/aphasia-apps/coreLexicon

Cavanaugh, R., Richardson, J., & Dalton, S. G. (2021). *Main Concept: An open-source web app for scoring main concept analysis.* R package version 0.0.1.0000. https://github.com/aphasia-apps/mainConcept

Chandregowda, A. (2020). Incidental diagnosis of primary progressive aphasia in the inpatient setting: A note to raise clinical awareness. *Perspectives of the ASHA Special Interest Groups, 5*(6), 1422–1426. https://doi.org/10.1044/2020_PERSP-20-00103

Cress, C., & King, J. (1999). AAC strategies for people with primary progressive aphasia without dementia: Two case studies. *Augmentative and Alternative Communication, 15*(4), 248–259. https://doi.org/10.1080/07434619912331278785

Croot, K. (2018). Treatment for lexical retrieval impairments in primary progressive aphasia: A research update with implications for clinical practice. *Seminars in Speech and Language, 39*(03), 242–256. https://doi.org/10.1055/s-0038-1660783

Dalton, S. G. H., Hubbard, H. I., & Richardson, J. D. (2020). Moving toward non-transcription-based discourse analysis in stable and progressive aphasia. *Seminars in Speech and Language, 41*(1), 32–44. https://doi.org/10.1055/s-0039-3400990

Dalton, S. G. H., Kim, H., Richardson, J. D., & Wright, H. H. (2020). A compendium of core lexicon checklists. *Seminars in Speech and Language, 41*(1), 45–60. https://doi.org/10.1055/s-0039-3400972

Dalton, S. G. H., Shultz, C., Henry, M. L., Hillis, A. E., & Richardson, J. D. (2018). Describing phonological paraphasias in three variants of primary progressive aphasia. *American Journal of Speech-Language Pathology, 27*(1S), 336–349. https://doi.org/10.1044/2017_AJSLP-16-0210

Duffy, J. R., Strand, E. A., & Josephs, K. A. (2014). Motor speech disorders associated with primary progressive aphasia. *Aphasiology, 28*(8–9), 1004–1017. https://doi.org/10.1080/02687038.2013.869307

Faroqi-Shah, Y., Treanor, A., Ratner, N. B., Ficek, B., Webster, K., & Tsapkini, K. (2020). Using narratives in differential diagnosis of neurodegenerative syndromes. *Journal of Communication Disorders, 85*, 105994. https://doi.org/10.1016/j.jcomdis.2020.105994

Gorno-Tempini, M. L., Brambati, S. M., Ginex, V., Ogar, J., Dronkers, N. F., Marcone, A., . . . Miller, B. L. (2008). The logopenic/phonological variant of primary progressive aphasia. *Neurology, 71*(16), 1227–1212. https://doi.org/10.1212/01.wnl.0000320506.79811.da

Gorno-Tempini, M. L., Hillis, A. E., Weintraub, S., Kertesz, A., Mendez, M., Cappa, S. F., . . .

Grossman, M. (2011). Classification of primary progressive aphasia and its variants. *Neurology*, *76*(11), 1006–1014. https://doi.org/10.1212/WNL.0b013e31821103e6

Greenslade, K. J., Stuart, J. E., Richardson, J. D., Dalton, S. G., & Ramage, A. E. (2020). Macrostructural analyses of *Cinderella* narratives in a large nonclinical sample. *American Journal of Speech-Language Pathology*, *29*(4), 1923–1936. https://doi.org/10.1044/2020_AJSLP-19-00151

Grossman, M. (2010). Primary progressive aphasia: Clinicopathological correlations. *Nature Reviews Neurology*, *6*(2), 88–97. https://doi.org/10.1038/nrneurol.2009.216

Henry, M. L., Hubbard, H. I., Grasso, S. M., Dial, H. R., Beeson, P. M., Miller, B. L., & Gorno-Tempini, M. L. (2019). Treatment for word retrieval in semantic and logopenic variants of primary progressive aphasia: Immediate and long-term outcomes. *Journal of Speech, Language, and Hearing Research*, *62*(8), 2723–2749. https://doi.org/10.1044/2018_JSLHR-L-18-0144

Henry, M. L., Hubbard, H. I., Grasso, S. M., Mandelli, M. L., Wilson, S. M., Sathishkumar, M. T . . . Gorno-Tempini, M. L. (2018). Retraining speech production and fluency in non-fluent/agrammatic primary progressive aphasia. *Brain*, *141*(6), 1799–1814. https://doi.org/10.1093/brain/awy101

Henry, M. L., Meese, M. V., Truong, S., Babiak, M. C., Miller, B. L., & Gorno-Tempini, M. L. (2013). Treatment for apraxia of speech in nonfluent variant primary progressive aphasia. *Behavioral Neurology*, *26*(1, 2), 77–88. https://doi.org/10.3233/BEN-2012-120260

Hilger, A., Ramsberger, G., Gilley, P., Menn, L., & Kong, A. (2014). Analyzing speech problems in a longitudinal case study of logopenic variant PPA. *Aphasiology*, *28*(7), 840–861. https://doi.org/10.1080/02687038.2014.895974

Hubbard, H. I., Nelson, L. A., & Richardson, J. D. (2020). Can script training improve narrative and conversation in aphasia across etiology? *Seminars in Speech and Language*, *41*(1), 99–124. https://doi.org/10.1055/s-0039-3401030

Kim, M., (2017). Effect of lexical retrieval cascade treatment on naming and discourse of individuals with logopenic variant of primary

progressive aphasia (lvPPA). *Clinical Archives of Communication Disorders*, *2*(3), 197–208. https://doi.org/10.21849/cacd.2017.00171

King J., Alarcon N., & Rogers M. (2007). Primary progressive aphasia. In D. Beukelman, K. Garrett, & K. Yorkston (Eds.), *Augmentative communication strategies for adults with acute or chronic medical conditions* (pp. 207–242). Brookes.

Kong, A. P. H. (2009). The use of main concept analysis to measure discourse production in Cantonese-speaking persons with aphasia: A preliminary report. *Journal of Communication Disorders*, *42*(6), 442–464. https://doi.org/10.1016/j.jcomdis.2009.06.002

Lambon-Ralph, M. A., Sage, K., Heredia, C. G., Berthier, M. L., Martínez-Cuitiño, M., Torralva, T., . . . Patterson, K. (2011). El-La: The impact of degraded semantic representations on knowledge of grammatical gender in semantic dementia. *Acta Neuropsychologica*, *9*(2), 115–131. http://1035.indexcopernicus.com/fulltxt.php?ICID=969706

Mooney, A., Bedrick, S., Noethe, G., Spaulding, S., & Fried-Oken, M. (2018). Mobile technology to support lexical retrieval during activity retell in primary progressive aphasia. *Aphasiology*, *32*(6), 666–692. https://doi.org/10.1080/02687038.2018.1447640

Neophytou, K., Wiley, R. W., Rapp, B., & Tsapkini, K. (2019). The use of spelling for variant classification in primary progressive aphasia: Theoretical and practical implications. *Neuropsychologia*, *133*, 107157. https://doi.org/10.1016/j.neuropsychologia.2019.107157

Nicholas, L. E., & Brookshire, R. H. (1995). Presence, completeness, and accuracy of main concepts in the connected speech of non-brain-damaged adults and adults with aphasia. *Journal of Speech, Language, and Hearing Research*, *38*(1), 145–156. https://doi.org/10.1044/jshr.3801.145

Pressman, P. S., & Miller, B. L. (2014). Diagnosis and management of behavioral variant frontotemporal dementia. *Biological Psychiatry*, *75*(7), 574–581. https://doi.org/10.1016/j.biopsych.2013.11.006

Pritchard, M., Hilari, K., Cocks, N., & Dipper, L. (2018). Psychometric properties of discourse measures in aphasia: Acceptability, reliability, and validity. *International Journal of Language and Communication Disorders, 53*(6), 1078–1093. https://doi.org/10.1111/1460-6984.12420

Richardson, J. D., & Dalton, S. G. (2016). Main concepts for three different discourse tasks in a large non-clinical sample. *Aphasiology, 30*(1), 45–73. https://doi.org/10.1080/02687038.2015.1057891

Richardson, J. D., Dalton, S. G., Greenslade, K. J., Jacks, A., Haley, K. L., & Adams, J. (2021). Main concept, sequencing, and story grammar analyses of *Cinderella* narratives in a large sample of persons with aphasia. *Brain Sciences, 11*(1), 110. https://doi.org/10.3390/brainsci11010110

Riello, M., Faria, A. V., Ficek, B., Webster, K., Onyike, C. U., Desmond, J., . . . Tsapkini, K. (2018). The role of language severity and education in explaining performance on object and action naming in primary progressive aphasia. *Frontiers in Aging Neuroscience, 10*, 346. https://doi.org/10.3389/fnagi.2018.00346

Rogalski, Y., & Edmonds, L. A. (2008). Attentive Reading and Constrained Summarization (ARCS) treatment in primary progressive aphasia: A case study. *Aphasiology, 22*(7–8), 763–775. https://doi.org/10.1080/02687030701803796

Rogers, M., King, J., & Alarcon, N. (2000). Proactive management of primary progressive aphasia. In D. Beukelman, K. Yorkston, & J. Reichle (Eds.), *Augmentative and alternative communication for adults with acquired neurological disorders* (pp. 305–337). Brookes.

Ruggero, L., Croot, K., & Nickels, L. (2020). How evidence-based practice (E3BP) informs speech-language pathology for primary progressive aphasia. *American Journal of Alzheimer's Disease and Other Dementias, 35*, 1–8. https://doi.org/10.1177/1533317520915365

Schneider, S. L., Thompson, C. K., & Luring, B. (1996). Effects of verbal plus gestural matrix training on sentence production in a patient with primary progressive aphasia. *Aphasiology, 10*(3), 297–317. https://doi.org/10.1080/02687039608248414

Thompson, C. K., Ballard, K. J., Tait, M. E., Weintraub, S., & Mesulam, M. (1997). Patterns of language decline in non-fluent primary progressive aphasia. *Aphasiology, 11*(4–5), 297–321. https://doi.org/10.1080/02687039708248473

Tsapkini, K., & Hillis, A. E. (2013). Spelling intervention in poststroke aphasia and primary progressive aphasia. *Behavioral Neurology, 26*(1, 2), 55–66. https://doi.org/10.3233/BEN-2012-110240

Whitworth, A., Cartwright, J., Beales, A., Leitão, S., Panegyres, P. K., & Kane, R. (2018). Taking words to a new level: A preliminary investigation of discourse intervention in primary progressive aphasia. *Aphasiology, 32*(11), 1284–1309. https://doi.org/10.1080/02687038.2017.1390543

Wilson, S. M., Henry, M. L., Besbris, M., Ogar, J. M., Dronkers, N. F., Jarrold, W., . . . Gorno-Tempini, M. L. (2010). Connected speech production in three variants of primary progressive aphasia. *Brain, 133*(7), 2069–2088. https://doi.org/10.1093/brain/awq129

14 What Discourse Analysis Reveals About Conversation and Language Processing in the Context of Dementia of the Alzheimer's Type

Jackie Guendouzi

Introduction: Discourse Analysis and Dementia

Qualitative research, particularly discourse analysis, is now widely accepted as a method of analysis in the field of communication disorders (Guendouzi, 2014). It has yielded a wealth of information that adds to the knowledge base of communication disorders. In the case of people living with dementia, discourse approaches have identified a range of sociopragmatic features that have helped both researchers and clinicians to better understand how this disease affects communication (e.g., Burshnic & Bourgeois, 2020; Davis, 2005; Davis & Maclagan, 2010, 2018; Guendouzi & Davis, 2013; Guendouzi et al., 2015; Hamilton, 1994; Orange et al., 1996; Plejert et al., 2017; Sabat, 2001; Schrauf & Müller, 2014; Shadden, 1996; Wray, 2013). For example, people with dementia of the Alzheimer's type (DAT) may exhibit the overuse of the following conversational features: formulaic language, repetitions, politeness markers, and minimal responses (Guendouzi & Müller, 2002; Guendouzi & Pate, 2014).

It is important to note that, although this chapter focuses on a case study involving a woman with a diagnosis of Alzheimer's disease, different types of dementia may affect communication in different ways. For example, frontotemporal dementia (FTD) may result in changes in impulse control or alter the person's social behaviors (Mikesell, 2014). Therefore, in addition to identifying sociopragmatic features of talk, discourse analysis also can reveal how different cognitive deficits may affect conversational patterns in various forms of dementia.

This chapter considers conversational data through the lens of psycholinguistic theories. The analysis suggests that people with DAT may express meaning through patterns of talk that are different from the structures identified through traditional discourse analysis methods (e.g., see Chapter 17). Reconsidering the ways in which we approach the analysis of discourse samples has implications for clinicians who may use these methods to assess language skills and identify conversational patterns in people with dementia. Discourse analysis (Schiffrin, 1994) and conversational analysis (Sacks et al., 1974; see also Chapter 7) are methodological tools rather than theories of language processing. Restricting our toolkit to discrete units of conversation (e.g., adjacency pairs) may limit our ability to see the larger picture that is the discourse of dementia.

Dementia and Communication Deficits

The Diagnostic and Statistical Manual of Mental Disorders (5th ed.; *DSM-5*; American Psychiatric Association, 2013) classifies dementia types under neurocognitive disorders and characterizes them as conditions that result in a decline of intellectual functioning and memory loss that impedes acts of daily living. DAT is a disease that progresses over time in stages from mild to mild-moderate, moderate-severe, and severe. However, the *DSM-5* itself differentiates neurodegenerative diseases such as dementias by classifying them as major or mild. There are a range of instruments used to assess dementia (Sheehan, 2012). These include the Alzheimer's Disease Assessment Scale–Cognitive Subscale (ADAS-Cog; Rosen et al., 1984), the Mini-Mental State Examination (MMSE; Folstein et al., 1975), and the Clinical Dementia Rating Scale (CDR-SOB; Morris, 1992). Such assessments have identified six cognitive domains that can be impaired in dementia and may

affect discourse comprehension and production. The most notable impairments are deficits in learning and memory that include problems with free recall, cued recall, object recognition, semantic and autobiographical memory, long-term memory, and implicit learning. In addition, people with dementia may have difficulty with attention, processing speed, and executive function skills that include planning, decision making, working memory, responding to feedback, inhibition, and flexibility. Deficits in perceptual-motor function can include difficulty with visual perception, visuoconstructional reasoning, and perceptual-motor coordination.

Typically, a neurologist makes the initial diagnosis of dementia; however, speech-language pathologists (SLPs) are often involved in the differential diagnosis of language skills. Deficits in language may be exhibited in the form of problems with object naming, word finding, fluency, grammar and syntax, and receptive language. It also has been suggested that social cognition (including theory of mind) may be affected (Sachdev et al., 2014). As communication skills progressively decline in the early clinical stage profile, the functional use of language, comprehension, and writing skills becomes compromised (Woodward, 2013).

Although SLPs are most familiar with tests such as the Boston Diagnostic Aphasia Examination (3rd ed.) (BDAE; Goodglass et al., 2001) or the Western Aphasia Battery–Revised (WAB-R; Kertesz, 2006), these are of limited value to the clinician when assessing people with DAT. Although these assessments may help to identify specific linguistic features such as word recall and picture description, they do not provide a clear picture of the person with dementia's ability to communicate in everyday situations. Other tests more specific to dementia are the Arizona Battery for Cognitive-Communication Disorders (2nd ed.; ABCD-2;

Bayles & Tomoeda, 2005) and the Functional Linguistic-Communication Inventory (3rd ed.) (FCLI-3; Bayles & Tomoeda, 2020). The ABCD includes a story retelling to elicit a discourse sample. Although this helps determine the ability of persons with DAT to link language cohesively in larger samples, it does not draw on the same interactional or cognitive skills needed to hold a conversation.

In the more advanced stages, people with DAT may not recognize family members, their surroundings, or the purpose of an interaction (Hassenstab et al., 2013). The person may appear mute or engage in echolalia or utter words or empty phrases that do not appear to carry meaning. Hassenstab et al. (2013) suggest that these deficits lead to an inability to convey meaning, an effect that severely limits communication between the people with DAT and their care partners. However, research suggests that lack of access to a fully functioning cognitive system can result in people with DAT using alternate ways to express themselves (Davis & Maclagan, 2013; Guendouzi & Müller, 2006).

Pragmatic disorders are communication differences that impede a person's ability to carry out satisfactory social interactions in a manner that members of a particular speech community perceive as normal. Pragmatic disorders are often viewed as an integral part of the clinical diagnosis of persons with DAT, a symptom of their condition. The reality is that pragmatic disorders emerge in interactions because of misunderstanding on the part of *all* interlocutors, both the neurotypical person and those who have a clinical label such as dementia. It is important to remember that when we approach an interaction, we do so with expectations of the pragmatic norms of our speech community. We have expectations of how conversations involving people from similar linguistic, cultural, or social backgrounds should proceed. When those expectations are not met, communication breakdowns occur.

Sherratt (2007) notes the difficulties in pinpointing "the impaired processes in any clinical population if the influence of other processes is not known" (p. 376). She also affirms the need for a multilevel approach to discourse to explore the cognitive mechanisms that support language processing structures. Without such an approach, it is difficult to begin to understand the language difficulties associated with DAT. Sherratt (2007) proposed a multilevel model of discourse processing begins with an input trigger that generates a frame or schema into which the interlocutor(s) will insert semantic information. This trigger typically takes the form of a direct request or the presentation of a visual cue (e.g., picture). However, Sherratt's model did not explore the role of given information (Halliday, 1985), nor were other preutterance cognitive mechanisms or triggers considered in her model. Her study involved use of narrative and procedural discourse samples elicited from 32 non-brain-injured adult males. These tasks do not reflect the type of discourse that emerges from conversations.

By collecting conversational samples, we can begin to recognize the patterns that emerge in the discourse of people with DAT. This chapter examines one neglected dimension of language processing—given information—and explores its role in the discourse of DAT.

Given Information

The neurotypical adult has a language processing system that supports rapid contextualization of information and other associated stimuli. This ability to process and frame interactions develops over time through repeated social interactions; it can be thought of as a process that is similar to self-learning software. Given information functions in a way like procedural memory; it is information we process rapidly and often automatically with little overt cognitive planning. It is the semantic, experiential, or contextual information shared by interlocutors that helps to establish shared mental referents to scaffold a conversation. Speakers typically expect that their interlocutors are able to recover a particular meaning based on their choice of words, grammatical structures, and shared common knowledge. Interlocutors assume that, within a specific context, participants from the same cultural and linguistic background will interpret an interaction in a distinctive way. Even in the case of an interaction with a total stranger, there are certain expectations about how such conversations might proceed. Given information can be general information that is understood by all members of a particular speech community or it might be specific information shared between friends, family, or close acquaintances. It also allows for the process of ellipsis (Leech & Short, 2007), whereby speakers can reduce redundancy in their conversational turns by omitting the need to verbally offer background information to their utterance.

For example, consider the following scenario set in a long-term care facility. A cousin of a person with DAT comes into the room to visit. The person with DAT had undergone a surgical procedure the previous day, and upon entering the room the cousin remarks, "Well, how did it go"? The pronoun *it* is an exophoric referent; it is not referencing something visible in the current situation or information that is easily recoverable from the words spoken with-

out prior knowledge. If this scenario had involved a neurotypical patient in a hospital, both participants would understand that the pronoun *it* refers to the procedure and the likely response would be "not so well" or "fine; they think it went well."

However, a person with DAT might not be able to access or activate the appropriate schema needed to interpret their cousin's request for information. The person with DAT may perceive the cousin as a stranger who seems to be asking them a personal question, and their reaction could range from anger to confusion. This type of reaction is common in the case of DAT and results in an unsatisfactory exchange for both participants. Given information is a feature of language that functions reflexively and at a lower level than higher-order language processing, but it is a key feature of social interactions.

Cognitive Structures: Scripts and Schemas

Since Bartlett (1932) originally posited his theory of schemata, there has been a great deal of debate regarding how cognitive schemas develop over time and how they interact with long-term memory to support language processing (Fillmore, 1982; Labov, 1980; Lakoff, 1987; Langacker, 2000; Minsky, 1975). However, despite the differences in theoretical approaches, most researchers accept the notion of a cognitive schema or semantic frame in some form. For further reading on this topic, Evans (2019) provides an excellent discussion of the different theoretical conceptualizations of frames and schemas.

The most easily understood description of schemas is that they are cognitive mechanisms created over time that help our brain to store, categorize, and organize information about the physical and social world around us. Schemas are thus part of the "software" structure that allows us to use our language processes more economically because we are not required to put together information in a linear unit-by-unit fashion. One of the key points of such theories is the notion of information being grouped together into categories. These categories share common or similar features such as phoneme sequences (Marslen-Wilson & Welch, 1978) or physical features such as color or shape (Rosch & Mervis, 1975). Rosch's prototype theory (1973) incorporated the idea that we store a core concept of an object or event at the center of a schema (e.g., a robin might represent a prototype in a "bird" schema). Such prototypes would not be universal because they are regionally or culturally determined. For instance, the prototypical representation of a bird is not likely to be a robin in the case of Inuit people living in the Arctic regions. Similar linguistic distinctions are discussed in Chapter 8.

Schemas help the brain to manage and organize the information that we use within our daily interactions when we encounter both new and familiar situations. As Piaget (1977) suggested, we assimilate information from new situations into the existing knowledge structures or cognitive schemas that we have stored over a lifetime. If I walk into a doctor's office, the physical environment triggers a generic schema of medical visits in my mind. This schema is triggered by all the environmental cues that I see or experience (e.g., reception desk, medical charts, nurses, doctors, thermometers, odors, uniforms).

Scripts are a specific subtype of schemas (Schank & Abelson, 1977) that refer to the expected verbal conversational features that become routinized over time and are associated with that particular schema. For example, the script associated with a medical setting schema in the U.S. includes the receptionist using interactional routines by asking how they can help me and transactional routines such as questions about my insurance coverage. I will likely respond to these questions in a predictable manner by showing my insurance card and driver's license, filling out an intake form, and paying my fee. I will then sit in a waiting room until a nurse comes to get me and carry out the initial health checks such as checking weight and blood pressure. This routine sequence of actions is accompanied by familiar utterances such as "How are you feeling today?" or "Take your jacket off so I can listen to your chest." Indeed, we may feel uncomfortable if events and conversations do not match the expectations of our established transactional and interactional routines (Brown & Yule, 1983).

Scripts, Schemas, and DAT

The contextual or conversational cues that trigger the activation of a schema or script can be highly problematic for people with DAT because they no longer remember or recognize the cues (e.g., people, environmental stimuli, or key words) that help to contextualize their daily interactions. Schemas are linked to long-term memory. They are structures of information that do not need to be newly constructed and processed online. Due to memory deficits, a person with DAT may experience difficulty accessing or activating prior knowledge and therefore may misinterpret a situation. They may not recognize information that their interlocutor may assume is given (e.g., the person's identity and reason for the interaction). If the person with dementia is unsure of a person's identity or the reason for their conversation with that person, they may become fixated on continually establishing this information. As described elsewhere (Guendouzi, 2013), people with DAT may repeatedly ask who they are talking to in an effort to establish relevance within the conversation (Wilson & Sperber, 2006).

Perseveration on establishing relevance may interfere with the interaction in two ways. First, it may interrupt the person with dementia's ability to hold current information (i.e., an interlocutor's utterance) in their working memory, thus creating a stalling effect on the conversation (Guendouzi & Savage, 2017). Second, not being able to establish contextual information that is typically *given* may have a negative effect on the interaction because the person with DAT misinterprets the situation and becomes aggressive or confused (Guendouzi et al., 2016). The result is that the interaction may break down and the interlocutors (both with and without dementia) may give up on the conversation or become confused.

Entering into both new and familiar situations becomes extremely difficult for people with DAT. The cognitive mechanisms that access the schemas that provide the given information needed to participate in everyday interactions are inconsistent. They are not intact as a whole and therefore difficult to access. An analogy that best describes the situation in dementia is to imagine that your memory and knowledge structures are stored in a manuscript. The manuscript is then tossed up into the air and all the sheets land randomly on the floor with some missing altogether. The confusion and frustration we may feel trying to put the manuscript back in a coherent order is similar to the process going on in the mind of the person with dementia, who is anxiously trying to match pieces of information to create relevance for their current interaction. This effect results in conversations that are difficult to follow and frustrating for both people with DAT and their care partners.

We present evidence from conversations between the researcher and a woman with DAT called Flo. Findings indicate that, although inconsistent, Flo's access to certain cognitive schemas was still evident within the interaction but her language processor was functioning in a less efficient manner. The analysis examines the semantic and propositional links between utterances that are not located in close proximity within the conversation.

Conversational Interactions With Flo

These data come from a corpus of conversations between the author (J. G.) and 82-year-old Flo. Flo was a homemaker all her life but engaged in some dressmaking for the family and her neighbors. Both she and her husband came from large working-class families and did not have any connection with academic careers or teaching. They owned a house on the same road as J. G., and although Flo now lived permanently in the nursing home for people with moderate to severe dementia, her husband was still a neighbor of J. G. Flo was placed in a local Catholic nursing home run by nuns who were assisted by secular nursing assistants and medical staff. J. G. was introduced to Flo as a neighbor living on the same road who worked at the university and was writing a book on older people's experiences. The information given to the author by the nursing assistants suggested that Flo could not retain new information associated with introductions to new people (e.g., details of their name, profession, or relationship to Flo). Staff also suggested that Flo was very confused and not able to sustain lengthy conversations. Although Flo often slept through visits, when awake she often managed to hold conversations with the author that lasted between 45 minutes to an hour. At times when she was tired, Flo's speech would become unintelligible or slightly slurred, and it was difficult in real time to follow what she was saying. The author relied on the audio recordings, her ethnographic field notes, and observations of nonverbal behaviors to help interpret Flo's less intelligible remarks when analyzing the data.

J. G. collected the data in weekly visits to Flo at the nursing home. The author obtained permissions from the university Institutional Research Board (IRB), Flo's family, and the nursing home's management board prior to recording. Conversations were audio recorded on a small Sony digital audio recorder placed in the researcher's handbag. The recorded data were supported by extensive ethnographic notes and interviews with staff of the nursing home. The recorder was connected to a lapel microphone on J. G.'s jacket. This gave J. G. great flexibility to move from Flo's bedroom to the lounge or outside area with no need to adjust the recorder or microphone. In the following sections the analysis will focus on the evidence for two schemas (*academic writing* and *my dementia*) that seemed to reoccur within conversations with Flo. Common transcription conventions are shown in Box 14–1.

Academic Writing Schema

J. G. entered the room and smiled at Flo, who was fiddling with a thread on her

> ### BOX 14–1. Transcription Conventions
>
> Transcription conventions were kept to a minimum for ease of reading but include the following:
>
> *Italics* = nonverbal or contextual information
>
> (.) = minimal pause
>
> (2 sec) = 2-second pause
>
> ? = indicates rising intonation associated with requests for further information
>
> : = lengthening of vowel phoneme
>
> ! = emphasis

sweater. She looked up at J. G. as she sat down beside Flo's bed.

Excerpt 1

1. J. G.: Hi, how are you today, Flo?

2. Flo: Oh the typewriter (*smiles and nods her head*)

3. J. G.: Mhm? It's noisy again (*noise of vacuuming in background*). Let me shut this, we have to wait until they finish the hoovering (*vacuuming*).

4. Flo: Pardon?

5. J. G.: (*R. notes some new items in Flo's room*) Does your husband take you to the shops?

As noted above, the staff in the nursing home often suggested that J. G. might find it difficult to have a conversation with Flo because she did not remember people. However, when reviewing lengthy exchanges in the transcripts, an interactional pattern emerged that suggested Flo had assimilated the researcher into a schema that was associated with education, books, and writing (in this case the use of the term *typewriter*). This not only provided a recognized identity for the researcher but also appeared to give Flo a context of relevance for their relationship. During the real-time conversations, J. G. did not initially notice the significance of these intermittent remarks because they randomly occurred within lengthy conversations when the researcher was attempting to pursue other topics with Flo. In Excerpt 1, J. G. did not overtly react to Flo's use of the term typewriter; instead, she commented on the noise of cleaners and asked Flo about going shopping.

The conversation then continued for another 218 turns at talk with no further mention of anything associated with writing or education until Flo looked at J. G. and asked about her "poem" (turn 219). The conversational turns prior to these utterances were about the weather, walking along the nearby riverbank, and the countryside surrounding the area. The content of the conversation leading up to the comment about the poem did not contain vocabulary that might have activated a question associated with an academic schema. On each occasion that Flo uttered comments associated with the academic writing schema, she looked directly at J. G., smiled, then nodded as if to say "we know each other." Flo's nonverbal behaviors suggested she might have felt there was some common ground between herself and the author.

The segment in Excerpt 2 occurred 15 minutes into a conversation regarding shopping in the city center and how it had changed over the past 5 years.

Excerpt 2

219. Flo: *(looks at J. G. and smiles)* And what about my poem? Has it come to a stop or *(unintelligible word possibly is it finished)* soon?

220. J. G.: Oh! It's still going *(laughs)*.

(2.5-second silence)

221. Flo: Am I in? *(smiling)*

222. J. G.: Yes, do you like poetry?

223. Flo: There's some kind of pieces (books) I like but I don't seem to be interested in anything lately.

224. J. G.: Do you like reading? (2 s) Did you used to like reading?

Flo's comment on turn 219 appeared to be randomly thrown in. However, when linked back to her greeting when she addressed J. G. with the words "oh the typewriter," it can be seen as an extension or return to that topic. The comment appeared to be both a greeting and a means for Flo to contextualize J. G.'s visit and their relationship. Although the earlier segments of the conversation did not include any references to J. G.'s research or work, it appeared that Flo had assimilated J. G. into this schema and it had become an important element in their conversations. Flo's choice of words and the nonverbal behaviors that accompanied them appeared to suggest that she assumed they conveyed shared *given* information and that J. G. would recover her implied meaning.

A further example took place a week later during a conversation about grandchildren while J. G. and Flo were looking at Flo's family photos. Flo made a remark relating to homework (turn 112) when J. G. asked Flo to identify the children in the photos.

Excerpt 3

110. Flo: She's in Australia.

111. J. G.: And this one? *(pointing at a photo)*

112. Flo: Oh I didn't do my homework, that loses me points does it? *(smiles and tilts her her head to one side).*

113. J. G.: No, why?

It was a point of interest for the researcher that Flo discursively positioned herself in the role of a student on several occasions during their interactions. The association of J. G. with a schema of education and writing was easy to explain. The initial introduction of J. G. as a university lecturer writing a book likely activated representations of items or activities associated with teaching or writing in Flo's cognitive schema. However, the question that arose was why Flo asked if she had lost points or whether she was still in the poem. For the care partners and nursing assistants, taken at face value, these remarks appeared to be oddly random and reflected the confusion of the person with dementia. The nursing assistant who overheard some of these remarks noted they reflected how far gone Flo might be.

However, if we consider the conversational data in relation to cognitive schemas that have become unstable rather than examining these data on a turn-by-turn basis, there is an alternate explanation. Flo's remark about losing points suggests she did know who the researcher was despite not remembering her name. Combined with her nonverbal behaviors, Flo's comment was interpreted by the researcher as an attempt at teasing. Instead, Flo was acknowledging their relationship by joking about her role in J. G.'s work. Her comments suggest she was aware who J. G. was and, more specifically, was at some level aware of J. G.'s occupation and work as a university educator and writer.

Due to her dementia, Flo's cognitive abilities did not allow her to construct the type of question a neurotypical person would produce to query how J. G.'s research was going or to ask about their part in the project. Yet by accessing parts of an academic schema, albeit one that was inconsistently available, Flo was able to contribute to the conversation in ways that were relevant to J. G. insofar as J. G. helped cocreate the shared mental referent of academic work between Flo and herself. Flo was attempting to engage in a topic that reflected her recognition of J. G. and acknowledgment of the work J. G. was engaged with, also accompanied by some humor. Traditional analytical constructs associated with conversational analysis (e.g., adjacency pairs) might have missed the connection between these utterances because they were isolated from each other over the course of the conversation. However, by examining the transcripts of the conversation as a larger whole and by identifying patterns of language that fit within a covalidated schema related to academics, we can see that Flo is attempting to convey meaning.

My Dementia Schema

The conversation below took place 2 days after the Christmas holiday. J. G. attempted to engage Flo in a conversation about Christmas activities. Prior to turn 21, J. G. asked Flo what presents she had received. Flo then changed the topic to imply that she had been left alone during the holiday period.

Excerpt 4

21. F: No:: we've (.) we're just left here dead.

21. J. G.: Mhm

22. Flo: Oh:: wha what I want is to (4.5 sec) I don't know, what you call it. (2 sec) I call it when something changes on your own brain.

. . . *(redacted text; J. G. changes the topic to Flo's family)*

33. Flo: That's it (2 sec) he wants me to be just kept here.

. . . *(redacted text; J. G. steered talk back to family and Christmas)*

47. Flo: No? (2 sec) *(unintelligible word)* there (3 sec) oh it had been taken away with me and they want me to (1 second pause) make me took

. . . *(redacted text; J. G. continued asking questions about Christmas)*

57. Flo: *(unintelligible word)* my mind's *(light laugh)* way missing

. . . *(redacted text; the conversation about Christmas continued)*

67. J. G.:   What do they do at Christmas here? Do they have a pantomime?

Flo: Eh? (2 sec) me I think now (1 sec) I feel awfully that I am 'ere

. . . *(redacted text; Flo and J. G. continue talking about family coming from Australia to visit)*

98. Flo: Ah well mhm things have been bakin (1 sec) anyway she'll be getting so excited (.) I can't be bothered with anybody or things and I don't want to grieve, it would be awful, but how can I when they don't want me here *(Flo is tearful)*.

99. J. G.:   Who doesn't want you here? *(repeats more loudly)* Who doesn't want you here? You don't want to be here?

100. Flo: No:: I would like to be *(unintelligible sound)* I would like to live outside and as a normal person.

111. J. G.:   You are a normal person (1 sec). Yes you are, you're a normal person, of course you are!

In this particular segment of the conversation, Flo appeared to resist J. G.'s attempt to create a more positive topic focusing on family, Christmas activities, and baking. Flo appeared to be more fixated on the topics relating to her dementia, her loss of independence, and her life in the nursing home. When Flo declared she had been "left for dead" during the Christmas period, J. G. attempted to deflect the topic back to the festivities because Flo appeared to be getting upset. J. G. was initially successful in steering the thread of conversation back to Flo's family. However, approximately every 10 to 20 turns at talk, Flo responded with a comment that appeared to be associated with her dementia schema. Box 14–2 shows that by redacting the utterances that occurred between the comments transcribed in Excerpt 4, it is possible to see eight propositions that are related to the particular meaning that Flo was conveying to J. G.

BOX 14–2. Propositions Related to My (Flo's) Dementia

1. Turn 21 = I am alone and no one comes to visit me
2. Turn 22 = it's because of my dementia
3. Turn 33 = my family (husband) want me to remain here
4. Turn 47 = because I have memory problems, they left me here
5. Turn 57 = it's because I get confused
6. Turn 67 = I am unhappy here
7. Turn 98 = I can't manage to do things (bake), I try not to grieve, it is awful when they don't want me here (tearful)
8. Turn 100 = I want to be (1-second pause) live in my own home like a normal person

Flo was visibly very upset at the point where she said, "They don't want me here." Her tears in conjunction with the use of the verb *grieve* suggested to J. G. that when Flo said "gone," she might be implying they would prefer she was dead. Flo's family were devoted and did come to see her each day, but they did not remain for long periods unless they were taking her out for a walk or outing. Most of Flo's care partners (family and professional) found that sustaining a lengthy conversation with Flo was confusing or emotionally upsetting. Hence, person-centered conversational discourse education and training of care providers is of paramount importance, even for family members who possess a great deal of shared knowledge, schemas, scripts, and mental referents with their relatives living with dementia. Clinicians can leverage the shared schemas and scripts, showing family and professional care providers the retained language and conversational skills among persons living with dementia that might help initiate more rewarding conversations.

Conclusions

As noted above, English language-based conversational norms develop over time and become socialized behavioral habits that we often take for granted. When in a conversation, it is not always possible to pick out the interactional patterns, such as those discussed in this chapter. It is difficult to suspend adherence to the normal patterns that we take for granted in a conversation. Typically, we assume certain interactional patterns are given conversational procedures understood by all the participants. For example, most people will assume the primacy of adjacency pairs (e.g., question and answer) and relate the propositional content of an utterance to either the utterance that came before it or to a new topic. The new topic would be introduced in a way that contextualizes its relevance to the conversation. However, in the case of conversations with persons living with dementia, viewing conversations rigidly on a turn-by-turn basis limits our ability to notice nuances of meaning; as a result, the message that might be fragmented within the overall discourse is missed.

The analysis of the conversations with Flo showed that she appeared to know who the researcher was, not by name but possibly by her role in both society and in Flo's life at that moment. Accommodating J. G. into a schema that included items and activities associated with academia or education helped Flo create a meaning for their relationship; one where she was an active participant in the conversations. Flo was aware at some level that J. G. was writing something that was important and that she was involved in some way in J. G.'s project. Box 14–3 highlights two points that emerged from the study and are important for future considerations.

Many clinicians or care partners may ask how close analysis of conversational patterns helps us on a daily basis and whether it is even possible to notice in real time meanings that may be threaded throughout a conversation with someone with dementia. As a linguist, J. G. was better equipped to notice patterns of difference that emerged in her conversations with Flo than were Flo's formal care partners. However, it was less J. G.'s ability as a linguist than her opportunity to hear replays of the conversations that allowed her to put together the schema and script pieces. During the COVID-19 pandemic, interactions often have been carried out using video conferencing programs due to the lockdowns in nursing homes. Therefore, with the rapidly growing use of

---

BOX 14–3. Future Considerations

(a) By using different theoretical approaches (e.g., schemas/cognitive frames) to analyze discourse data, we gain knowledge about how our brains process information in real time rather than relying on clinical or experimental contexts where elicitation tasks are likely to reveal weaknesses rather than the strengths of persons living with dementia.

(b) Researchers must look beyond traditional discourse analysis methods that rigidly examine data on a turn-by-turn basis because it does not reveal potential strengths people with DAT may retain, thus constraining our ability to recognize the meanings that people with dementia may be trying to assert within their interactions.

---

telehealth modalities, it would not be difficult or necessarily intrusive to record our daily conversations with people with dementia (and indeed other communication disorders; see Chapter 12). Being able to go back and find the key to the conversational style of a person with dementia may assist in helping care partners to develop communicative skills more adapted to interacting with those whose conversational patterns do not fall within our established social norms.

Wittgenstein (1958) asked whether it is always an advantage to replace an indistinct picture with a sharp one. Clinicians and researchers typically have clearly defined goals they seek to achieve; it is what they are trained to do—to assess and to help remediate. However, the *indistinct picture* may be all we can ever have when interacting with people with DAT. We rarely find distinct, neatly structured patterns in the discourse of people with dementia, but the indistinct remnants are still present in their language-processing systems and can function in a way that allows them and their conversational partners to create meaning. We just have to take the time to seek out and to put together the subtle pieces of the conversational puzzle, and begin to recog-

nize, as we do with cultural differences, that not only do languages and dialects differ but conversational structures vary too. Our conversational patterns have emerged over time through social use, driven by fully functioning cognitive systems (e.g., memory, attention, inhibition, executive function). When, as in the case of persons living with DAT, we lose some of the parts necessary to operate that language system, it is not simply the case that the language system completely breaks down. Rather, as Sperber and Wilson (2002) noted, it adapts and attempts to seek relevance and generate meaning regardless of the incomplete information.

Morris et al. note that "it is possible to improve carers' knowledge of communication strategies and skills" (2020, p. 1740) but knowledge does not always translate into practice. Although many approaches to care (e.g., Kitwood, 1997; Mitchell & Agnelli, 2015) are person centered, they are "insufficiently underpinned by an understanding of what is required to achieve" their aims (Morris et al., 2020, p. 1741). In their own work, Morris et al. attempt to combine multiple theoretical perspectives to provide a framework for targeting the training of care partners that stresses "cognitive flexibility"

(2020, p. 1752). However, it is not enough to discuss cognitive theories that underpin approaches to dementia care. We also need to identify the differences in interactional norms and conversational structures that emerge from a language processing system stressed by cognitive limitations. Therefore, we need to use discourse analysis as a regular clinical tool to help identify the conversational dialects of dementia and use our findings to create programs that educate and train all care partners (professional and nonprofessional) on how to adapt and to communicate with people with dementia. Indeed, perhaps we need to teach courses focused on the discourses of disorders that start with no preconceptions and commence by examining conversational patterns beyond those we take for granted.

Traditional language and communication assessment protocols by their nature are designed to identify the deficits in people's communication skills. What they often miss are the strengths of those whom we serve. We need to be able to identify what remains of the language processing system of the person with dementia, establish how it appears to be functioning, and explore whether there are similarities across groups of people with dementia and other cognitive disorders. Discourse analysis informed by a range of theoretical perspectives has the power to assist clinicians, care partners, and people with DAT to identify discourse strengths and find ways to connect and to communicate.

References

American Psychiatric Association. (2013). *Diagnostic and statistical manual of mental disorders* (5th ed.). https://doi.org/10.1086/399084

Bartlett, F. C. (1932). *Remembering: A study in experimental and social psychology.* Cambridge University Press.

Bayles, K. A., & Tomoeda, C. K. (2005). *Arizona Battery for Cognitive-Communication Disorders (ABCD-2)* (2nd ed.). Pro-Ed.

Bayles, K. A., & Tomoeda, C. K. (2020). *Functional Linguistic Communication Inventory (FLCI-3)* (3rd ed.). Pro-Ed.

Brown, G., & Yule, G. (1983). *Discourse analysis.* Cambridge University Press.

Burshnic, V., & Bourgeois, M. (2020). A seat at the table: Supporting persons with severe dementia in communicating their preferences. *Clinical Gerontologist, 43*(1). https://doi.org/10.1080/07317115.2020.1764686

Davis, B. (2005). *Alzheimer talk, text, and context.* Palgrave MacMillan.

Davis, B. H., & Maclagan, M. (2018). Narrative ageing: Exploring the range of narrative types in dementia conversation. *European Journal of English Studies, 22*(1), 76–90. https://doi.org/10.1080/13825577.2018.1427198

Davis, B., & Maclagan, M. (2013). Talking with Maureen: Pauses, extenders, and formulaic language in small stories and canonical narratives by a woman with dementia. In R. W. Schrauf & N. Müller (Eds.), *Dialogue and dementia: Cognitive and communicative resources for engagement* (pp. 87–121). Psychology Press. https://doi.org/10.4324/9781315851747

Davis, B., & Maclagan, M. (2010). Pauses, placeholders and fillers in Alzheimer's discourse: Gluing relationships as impairment increases. In N. Amiridze, B. Davis, & M. Maclagan (Eds.), *Fillers, pauses and placeholders in discourse and grammar* (pp. 189–215). John Benjamins. https://doi.org/10.1075/tsl.93

Evans, V. (2019). *Cognitive linguistics: A complete guide.* Edinburgh University Press.

Fillmore, C. (1982). Frame semantics. In Linguistic Society of Korea (Ed.), *Linguistics in the morning calm* (pp. 111–137). Hanshin.

Folstein, M., Folstein, S., & McHugh, P. (1975). Mini-mental state: A practical method for grading the cognitive state of patients for the clinician. *Journal of Psychiatry Research, 12,*

189–198. https://doi.org/10.1016/0022-3956 (75)90026-6

Goodglass, H., Kaplan E., & Barresi B. (2001). *The Boston Diagnostic Aphasia Examination* (3rd ed.). Lippincott Williams & Wilkins.

Guendouzi, J. (2014). Qualitative research revisited. In M. J. Ball, N. Müller, & R. Nelson (Eds.), *The handbook of qualitative research in communication disorders* (pp. 353–364). Psychology Press. https://doi.org/10.4324/97 80203798874

Guendouzi, J. (2013). So what's your name? Relevance in dementia. In B. Davis & J. Guendouzi (Eds.), *Pragmatics in dementia discourse* (pp. 29–54). Cambridge Scholars Publishing.

Guendouzi, J., & Davis, B. (2013). Dementia, discourse and pragmatics. In B. Davis & J. Guendouzi (Eds.), *Pragmatics in dementia discourse: Applications and issues* (pp. 1–28). Cambridge Scholars Publishing.

Guendouzi, J., Davis, B., & Maclagan, M. (2015). Listening to narratives from people recently diagnosed with dementia. *Topics in Language Disorders, 35*(3), 237–257. https://doi.org/10 .1097/TLD.0000000000000061

Guendouzi, J., Meaux, A., & Müller, N. (2016). Avoiding interactional and cognitive conflict in dementia. *Journal of Language Aggression and Conflict, 4*(1), 8–34. https://doi.org/10 .1075/jlac.4.1.01gue

Guendouzi, J., & Müller, N. (2006). *Approaches to discourse in dementia.* Lawrence Erlbaum Associates.

Guendouzi, J., & Müller, N. (2002). Defining trouble sources in dementia: Repair strategies and conversational satisfaction in interactions with an Alzheimer's patient. In F. Windsor, M. L. Kelly, & N. Hewlett (Eds.), *Investigations in clinical phonetics and linguistics* (pp. 15–30). Lawrence Erlbaum Associates.

Guendouzi, J., & Pate, A. (2014). Interactional and cognitive resources in dementia: A perspective from politeness theory. In R. Schrauf & N. Müller (Eds.), *Dialogue and dementia: Cognitive and communicative resources for engagement* (pp. 121–146). Blackwell.

Guendouzi, J., & Savage, M. (2017). Alzheimer's disease. In L. Cummings (Ed.), *Research in clinical pragmatics.* Springer.

Halliday, M. A. K. (1985). *An introduction to functional grammar.* Edward Arnold.

Hamilton, H. E. (1994). *Conversations with an Alzheimer's patient: An interactional sociolinguistic study.* Cambridge University Press. https://doi.org/10.1017/CBO9780511627774

Hassenstab, J., Burns, J., & Morris, J. (2013). Clinical and neuropsychological features of Alzheimer's disease. In D. Charney, J. G. Buxbaum, & P. Sklar (Eds.), *Neurobiology of mental illness* (4th ed., pp. 791–804). Oxford University Press.

Kertesz, A. (2006). *Western Aphasia Battery–Revised.* Pearson.

Kitwood, T. (1997). *Dementia reconsidered: The person comes first.* Open University.

Labov, W. (1980). The social origins of sound change. In W. Labov (Ed.), *Locating language in time and space* (pp. 251–266). Academic Press.

Lakoff, G. (1987). *Women, fire and dangerous things: What categories reveal about the mind.* University of Chicago Press.

Langacker, R. (2000). A dynamic usage-based model. In M. Barlow and S. Kemmer (Eds.), *Usage-based models of language* (pp. 1–64). Stanford: CSLI.

Leech, G., N., & Short, M. H. (1983/2007). *Style in fiction: Linguistic introduction to English fictional prose.* Routledge.

Marslen-Wilson, W. D., & Welsh, A. (1978). Processing interactions and lexical access during word recognition in continuous speech. *Cognitive Psychology, 10*(1), 29–63. https://doi .org/10.1016/0010-0285(78)90018-X

Mikesell, L. (2014). Conflicting demonstrations of understanding in the interactions of individuals with frontotemporal dementia: Considering cognitive resources and their implications for caring and communication. In R. W. Schrauf & N. Müller (Eds.), *Dialogue and dementia: Cognitive and communicative resources for engagement* (pp. 147–180). Psychology Press.

Minsky, M. (1975). A framework for representing knowledge. In P. H. Winston (Ed.), *The psychology of computer vision* (pp. 211–277). McGraw-Hill.

Mitchell, G., & Agnelli, J. (2015). Person-centered care for people with dementia: Kitwood reconsidered. *Nursing Standard*, *30*(7), 46–50. https://doi.org/10.7748/ns.30.7.46.s47

Morris, J. C. (1992). The Clinical Dementia Rating (CDR): Current vision and scoring rules. *Neurology*, *43*(11), 2412–2414.

Morris, L., Mansell, W., Williamson, T., Wray, A., & McEvoy, P. (2020). Communication empowerment framework: An integrative framework to support effective communication and interaction between carers and people living with dementia. *Dementia*, *19*(6), 1739–1757. https://doi.org/10.1177/14713012188 05329

Orange, J. B., Lubinski, R. B., & Higginbotham, J. (1996). Conversational repair by individuals with dementia of the Alzheimer's type. *Journal of Speech and Hearing Research*, *39*(4), 881–895.

Piaget, J. (1977). The role of action in the development of thinking. In W. F. Overton & J. M. Gallager (Eds.), *Knowledge and development* (pp. 17–42). Springer.

Plejert, C., Lindholm, C., & Schrauf, R. W. (Eds.). (2017). *Multilingual interaction and dementia*. Multilingual Matters. https://doi .org/10.21832/9781783097678

Rosch, E. (1973). Natural categories. *Cognitive Psychology*, *4*(3), 328–350. https://doi.org/10 .1016/0010-0285(73)90017-0

Rosch, E., & Mervis, C. B. (1975). Family resemblances: Studies in the internal structure of categories. *Cognitive Psychology*, *7*(4), 573–605. https://doi.org/10.1016/0010-0285(75) 90024-9

Rosen, W. G., Mohs, R. C., & Davis, K. L. (1984). A new rating scale for Alzheimer's disease. *American Journal of Psychiatry*, *141*, 1356–1364. https://doi.org/10.1176/ajp.141.11.1356

Sabat, S. R. (2001). *The experience of Alzheimer's disease: Life through a tangled veil*. Blackwell Publishers.

Sachdev, P. S., Blacker, D., Blazer, D. G., Ganguli, M., Jeste, D. V., Paulsen, J. S., & Petersen, R. C. (2014). Classifying neurocognitive disorders: The DSM-5 approach. *Nature Reviews Neurology*, *10*(11), 634–642. https://doi.org/ 10.1038/nrneurol.2014.181

Sacks, H., Schegloff, E., & Jefferson, G. (1974). A simplest systematics for the organization of turn taking for conversation. *Language*, *50*(4), 696–735. httpu://doi.org/10.2307/412243

Schank, R. C., & Abelson, R. (1977). *Scripts, plans, goals, and understanding*. Erlbaum.

Schiffrin, D. (1994). *Approaches to discourse: Language as social interaction*. Blackwell.

Schrauf, R., & Müller, N. (Eds.), (2013). *Dialogue and dementia: Cognitive and communicative resources for engagement*. Blackwell.

Shadden, B. (1996). Dementia and communication. *Topics in Language Disorders*, *16*(3), 77–78.

Sheehan, B. (2012). Assessment scales in dementia. *Therapeutic Advances in Neurological Disorders*, *5*(6), 349–358. https://doi.org/10.11 77/1756285612455733

Sherratt, S. (2007). Multi-level discourse analysis: A feasible approach. *Aphasiology*, *21*(3/4), 375–393. https://doi.org/10.1080/026870306 00911435

Sperber, D., & Wilson, D. (2002). Pragmatics, modularity and mind-reading. *Mind and Language*, *17*(1–2), 3–23. https://doi.org/10 .1111/1468-0017.00186

Wilson, D., & Sperber, D. (2006). Relevance theory. In L. Horn & G. Ward (Eds.), *The handbook of pragmatics* (pp. 607–632). Wiley-Blackwell.

Wittgenstein, L. (1958). *Philosophical investigations*. Blackwell.

Woodward, M. (2013). Aspects of communication in Alzheimer's disease: Clinical features and treatment options. *International Psychogeriatrics*, *25*(6), 877–885. https://doi .org/10.1017/S1041610213000318

Wray, A. (2013). Mislaying compassion: Linguistic triggers for inadequate caregiving in Alzheimer's disease care. In B. Davis & J. Guendouzi (Eds.), *Pragmatics in dementia discourse* (pp. 125–152). Cambridge Scholars Publishing.

15 Multilevel Discourse Analysis in Parkinson's Disease and Related Disorders

Katharine Aveni and Angela Roberts

Introduction

Parkinson's disease (PD) is the second-most common neurodegenerative disease worldwide with prevalence estimates of 572 per 100,000 for persons 45 years or older living in the United States and Canada (Marras et al., 2018). This equates to an estimated 930,000 cases in the United States currently, which could rise to approximately 1.2 million cases by the year 2030 (Marras et al., 2018). With steep rises in the number of PD cases, clinicians are increasingly called upon to support the communication needs of people living with PD. Yet, speech-language pathology (SLP) services are underutilized compared to physical therapy, even in PD expert care centers (Roberts, Rafferty, et al., 2021). One reason is that current SLP practices may not address the complex communication needs of people with PD (Johansson et al., 2020). These complexities, and their linkages to underlying motor and cognitive changes, manifest uniquely in spoken discourse, highlighting its importance in clinical care and research (Roberts & Orange, 2013). The primary aims of this chapter are to expand clinicians' and researchers' understanding of PD communication difficulties and to support the development of discourse assessments and communication interventions for persons with PD.

Parkinson's Disease Overview

Motor and Cognitive Impairments

PD falls under the umbrella of Lewy Body Spectrum Disorders (LBSD), a group of neurodegenerative conditions sharing underlying neuropathology including Parkinson's disease dementia (PDD) and dementia with Lewy bodies (DLB; Lippa et al., 2007). PD is characterized by bradykinesia (e.g., slowed and reduced amplitude of movement), rigidity, and gait abnormalities (Gelb et al., 1999). Tremor, while often present, is not essential for a PD diagnosis (Gelb et al., 1999). Motor speech impairments, consistent with a hypokinetic dysarthria profile, are ubiquitous in PD (Ho et al., 1999) and can affect spoken discourse performance. These include reduced lung volume initiation and termination that can impact utterance length, pausing, and stamina when speaking (Huber & Darling-White, 2017). Persons with PD also demonstrate impaired articulatory precision and speed in connected speech (Ho et al., 1999).

Cognitive impairments typically develop later in PD and in those who are older at disease onset (Aarsland et al., 2021). However, the finding that cognitive changes manifest at diagnosis for around one third of patients underscores the importance of considering spoken discourse impairments at all disease stages (Aarsland et al., 2021). PD commonly affects working memory (e.g., Dubois & Pillon, 1997), procedural memory and learning (Muslimović et al., 2007), selective attention (e.g., Zhou et al., 2012), executive control (e.g., Dubois & Pillon, 1997), and visuospatial domains (e.g., Dubois & Pillon, 1997). Over time, the PD cognitive phenotype has evolved to include impairments in action semantics (e.g., Fernandino et al., 2013; Roberts et al., 2017), verb retrieval (e.g., Herrera et al., 2012), and complex syntax processing (e.g., Grossman, 1999; Hochstadt, 2009). Impaired verb retrieval and action knowledge have the potential to impact microstructural and macrostructural features in PD discourse (e.g., information content, event structure) (Godbout & Doyon, 2000; Roberts & Post, 2018). Converging evidence from language comprehension studies also shows that working memory and executive function abilities are associated with impaired comprehension of complex syntax in PD (Grossman, 1999; Lieberman et al., 1992), which may also contribute to syntax production impairments in spoken discourse.

Spoken discourse challenges in PD are compounded by social cognition impairments. These include difficulties perceiving and interpreting emotion information from faces, speaker intentions, and prosodic cues (Schwartz & Pell, 2017) and theory of mind deficits (Freedman & Stuss, 2011). When combined with hypomimia (i.e., flattened facial expressions) and reduced spontaneous limb movements that affect gesturing, social cognition deficits—one of several diagnostic criteria of dementia—contribute significantly to communication challenges in PD (Prenger et al., 2020). Recent evidence indicates that social cognition impairments are common in PD, independent of more general cognitive impairments (e.g., executive function), and can appear within 4 years of diagnosis (Czernecki et al., 2021).

Collectively, these studies highlight the complexity of motor and cognitive impairments in PD that have cascading effects on spoken discourse. These multidimensional impairments can affect spoken discourse at multiple levels from conceptualization to articulation (Sherratt, 2007). They can also affect interactional abilities.

Perspectives of People Living With Parkinson's Disease

Family care partners and persons with PD are sensitive to motor and cognitive changes and their wide-ranging effects on spoken discourse abilities, quality of life, and communication participation (Johansson et al., 2020; McAuliffe et al., 2017; Miller et al., 2006). In addition to speech and voice changes, communication partners and persons with PD report that frequent pauses, abandoned utterances, difficulty starting and maintaining conversation turns, slowed processing, misperceptions of speaker intentions, and cognitive fatigue negatively affect communication participation and quality of life (Johansson et al., 2020; McAuliffe et al., 2017; Miller et al., 2006). When asked to compare feelings about their communication to before their diagnosis, persons with PD reported loss of control during communication events, frustration in communicating intended messages, and reduced confidence (Johansson et al., 2020; Miller et al., 2007). Consequently, spoken discourse challenges can contribute to a perceived loss of independence (Miller et al., 2007; Schalling et al., 2017) and to stigmatization and dehumanization of people with PD (Prenger et al., 2020).

BOX 15–1

Motor and cognitive impairments in PD, and their cascading effects on spoken discourse, deleteriously affect communication participation and quality of life for persons with PD and their care partners. This highlights the importance of assessing spoken discourse impairments and their impact as part of routine clinical practice.

Parkinson's Disease-Related Changes in Conversation

Surprisingly, there are few objective studies of conversation abilities in PD. Anchored in conversation analysis methods, Trouble-Source Repair analysis (TSR) (Sacks et al., 1974) can inform how misunderstandings, or failed message exchanges, in conversation occur (i.e., trouble sources) and the subsequent communication actions undertaken by interlocutors to signal (i.e., repair initiators) and to correct or mend those breakdowns (i.e., repairs). TSR analysis can reveal patterns of difficulties in PD that are addressable by conversation strategies (Forsgren et al., 2013; Holtgraves & Cadle, 2016).

Our research highlights the heterogeneity of trouble source behaviors in conversations between persons with PD and their primary care partners (Rinne & Roberts, 2019). We examined conversations in eight dyads made up of a person with PD and their primary family care partner using data collected with a mealtime conversation protocol described previously by Orange et al. (1996). Conversations were transcribed orthographically and segmented into turn construction units (Ford & Thompson, 1996), then TSR sequences were annotated (Sacks et al., 1974).

We found that 64.8% of conversation breakdowns in PD dyads resulted from trouble sources unrelated to reduced speech intelligibility or hypophonia (Figure 15–1). Two findings are worth highlighting. First, sources of breakdowns in PD conversations are myriad and include issues with topic and turn management, as well as language form and content (e.g., verb tense and word-retrieval errors). Second, conversation breakdowns were attributed to both the person with PD and to their family care partner (CP). The latter finding is important because it affirms the need for interventions that address the dyad as the central therapeutic unit, in contrast to prevailing SLP interventions that focus on the person with PD exclusively (Forsgren et al., 2013; Johansson et al., 2020).

Our findings are consistent with other studies reporting a high frequency of overlapping talk (i.e., two speakers talking simultaneously) in PD conversations (Griffiths et al., 2012). These researchers also found that sources of conversation breakdowns were both motoric in the case of low voice volume (Griffiths et al., 2012) and linguistic, including word errors and nonspecific references (Saldert & Bauer, 2017; Saldert et al., 2014). Griffiths (2013) further observed that conversation partners of persons with PD often initiated restricted topics that constrained the person with PD's responses, concluding that such deterministic topic-management

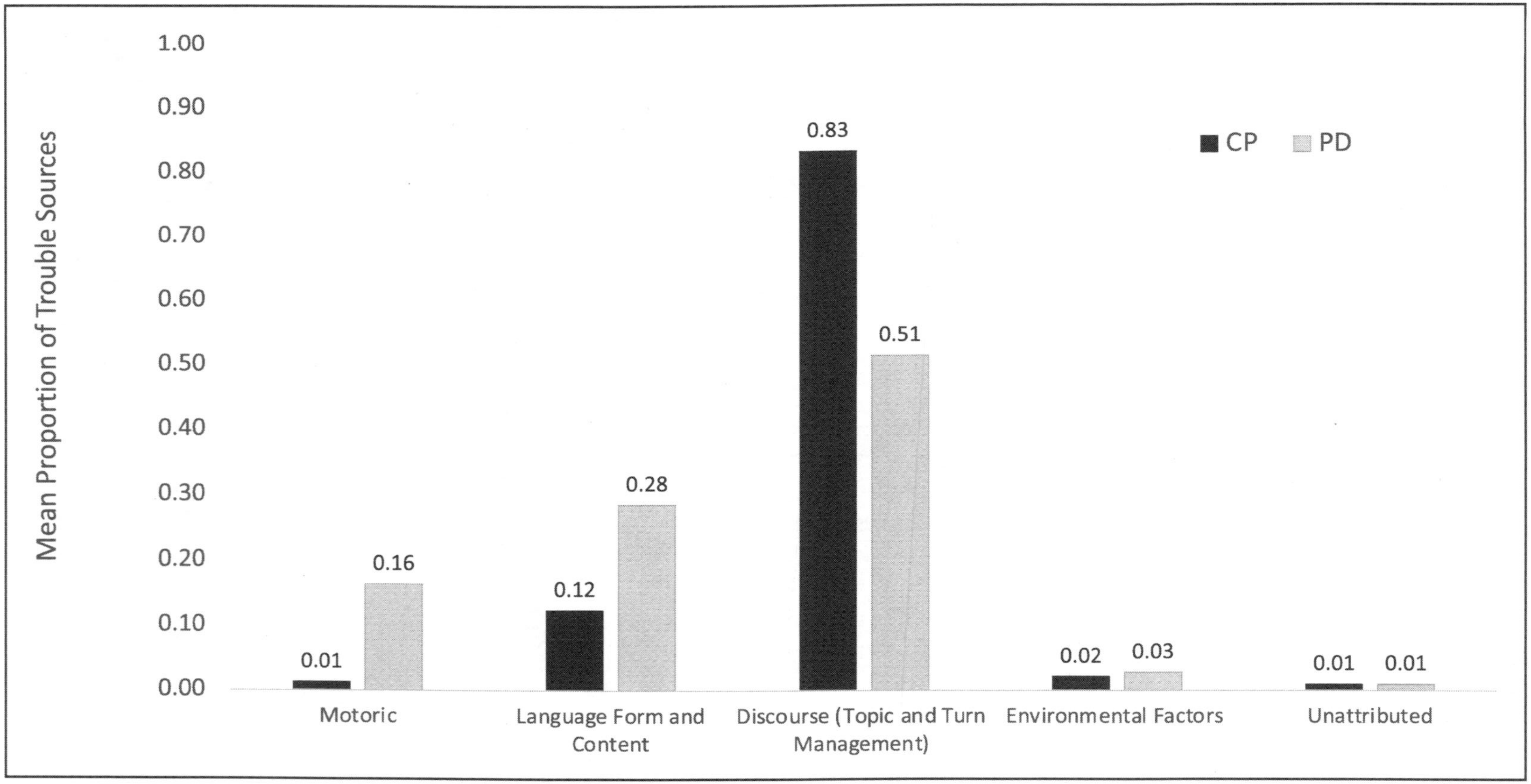

Figure 15–1. Distribution of trouble source types for person with Parkinson's disease (PD) and their family care partner (CP).

behaviors limited the PD interlocutor's ability to contribute to conversation.

Conversation difficulties in PD also extend to repair behaviors. In our research, we found that the proportion of complex repairs in PD conversations (i.e., those where embedded or secondary conversation breakdowns occur in the attempt to repair a primary trouble source) was similar to that reported in Alzheimer's dementia (AD) conversations (Orange et al., 1996; Rinne & Roberts, 2019). Consistent with our findings, Griffiths et al. (2015) observed that conversation breakdowns were frequently left unrepaired by the conversation partner, which ultimately led to decreased engagement by the person with PD. Moreover, care partners frequently used repair strategies shown to be ineffective (Savundranayagam & Orange, 2014), such as nonspecific repair initiators as in the use of "what?" or "huh?" (Griffiths et al., 2015).

BOX 15–2

Conversation behaviors and pragmatic abilities can interact with other factors such as sex and gender, cultural and linguistic diversity, the presence of dementia, hearing loss, and caregiving relationship and family roles (e.g., spouse versus child; formal versus informal caregiver). To date, few studies of PD discourse have considered these factors, leaving significant gaps in the spoken discourse research.

In summary, differences in study methodologies, and the high heterogeneity and day-to-day variability of PD symptoms, create challenges in synthesizing data across studies to create a comprehensive portrait of conversation difficulties in PD. However, these literatures converge on the point that motor impairments do not account fully for difficulties in everyday conversations for persons with PD. Another consistent finding is that the actions of both the person with PD and their communication partners contribute to conversation difficulties. These findings highlight key limitations in current PD interventions, which focus almost exclusively on motor symptoms and only rarely are centered on the dyad (Forsgren et al., 2013; Holtgraves & Cadle, 2016).

Parkinson's Disease-Related Changes in Monologue Discourse

In 2013, when the first comprehensive review of spoken discourse in LBSD was written, there were only a handful of studies in this area (Roberts & Orange, 2013). Since then, there has been rapid growth in spoken discourse research in PD and PD-related cognitive impairment, largely driven by the need for diagnostic and disease-progression monitoring tools. In the sections that follow, the literature on monologue discourse task performance in PD is reviewed within a multilevel discourse analysis framework (Frederiksen et al., 1990; Sherratt, 2007).

BOX 15–3

Contrasted with some conversation tasks (e.g., dialogue), monologue elicitation tasks can provide a higher degree of experimental control and language sample consistency across speakers and across time points. These tasks also provide opportunities to systematically manipulate language planning and cognitive load through gross and subtle task manipulations (Shadden, 1998).

Microstructural Changes

Productivity and Speech Rate

Despite motor deficits in PD, discourse productivity (e.g., number of words, utterances) is often found to be similar between healthy adults and PD participants with age-normal cognition (Ash, McMillan, et al., 2012; Lee et al., 2019; Murray, 2000; Reddy et al., 2016; Roberts & Post, 2018). Only rarely have studies reported that persons with PD without cognitive impairment produce fewer total words (McNamara et al., 1992) or fewer total utterances (Reddy et al., 2016) than controls. While persons with PD generally produce the same amount of language as controls, studies often report that they produce fewer words or syllables per minute (Ash et al., 2017; Cummings et al., 1988; Illes et al., 1988). These speaking rate differences may be driven primarily by unfilled speech pauses (Roberts & Post, 2018) typically located between utterances and at grammatical boundaries (Ash, McMillan, et al., 2012; Illes, 1989; Illes et al., 1988).

Productivity impairments in persons with PD often are exaggerated in the context of cognitive impairment. When compared with persons who have age-normal cognition, those with PD-related dementia showed slower rates of speech and longer between-utterance pause durations (Ash et al., 2017; Ash, McMillan, et al., 2012; Ash et al., 2011). Specifically, participants with DLB demonstrated lower word-productivity rates compared to controls and those with PD and PDD, even when pause time was excluded (Ash, McMillan, et al., 2012). Interestingly, DLB participants' total word and utterance counts may rival or exceed those of healthy controls and in some cases participants with PD and PDD (Ash, McMillan, et al., 2012), suggesting

that these impairments may reflect longer planning times, but not overall differences in language output.

Fluency

Fluency disruptions in spoken discourse can be important signals of underlying disruptions to sensorimotor feedback and/or cognitive monitoring systems during language planning and speech production (e.g., Postma, 2000). Persons with PD produce a broad range of fluency disrupting behaviors in spoken discourse (e.g., filled and unfilled pauses, partial and whole-word repetitions, reformulations). Rates of fluency disruptions in persons with PD who have age-normal cognition are typically reported as equivalent to healthy controls (Ash, McMillan, et al., 2012; Roberts, 2014). However, differences are often reported for individual fluency behaviors such as pausing. While several studies found no PD versus control differences for silent pauses in earlier-stage disease (Illes, 1989; Lee et al., 2019; Roberts, 2014), increased pause rates are reported in advanced disease (Illes, 1989) and in the context of PD-related dementia (Ash, McMillan, et al., 2012). Interestingly, rates of filled pauses (e.g., *uh* and *um*) do not typically differ from controls, except in the context of dementia or advanced disease, where filled pause rates tend to be lower than controls and persons with PD (Ash, McMillan, et al., 2012; Illes et al., 1988). Increased rates of sound and word level disfluencies in spoken discourse are often reported in PD cognitive impairment, but in the absence of cognitive impairment persons with PD perform similarly to controls (Ash et al., 2010; Ash, McMillan, et al., 2012).

Interpreting disfluency behaviors in PD is complex. Shifts in both the number and pattern of verbal disfluencies are important considerations. For example, some behaviors increase in frequency/rate as a function of increased cognitive impairment (e.g., silent pauses; reformulated utterances) while others appear to decrease in frequency as an indicator of discourse impairment (e.g., filled pauses). The nature of disfluency patterns in the discourse of persons with PD creates challenges in using total disfluency counts as a marker of impaired discourse. This is further complicated by spoken discourse studies reporting that persons with PD were more likely to show undetected language errors (McNamara et al., 1992). As a result, they may generate fewer self-correction behaviors (Illes, 1989), resulting in a bias toward lower disfluency rates, but higher errors in PD language production. However, overall, these studies suggest that fluency-related spoken discourse impairments likely result from challenges managing task demands within available cognitive resources for language planning and speech production.

Information Content

Information content is impaired in PD relatively early in the disease course and in the absence of dementia. Persons with PD produce lower percentages of correct information units (CIUs; Nicholas & Brookshire, 1993) as well as fewer CIUs per minute compared to healthy adults (Lee et al., 2019; Murray, 2000; Reddy et al., 2016; Roberts & Post, 2018). Deficits in information content are not limited to CIU measures. There is also reduced information content, compared to controls, for proposition and utterance units (Cummings et al., 1988; Holtgraves et al., 2013; Murray, 2000; Reddy et al., 2016). Not surprisingly, information content is further impaired in people with PD-related cognitive impairment,

with some researchers finding information content deficits only in PD participants with dementia (Ash et al., 2017).

The source of information content impairments in PD is not altogether clear. PD may impair the ability to inhibit irrelevant word meanings (e.g., Copland, 2003; Copland et al., 2001), which could affect lexical retrieval and information content in spoken discourse. Similarly, poorer executive function in PD may contribute to impaired selection and sequencing of information and events (Godbout & Doyon, 2000). Consistent with this hypothesis, previous studies reported that poorer executive function is associated with lower information content (Holtgraves et al., 2013). While possibly attributable to motor speech difficulties and their impact on discourse production, motor disease may also disrupt the representation of action and event knowledge in PD (e.g., Cardona et al., 2013), leading to impairments in information content in discourse (Garcia et al., 2016; Godbout & Doyon, 2000; Roberts & Post, 2018).

Syntax and Grammar

Syntax and grammar impairments in persons with PD are not limited to comprehension, with several studies finding impairments in sentence production (e.g., Troche & Altmann, 2011; Ullman et al., 1997). Thus, it is perhaps not surprising that studies of spoken discourse in PD have largely focused on characterizing syntax and grammar impairments. Syntax complexity in PD spoken discourse is typically examined with mean length of utterance (MLU) or clause count and structure measures. Persons with PD without cognitive impairment generally perform similarly to healthy adults on measures of syntax complexity (Ash et al., 2017; Ash, McMillan, et al., 2012; Lee et al., 2019;

Murray, 2000). However, a handful of studies report more severe impairments (Cummings et al., 1988; Reddy et al., 2016) that appear to worsen in the presence of cognitive impairment and in advanced disease (Ash et al., 2017; Ash et al., 2011; Murray, 2000; Murray & Lenz, 2001).

Syntactic impairments in PD also may affect the production of grammatical morphology and functor words. An increased proportion of optional open-class phrases has been reported (Illes, 1989; Illes et al., 1988) but not replicated in a later study (Ash, McMillan, et al., 2012). Garcia et al. (2016) found higher numbers of subordinating conjunctions, dependent clauses, and negation markers in persons with PD. This finding supports Illes et al.'s (1988) conclusion that persons with PD include more peripheral information than healthy adults, perhaps as a subconscious strategy for maintaining the forward flow of spoken language (Garcia et al., 2016). A recent cross-linguistic study demonstrated that automatic analyses of morphological patterning also can differentiate between persons with PD and controls (Eyigoz et al., 2020).

In contrast, reduced proportions of grammatically well-formed utterances in narrative discourse may appear earlier in PD (Murray, 2000; Roberts, 2014). However, not all investigators have found this effect, with some reporting no differences in grammaticality between PD and control groups (Lee et al., 2019; Reddy et al., 2016). Zanini et al. (2010) conducted one of the few cross-linguistic studies of bilingual speakers with PD. They found that bilingual Friulian (L1)-Italian (L2) speakers with PD produced increased grammatical errors in spoken discourse, but only in their L1. The opposite pattern was observed for non-PD controls. Like many discourse behaviors in PD, syntax and grammaticality impairments are exaggerated in DLB, with studies showing impaired syntactic complexity and grammaticality in persons with DLB compared to PD and healthy controls (Ash, McMillan, et al., 2012; Ash et al., 2011).

Variability in the precise nature and extent of reported syntax and grammar impairments in PD may be attributed in part to differing study methods and the measures used to examine syntax. Whereas some studies assess syntax complexity and grammaticality separately, others assess only one of these domains or collapse aspects of both complexity and grammaticality into composite measures (e.g., Ash, McMillan, et al., 2012). As a result, it can be difficult to compare findings across studies, even when PD participants are otherwise similar in motor and cognitive disease severity. As with other discourse measures, small numbers of participants and small discourse samples further complicate the interpretation of conflicting findings.

The choice of segmentation conventions can influence syntax findings in PD. Box 15–4 shows the same language sample that is elicited using a sequenced-story picture stimulus (Brookshire & Nicholas, 1994). However, syntax complexity scores are affected by the choice of utterance segmentation rules. Typical of speakers with PD (Illes et al., 1988), in this sample the subject is produced explicitly only once and then omitted from subsequent predicate clauses that are produced serially with or without a coordinating conjunction.

Example 1 is segmented using the monolingual English-speaker C-unit segmentation rules from the Systematic Analysis of Language Transcripts (SALT) manual that require an utterance to have a subject and a predicate (SALT, 2020). By contrast, Example 2 is segmented using T-unit procedures (Hunt, 1965). The T-unit approach

---

BOX 15–4. Segmentation Conventions Influence Syntax Complexity

(1) C "The woman is standing in the living room, and bending over, and shaking her finger, and shouting at the husband very angrily."

   MLU (words) = 22; verb clauses/utterance = 4

(2) C "The woman is standing in the living room,

   C and bending over,

   C and shaking her finger,

   C and shouting at the husband very angrily."

   MLU = 5.5, verb clauses/utterance = 1

---

also requires that an utterance have a stated subject, except when the speaker introduces a new action and uses a coordinating conjunction (as in this example). In PD, the C-unit approach is biased toward higher-complexity scores when using MLU and verb clause count measures, while the T-unit approach is biased toward lower-complexity scores. Thus, clinicians and researchers should be consistent in the segmentation approach applied across samples and consider segmentation approach differences when integrating findings across studies. Caution also is warranted when using prosody and pause duration as segmentation markers because PD speakers often produce longer pauses and have flattened prosody that can create ambiguity in utterance boundaries when using these approaches.

The mechanistic underpinnings of syntax and grammar impairments in PD continue to be explored. Reduced syntax complexity often correlates with lower speech intelligibility and more severe motor disease severity in PD, leading researchers to posit that these impairments reflect linguistic adaptations to motor impairment (Illes et al., 1988; Murray & Lenz, 2001). In addition, disruptions to high-level conceptual and functional processing and/or impairments in synchronizing information across conceptual, functional, and/or positional levels (Garrett, 1989) are thought to cause downstream syntactic and grammatical deficits in PD (Altmann & Troche, 2011; Reddy et al., 2016). In support of this hypothesis, Troche and Altmann (2011) observed grammaticality impairments in PD participants in a sentence-generation task, which entailed conceptual and functional planning. This contrasted with adequate performance on a sentence-repetition task that required only positional and phonological/articulatory planning. However, the more robust hypothesis, based on the available experimental evidence, is that working memory, speed of processing, and executive function changes underlie syntactic and grammatical impairments in this population (see Grossman, 1999, for review).

Cohesion

Studies of narrative cohesion are extremely limited in LBSD. The available research suggests that while persons with early-stage PD tend to produce a similar number of cohesive ties (reference, conjunction, and lexical) as healthy controls, they also produce more erroneous cohesion devices, or omit them altogether, across utterances (Ellis et al., 2015). Ellis et al. found that 69% of all erroneous or incomplete cohesive devices were of the reference type, suggesting that PD has a particular impact on pronoun referencing. This finding is consistent with Illes et al. (1988) and is illustrated in the language sample provided earlier in Box 15–4. Cohesion measures sit at the interface of microstructural and macrostructural aspects of discourse. Macrostructural impairments in local connectedness and global coherence (discussed in the next section) can co-occur with, or even result from, microstructural impairments in discourse including referencing, lexical retrieval, and syntax.

Macrostructural Changes

Macrostructural discourse measures are some of the more common discourse measures applied in clinical settings (Pritchard et al., 2017). However, only rarely have these measures been examined in PD. Studies reported that persons with DLB have substantial impairments in maintaining local connectedness compared to healthy controls and persons with PD without dementia (Ash et al., 2011). In contrast, global coherence does not appear to differentiate between early-stage PD participants with age-normal cognition and healthy adults (Ellis et al., 2016). However, there is evidence to suggest that these deficits emerge with dementia in PD (Ash et al., 2011).

Ash, Xie, and colleagues (2012) reported that poorer search theme maintenance was moderately correlated with slower response latencies in a narrative discourse comprehension task and moderately to highly correlated with poorer performance on several measures of executive function. These impairments all related to atrophy in a right ventral lateral region of the frontal lobe (BA 47), suggesting that prefrontal cortical atro-

phy and subsequent cognitive changes in PD impair both comprehension and production of narrative organization (Ash, Xie, et al., 2012). Furthermore, and importantly from a clinical perspective, deficits in comprehension of narrative organization may indicate the presence of AD pathology as a contributing cause in some cases of PDD (Grossman et al., 2017).

Main event analyses that examine how individuals use linguistic and conceptual knowledge (i.e., event and world knowledge) to structure and sequence narrative events are potentially important markers of PD-related discourse impairments. Roberts and Post (2018) showed, in a well-characterized cohort with age-normal cognition, that persons with PD produced significantly lower proportions of correct story main events compared to healthy adults. However, these findings are countered by those of previous studies reporting no differences in numbers of propositions or major story themes in PD (Ash et al., 2017; Bayles, 1990; McNamara et al., 1992). Methodological differences may account for these discrepancies. First, in contrast to other studies, Roberts and Post (2018) used an event cast framework that is grounded in action concepts (Wright et al., 2005), which may be more sensitive to PD impairments in action semantics. Second, task differences may account for noted discrepancies, with single-picture descriptions (Bayles, 1990) promoting listlike descriptions of portrayed events, whereas picture sequences such as those used by Roberts and Post (2018) may encourage production of sequentially linked event casts grounded in the overarching story theme. These limited findings highlight the importance of considering task effects in spoken discourse, specifically in macrostructural analyses of PD discourse.

BOX 15–5. Summary

While research in this area is increasing, the majority of studies explore spoken discourse performance in persons with PD with little to no cognitive impairment and in those with relatively mild disease. Although motor speech impairments can account for some of these findings, other changes in discourse abilities in PD appear to be driven largely by changes in cognitive functions and disease progression.

Speech fluency, syntax complexity, cohesion, and macrolinguistic discourse measures may be particularly sensitive to cognitive impairments in PD. Impairments shared between monologue and dialogue spoken discourse include reduced information content, word-retrieval errors, long pauses, grammar and syntax errors, and difficulties maintaining a central theme and local connectedness in monologues that align with topic management difficulties observed in conversation.

A Multilevel Model Approach in Parkinson's Disease Spoken Discourse

PD can affect discourse performance at multiple levels, in multiple discourse genres (dialogue and monologue), and in differing severities, with increasing impairment as dementia emerges and disease severity progresses. Although rarely employed, these findings suggest that multilevel discourse analyses are an ideal approach to the study of spoken discourse deficits in this population. Multilevel analyses conducted within cognitivist frameworks of spoken discourse (Frederiksen et al., 1990; Sherratt, 2007) provide opportunities to examine the potential cognitive underpinnings of PD spoken language impairments (Garcia et al., 2016; Roberts, 2014). In a series of systematic studies, our research is advancing multilevel discourse analysis approaches to discover markers and predictors of cognitive impairment in PD (Roberts, 2014; Romana et al., 2021), and in other neurodegenerative disorders (Roberts, Aveni, et al., 2021), as part of a larger initiative to develop speech and language biomarkers for dementia.

Summarized in Figure 15–2 and further detailed in the companion website, our multilevel analysis approach is often applied to large data sets such as those collected in ongoing projects funded by the National Institutes of Deafness and Communicative Disorders (NIDCD 1R21DC017255-01) and the Ontario Neurodegenerative Disease Research Initiative (ONDRI; NCT0410 4373). The ONDRI study is an open science initiative with 520 participants across five cohorts, including PD, cerebrovascular disease, AD/mild cognitive impairment, amyotrophic lateral sclerosis, and frontotemporal dementia (Farhan et al., 2017; McLaughlin et al., 2021) that contains more than 4,000 spoken language samples. The spoken discourse data in ONDRI complement other spoken discourse data banks focusing on aging and dementia, including Dementia-Bank (see Chapter 17) and data from Boyd Davis and others available through the Carolina Conversations Collection.

The coding workflow followed by our lab and illustrated in Figure 15–2 progresses from transcribing orthographically

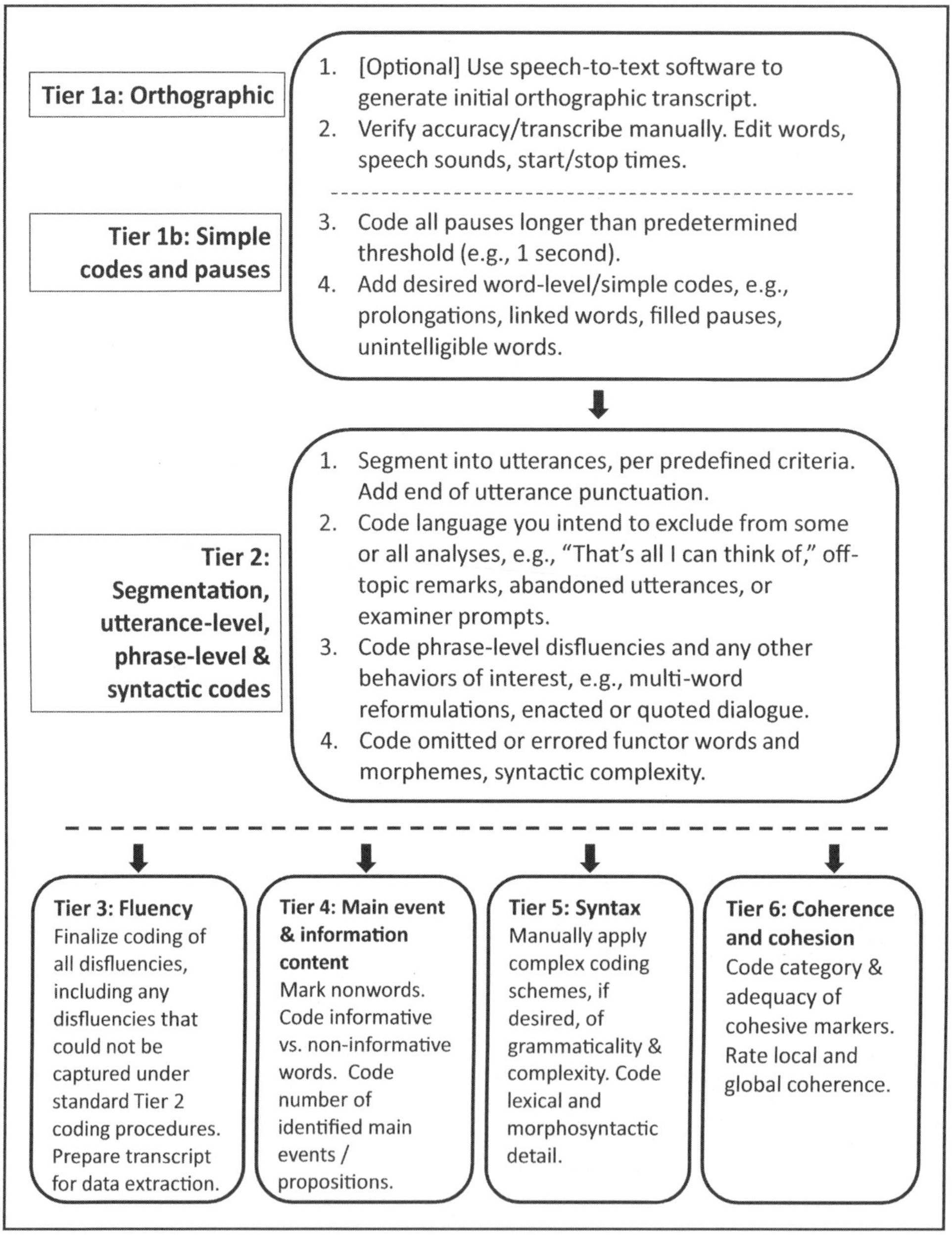

Tier 1a: Orthographic

1. [Optional] Use speech-to-text software to generate initial orthographic transcript.
2. Verify accuracy/transcribe manually. Edit words, speech sounds, start/stop times.

- -

Tier 1b: Simple codes and pauses

3. Code all pauses longer than predetermined threshold (e.g., 1 second).
4. Add desired word-level/simple codes, e.g., prolongations, linked words, filled pauses, unintelligible words.

Tier 2: Segmentation, utterance-level, phrase-level & syntactic codes

1. Segment into utterances, per predefined criteria. Add end of utterance punctuation.
2. Code language you intend to exclude from some or all analyses, e.g., "That's all I can think of," off-topic remarks, abandoned utterances, or examiner prompts.
3. Code phrase-level disfluencies and any other behaviors of interest, e.g., multi-word reformulations, enacted or quoted dialogue.
4. Code omitted or errored functor words and morphemes, syntactic complexity.

Tier 3: Fluency
Finalize coding of all disfluencies, including any disfluencies that could not be captured under standard Tier 2 coding procedures. Prepare transcript for data extraction.

Tier 4: Main event & information content
Mark nonwords. Code informative vs. non-informative words. Code number of identified main events / propositions.

Tier 5: Syntax
Manually apply complex coding schemes, if desired, of grammaticality & complexity. Code lexical and morphosyntactic detail.

Tier 6: Coherence and cohesion
Code category & adequacy of cohesive markers. Rate local and global coherence.

Figure 15–2. Language and cognition in aging and neurodegeneration tiered approach to multilevel discourse analysis. © Roberts, Aveni, Gutierrez, Basque, & Orange (2021). Reprinted under CC license CC BY-NC-SA.

(Tier 1a), to adding minimal codes primarily at the word level (Tier 1b), to inserting all necessary phrase- and utterance-level coding (Tier 2), and finally to specialized coding levels (Tiers 3+). In our workflow, the Tier 2 transcript becomes the base transcript and is a full representation of its source audio file (e.g., words, speech/vocal sounds, pause/prosody/fluency notations, and segmentation) upon which later analyses will be based. Quality assurance checks and reliability analyses are conducted on the Tier 2 transcript to minimize propagating errors to later tiers. Many microstructural features can be analyzed from the Tier 2 transcript on its own.

When analyzing large data sets, there are several advantages to completing multilevel discourse analyses in several distinct annotation tiers. First, it enables transcribers to manage conflicts between different annotation conventions. For example, contractions may be counted as two words under one convention but as only one word by others. Similarly, this system allows for differing segmentation conventions such as those that prioritize syntactic properties versus those that prioritize prosodic markers. Second, a multitier coding approach may improve annotation accuracy. The tiered workflow allows transcribers and coders to focus their attention on one aspect of discourse behavior at a time, generating fewer errors than when coding several behaviors simultaneously. While many discourse features can be analyzed using automatic speech recognition, some features, particularly those classified as macrostructural, require manual annotation. In our experience, splitting the workflow into separate tiers, each with its own annotated transcript, greatly improves a transcript's readability and thereby reduces the potential for transcription and interpretation errors for features that require manual annotation. Finally, in our experience we find that this workflow increases training efficiency, data accuracy, and inter- and intrarater reliability by training expert coders who specialize in working with a specific tier and who may be cross-trained on similar annotation conventions within a tier.

While our workflow was designed to ease the burden of analyzing larger data sets, it is adaptable for clinical contexts. For example, clinicians working within the same setting may wish to develop expertise in specific discourse coding levels and share the burden of analysis across their caseloads. Even in cases where there is a single clinician, annotation accuracy and ease of coding may benefit from this tiered approach, particularly when clinicians are focused on a more narrowed set of clinical outcomes (e.g., syntax complexity or information content) as part of their client's plan of care.

Summary, Clinical Implications, and Future Directions

Studies of spoken discourse in PD, PDD, and DLB provide a valuable window into how motor and cognitive systems interface in language planning and speech production. Collectively, this growing area of research converges on several key findings: (a) spoken discourse impairments in PD are manifested in both conversation and monologue tasks; (b) they are multidimensional, affecting discourse processes from conceptualization to articulation; and (c) while present in early-stage disease, they become more complex and severe as the disease progresses and cognitive impairments develop. The relevance of spoken discourse to clinical practice is high given its significant impact on quality of life and communication participation for people with PD. Clinically, findings to date suggest that spoken discourse measures are potentially valuable SLP assessment and outcome measures for persons with PD. As highlighted by the literature reviewed, it is important that clinicians and researchers consider developing holistic communication interventions for persons with PD that address a broad range of motor and linguistic impairments, in addition to conversation difficulties that affect participation in daily activities and social relationships with family and friends. While analyzing discourse can be time consuming, and concerns have been raised over its test–retest reliability in clinical practice (Stark et al., 2021), we offer a workflow solution that may address these concerns when considered alongside advances in automated and semiautomated discourse analysis software.

Despite the promising findings to date, more research is needed, including examining spoken discourse in culturally and linguistically diverse groups of persons with PD to reduce bias in, and increase the generalizability of, discourse measures and profiles in PD (see Chapter 8). Future studies also may wish to explore the close links among spoken discourse in persons with PD and genetic, cognitive, and neural underpinnings to advance theoretical and clinical models of both PD and discourse performance. Importantly, to increase the feasibility of using spoken discourse in PD clinical practice, more research is needed into the psychometric properties of spoken discourse in PD and the development of automated analytics solutions that are robust in PD given the added confound of motor speech issues (e.g., Eyigoz et al., 2020; Romana et al., 2021).

References

Aarsland, D., Batzu, L., Halliday, G. M., Geurtsen, G. J., Ballard, C., Chaudhuri, K. R., & Weintraub, D. (2021). Parkinson disease-associated cognitive impairment. *Nature Reviews Disease Primers*, 7(1), 1–21. https://doi.org/10.1038/s41572-021-00280-3

Altmann, L. J. P., & Troche, M. S. (2011). High-level language production in Parkinson's disease: A review. *Parkinson's Disease*, *2011*, 238956–12. https://doi.org/10.4061/2011/238956

Ash, S., Jester, C., York, C., Kofman, O. L., Langey, R., Halpin, A., . . . Grossman, M. (2017). Longitudinal decline in speech production in Parkinson's disease spectrum disorders. *Brain and Language*, *171*, 42–51. https://doi.org/10.1016/j.bandl.2017.05.001

Ash, S., McMillan, C., Gross, R. G., Cook, P., Gunawardena, D., Morgan, B., . . . Grossman, M. (2012). Impairments of speech fluency in Lewy body spectrum disorder. *Brain and Language*, *120*(3), 290–302. https://doi.org/10.1016/j.bandl.2011.09.004

Ash, S., McMillan, C., Gross, R. G., Cook, P., Morgan, B., Boller, A., . . . Grossman, M. (2011). The organization of narrative discourse in Lewy body spectrum disorder. *Brain and Language*, *119*(1), 30–41. https://doi.org/10.1016/j.bandl.2011.05.006

Ash, S., McMillan, C., Gunawardena, D., Avants, B., Morgan, B., Khan, A., . . . Grossman, M. (2010). Speech errors in progressive nonfluent aphasia. *Brain and Language*, *113*(1), 13–20. https://doi.org/10.1016/j.bandl.2009.12.001

Ash, S., Xie, S. X., Gross, R. G., Dreyfuss, M., Boller, A., Camp, E., . . . Grossman, M. (2012). The organization and anatomy of narrative comprehension and expression in Lewy body spectrum disorders. *Neuropsychology*, *26*(3), 368–384. https://doi.org/10.1037/a0027115

Bayles, K. A. (1990). Language and Parkinson disease. *Alzheimer Disease and Associated Disorders*, *4*(3), 171–180. https://doi.org/10.1097/00002093-199040300-00005

Brookshire, R. H., & Nicholas, L. E. (1994). Test-retest stability of measures of connected speech in aphasia. *Clinical Aphasiology*, *22*, 119–133. https://aphasiology.pitt.edu/163/1/22-09.pdf

Cardona, J. F., Gershanik, O., Gelormini-Lezama, C., Houck, A. L., Cardona, S., Kargieman, . . . Ibáñez, A. (2013). Action-verb processing in Parkinson's disease: New pathways for motor-language coupling. *Brain Structure and Function, 218*(6), 1355–1373. https://doi.org/10.1007/s00429-013-0510-1

Copland, D. A. (2003). The basal ganglia and semantic engagement: Potential insights from semantic priming in individuals with subcortical vascular lesions, Parkinson's disease, and cortical lesions. *Journal of the International Neuropsychological Society, 9*(7), 1041–1052. https://doi.org/10.1017/S1355617703970081

Copland, D. A., Chenery, H. J., & Murdoch, B. E. (2001). Discourse priming of homophones in individuals with dominant nonthalamtic subcortical lesions, cortical lesions and Parkinson's disease. *Journal of Clinical and Experimental Neuropsychology, 23*(4), 538–556. https://doi.org/10.1076/jcen.23.4.538.1233

Cummings, J. L., Darkins, A., Mendez, M., Hill, M. A., & Benson, D. F. (1988). Alzheimer's disease and Parkinson's disease: Comparison of speech and language alterations. *Neurology, 38*(5), 680–684. https://doi.org/10.1212/WNL.38.5.680

Czernecki, V., Benchetrit, E., Houot, M., Pineau, F., Mangone, G., Corvol, J. C., . . . Levy, R. (2021). Social cognitive impairment in early Parkinson's disease: A novel "mild impairment"? *Parkinsonism and Related Disorders, 85*, 117–121. https://doi.org/10.1016/j.parkreldis.2021.02.023

Dubois, B., & Pillon, B. (1997). Cognitive deficits in Parkinson's disease. *Journal of Neurology, 244*(1), 2–8. https://doi.org/10.1007/PL00007725

Ellis, C., Crosson, B., Gonzalez Rothi, L. J., Okun, M. S., & Rosenbek, J. C. (2015). Narrative discourse cohesion in early stage Parkinson's disease. *Journal of Parkinson's Disease, 5*(2), 403–411. https://doi.org/10.3233/JPD-140476

Ellis, C., Fang, X., & Briley, P. (2016). Temporal aspects of global coherence during discourse production in early stage Parkinson's disease. *Advances in Parkinson's Disease, 5*(3), 41–49. http://dx.doi.org/10.4236/apd.2016.53006

Eyigoz, E., Courson, M., Sedeño, L., Rogg, K., Orozco-Arroyave, J. R., Nöth, E., . . . Garcia, A. M. (2020). From discourse to pathology: Automatic identification of Parkinson's disease patients via morphological measures across three languages. *Cortex, 132*, 191–205. https://doi.org/10.1016/j.cortex.2020.08.020

Farhan, S. M., Bartha, R., Black, S. E., Corbett, D., Finger, E., Freedman, M., . . . Strong, M. J. (2017). The Ontario Neurodegenerative Disease Research Initiative (ONDRI). *Canadian Journal of Neurological Sciences, 44*(2), 196–202. https://doi.org/10.1017/cjn.2016.415

Fernandino, L., Conant, L. L., Binder, J. R., Blindauer, K., Hiner, B., Spangler, K., & Desai, R. H. (2013). Parkinson's disease disrupts both automatic and controlled processing of action verbs. *Brain and Language, 127*(1), 65–74. https://doi.org/10.1016/j.bandl.2012.07.008

Ford, C. E., & Thompson, S. A. (1996). Intonational and pragmatic resources for the management of turns. *Interaction and Grammar,* (13), 134–184. https://dept.english.wisc.edu/cecilia_e_ford/wp-content/uploads/2014/03/Ford_UnitsinConversation.pdf

Forsgren, E., Antonsson, M., & Saldert, C. (2013). Training conversation partners of persons with communication disorders related to Parkinson's disease—A protocol and a pilot study. *Logopedics Phoniatrics Vocology, 38*(2), 82–90. https://doi.org/10.3109/14015439.2012.731081

Frederiksen, C. H., Bracewell, R. J., Breuleux, A., & Renaud, A. (1990). The cognitive representation and processing of discourse: Function and dysfunction. In Y. Joanette & H. H. Brownell (Eds.), *Discourse ability and brain damage* (pp. 69–110). Springer. https://doi.org/10.1007/978-1-4612-3262-9_4

Freedman, M., & Stuss, D. T. (2011). Theory of mind in Parkinson's disease. *Journal of the Neurological Sciences, 310*(1–2), 225–227. https://doi.org/10.1016/j.jns.2011.06.004

Garcia, A. M., Carrillo, F., Orozco-Arroyave, J. R., Trujillo, N., Vargas Bonilla, J. F., Fittipaldi, S., . . . Cecchi, G. A. (2016). How language flows when movements don't: An automated analysis of spontaneous discourse in Parkinson's disease. *Brain and Language, 162*, 19–28. https://doi.org/10.1016/j.bandl.2016.07.008

Garrett, M. F. (1989). Processes in language production. *Linguistics: The Cambridge Survey, 3*, 69–96.

Gelb, D. J., Oliver, E., & Gilman, S. (1999). Diagnostic criteria for Parkinson disease. *Archives of Neurology, 56*(1), 33–39. https://doi.org/10.1001/archneur.56.1.33

Godbout, L., & Doyon, J. (2000). Defective representation of knowledge in Parkinson's disease: Evidence from a script-production task. *Brain and Cognition, 44*(3), 490–510. https://doi.org/10.1006/brcg.2000.1213

Griffiths, S. (2013). *Managing everyday participation in Parkinson's disease: A conversation analytic study* [Doctoral dissertation, Exeter and Plymouth Peninsula Medical School]. https://ethos.bl.uk/OrderDetails.do?uin=uk.bl.ethos.658027

Griffiths, S., Barnes, R., Britten, N., & Wilkinson, R. (2012). Potential causes and consequences of overlap in talk between speakers with Parkinson's disease and their familiar conversation partners. *Seminars in Speech and Language, 33*(1), 27–43. https://doi.org/10.1055/s-0031-1301161

Griffiths, S., Barnes, R., Britten, N., & Wilkinson, R. (2015). Multiple repair sequences in everyday conversations involving people with Parkinson's disease. *International Journal of Language and Communication Disorders, 50*(6), 814–829. https://doi.org/10.1111/1460-6984.12178

Grossman, M. (1999). Sentence processing in Parkinson's disease. *Brain and Cognition, 40*(2), 387–413. https://doi.org/10.1006/brcg.1999.1087

Grossman, M., Irwin, D. J., Jester, C., Halpin, A., Ash, S., Rascovsky, K., . . . McMillan, C. T. (2017). Narrative organization deficit in Lewy body disorders is related to Alzheimer pathology. *Frontiers in Neuroscience, 11*, 53–53. https://doi.org/10.3389/fnins.2017.00053

Herrera, E., Rodriguez-Ferreiro, J., & Cuetos, F. (2012). The effect of motion content in action naming by Parkinson's disease patients. *Cortex, 48*(7), 900–904. https://doi.org/10.1016/j.cortex.2010.12.007

Ho, A. K., Iansek, R., Marigliani, C., Bradshaw, J. L., & Gates, S. (1999). Speech impairment in a large sample of patients with Parkinson's disease. *Behavioral Neurology, 11*(3), 131–137. https://downloads.hindawi.com/journals/bn/1999/327643.pdf

Hochstadt, J. (2009). Set-shifting and the online processing of relative clauses in Parkinson's disease: Results from a novel eye-tracking method. *Cortex, 45*(8), 991–1011. https://doi.org/10.1016/j.cortex.2009.03.010

Holtgraves, T., & Cadle, C. (2016). Communication impairment in patients with Parkinson's disease: Challenges and solutions. *Journal of Parkinsonism and Restless Legs Syndrome, 6*(1), 45–55. https://doi.org/10.2147/JPRLS.S83164

Holtgraves, T., Fogle, K., & Marsh, L. (2013). Pragmatic language production deficits in Parkinson's disease. *Advances in Parkinson's Disease, 2*(1), 31–36. https://www.scirp.org/pdf/APD_2013021813330032.pdf

Huber, J. E., & Darling-White, M. (2017). Longitudinal changes in speech breathing in older adults with and without Parkinson's disease. *Seminars in Speech and Language, 38*(3), 200–209. https://doi.org/10.1055/s-0037-1602839

Hunt, K. (1965). *National Council of Teachers of English (NCTE) Research Report No. 3.* NCTE.

Illes, J. (1989). Neurolinguistic features of spontaneous language production distinguish three forms of neurodegenerative disease: Alzheimer's, Huntington's, and Parkinson's. *Brain and Language, 37*(4), 628–642. https://doi.org/10.1016/0093-934X(89)90116-8

Illes, J., Metter, E. J., Hanson, W. R., & Iritani, S. (1988). Language production in Parkinson's disease: Acoustic and linguistic considerations. *Brain and Language, 33*(1), 146–160. https://doi.org/10.1016/0093-934X(88)90059-4

Johansson, I. L., Samuelsson, C., & Muller, N. (2020). Patients' and communication partners' experiences of communicative changes in Parkinson's disease. *Disability and Reha-*

bilitation, 42(13), 1835–1843. https://doi.org/
10.1080/09638288.2018.1539875

Lee, J., Huber, J., Jenkins, J., & Fredrick, J. (2019). Language planning and pauses in story retell: Evidence from aging and Parkinson's disease. *Journal of Communication Disorders, 79*, 1–10. https://doi.org/10.1016/j.jcomdis.2019.02.004

Lieberman, P., Kako, E., Friedman, J., Tajchman, G., Feldman, L. S., & Jiminez, E. B. (1992). Speech production, syntax comprehension, and cognitive deficits in Parkinson's disease. *Brain and Language, 43*(2), 169–189. https://doi.org/10.1016/0093-934X(92)90127-Z

Lippa, C., Duda, J., Fahn, S., Farmer, J. M., Galasko, D., Galvin, J. E., . . . Wszolek, Z. K. (2007). DLB and PDD boundary issues: Diagnosis, treatment, molecular pathology, and biomarkers. *Neurology, 68*(11), 812–819. https://doi.org/10.1212/01.wnl.0000256715.13907.d3

Marras, C., Beck, J. C., Bower, J. H., Roberts, E., Ritz, B., Ross, G. W., . . . Tanner, C. M. (2018). Prevalence of Parkinson's disease across North America. *NPJ Parkinson's Disease, 4*(1), 21–27. https://doi.org/10.1038/s41531-018-0058-0

McAuliffe, M. J., Baylor, C. R., & Yorkston, K. M. (2017). Variables associated with communicative participation in Parkinson's disease and its relationship to measures of health-related quality of life. *International Journal of Speech Language Pathology, 19*(4), 407–417. https://doi.org/10.1080/17549507.2016.1193900

McLaughlin, P. M., Sunderland, K. M., Beaton, D., Binns, M. A., Kwan, D., Levine, B., . . . Troyer, A. K. (2021). The quality assurance and quality control protocol for neuropsychological data collection and curation in the Ontario Neurodegenerative Disease Research Initiative (ONDRI) study. *Assessment, 28*(5), 1267–1286. https://doi.org/10.1177/1073191120913933

McNamara, P., Obler, L. K., Au, R., Durso, R., & Albert, M. L. (1992). Speech monitoring skills in Alzheimer's disease, Parkinson's disease, and normal aging. *Brain and Language, 42*(1), 38–51. https://doi.org/10.1016/0093-934X(92)90055-J

Miller, N., Allcock, L., Jones, D., Noble, E., Hildreth, A. J., & Burn, D. J. (2007). Prevalence and pattern of perceived intelligibility changes in Parkinson's disease. *Journal of Neurology, Neurosurgery, and Psychiatry, 78*(11), 1188–1190. https://doi.org/10.1136/jnnp.2006.110171

Miller, N., Noble, E., Jones, D., & Burn, D. (2006). Life with communication changes in Parkinson's disease. *Age and Ageing, 35*(3), 235–239. https://doi.org/10.1093/ageing/afj053

Murray, L. L. (2000). Spoken language production in Huntington's and Parkinson's diseases. *Journal of Speech, Language, and Hearing Research, 43*(6), 1350–1366. https://doi.org/10.1044/jslhr.4306.1350

Murray, L. L., & Lenz, L. P. (2001). Productive syntax abilities in Huntington's and Parkinson's diseases. *Brain and Cognition, 46*(1), 213–219. https://doi.org/10.1016/S0278-2626(01)80069-5

Muslimović, D., Post, B., Speelman, J. D., & Schmand, B. (2007). Motor procedural learning in Parkinson's disease. *Brain, 130*(11), 2887–2897. https://doi.org/10.1093/brain/awm211

Nicholas, L. E., & Brookshire, R. H. (1993). A system for quantifying the informativeness and efficiency of the connected speech of adults with aphasia. *Journal of Speech and Hearing Research, 36*(2), 338–350. https://doi.org/10.1044/jshr.3602.338

Orange, J. B., Lubinski, R. B., & Higginbotham, D. J. (1996). Conversational repair by individuals with dementia of the Alzheimer's type. *Journal of Speech and Hearing Research, 39*(4), 881–895. https://doi.org/10.1044/jshr.3904.881

Postma, A. (2000). Detection of errors during speech production: A review of speech monitoring models. *Cognition, 77*(2), 97–132. https://doi.org/10.1016/S0010-0277(00)00090-1

Prenger, M., Madray, R., Van Hedger, K., Anello, M., & MacDonald, P. A. (2020). Social symptoms of Parkinson's disease. *Parkinson's Disease, 2020*. https://doi.org/10.1155/2020/8846544

Pritchard, M., Hilari, K., Cocks, N., & Dipper, L. (2017). Reviewing the quality of discourse information measures in aphasia. *International Journal of Language and Communication Disorders*, *52*(6), 689–732. https://doi.org/10.1111/1460-6984.12318

Reddy, M. S., Rao, A. P., & Narayanan, S. (2016). Narrative discourse in persons with Parkinson's disease. *Speech, Language and Hearing*, *19*(1), 1–9. https://doi.org/10.1179/2050572815Y.0000000007

Rinne, N., & Roberts, R. (2019). *Examining conversation breakdowns in Parkinson's disease versus Alzheimer's dementia* [Unpublished undergraduate thesis]. Northwestern University.

Roberts, A. (2014). *Characterizing spoken discourse in individuals with Parkinson disease without dementia* (Publication No. 2336) [Doctoral dissertation, Western University]. Electronic Thesis and Dissertation Repository. https://ir.lib.uwo.ca/cgi/viewcontent.cgi?article=3783&context=etd

Roberts, A., Aveni, K., Basque, S., Orange, J. B., McLaughlin, P., Ramirez, J., . . . Swartz, R. (2021). Predicting cognitive impairment in cerebrovascular disease using spoken discourse production. *Topics in Language Disorders*, *41*(1), 73–98. https://doi.org/10.1097/TLD.0000000000000242

Roberts, A., Nguyen, P., Orange, J. B., Jog, M., Nisbet, K. A., & McRae, K. (2017). Differential impairments of upper and lower limb movements influence action verb processing in Parkinson disease. *Cortex*, *97*, 49–59. https://doi.org/10.1016/j.cortex.2017.09.022

Roberts, A., & Orange, J. B. (2013). Discourse in Lewy body spectrum disorder. In H. B. Davis & J. Guendouzi (Eds), *Pragmatics in dementia discourse* (pp. 153–211). Cambridge Scholars Publishing.

Roberts, A., & Post, D. (2018). Information content and efficiency in the spoken discourse of individuals with Parkinson's disease. *Journal of Speech, Language, and Hearing Research*, *61*(9), 2259–2274. https://doi.org/10.1044/2018_JSLHR-L-17-0338

Roberts, A., Rafferty, M. R., Wu, S. S., Miao, G., Cubillos, F., . . . Simuni, T. . (2021). Patterns and predictors of referrals to allied health services for individuals with Parkinson's disease: A Parkinson's foundation (PF) QII study. *Parkinsonism and Related Disorders*, *83*, 115–122. https://doi.org/10.1016/j.parkreldis.2020.11.024

Romana, A., Bandon, J., Perez, M., Gutierrez, S., Richter, R., Roberts, A., & Provost, E. M. (2021). Automatically detecting errors and disfluencies in read speech to predict cognitive impairment in people with Parkinson's disease. *Interspeech 2021*, 1907–1911. https://www.isca-speech.org/archive/interspeech_2021/romana21_interspeech.html

Sacks, H., Schegloff, E. A., & Jefferson, G. (1974). A simplest systematics for the organization of turn taking for conversation. *Language*, *50*(4), 696–735. https://doi.org/10.2307/412243

Saldert, C., & Bauer, M. (2017). Multifaceted communication problems in everyday conversations involving people with Parkinson's disease. *Brain Sciences*, *7*(10), 123. https://doi.org/10.3390/brainsci7100123

Saldert, C., Ferm, U., & Bloch, S. (2014). Semantic trouble sources and their repair in conversations affected by Parkinson's disease. *International Journal of Language and Communication Disorders*, *49*(6), 710–721. https://doi.org/10.1111/1460-6984.12105

SALT Software, LLC. (2020). *C-unit segmentation rules*. Coding aids available from https://www.saltsoftware.com/resources/tranaids

Savundranayagam, M. Y., & Orange, J. B. (2014). Matched and mismatched appraisals of the effectiveness of communication strategies by family caregivers of persons with Alzheimer's disease. *International Journal of Language and Communication Disorders*, *49*(1), 49–59. https://doi.org/10.1111/1460-6984.12043

Schalling, E., Johansson, K., & Hartelius, L. (2017). Speech and communication changes reported by people with Parkinson's disease. *Folia Phoniatrica et Logopaedica*, *69*(3), 131–141. https://doi.org/10.1159/000479927

Schwartz, R., & Pell, M. D. (2017). When emotion and expression diverge: The social costs of Parkinson's disease. *Journal of Clinical and Experimental Neuropsychology*, *39*(3), 211–230. https://doi.org/10.1080/13803395.2016.1216090

Shadden, B. B. (1998). Obtaining the discourse sample. In L. R. Cherney, B. B. Shadden, & C. A. Coelho (Eds.), *Analyzing discourse in communicatively impaired adults* (pp. 9–34). Aspen Publishers.

Sherratt, S. (2007). Multi-level discourse analysis: A feasible approach. *Aphasiology, 21*(3–4), 375–393. https://doi.org/10.1080/026870 30600911435

Stark, B. C., Dutta, M., Murray, L. L., Fromm, D., Bryant, L., Harmon, T. G., . . . Roberts, A. C. (2021). Spoken discourse assessment and analysis in aphasia: An international survey of current practices. *Journal of Speech, Language, and Hearing Research, 64*(11), 4366–4389. https://doi.org/10.1044/2021_JSLHR-20-00708

Troche, M. S., & Altmann, L. J. P. (2011). Sentence production in Parkinson disease: Effects of conceptual and task complexity. *Applied Psycholinguistics, 33*(2), 225–251. https://doi.org/10.1017/S0142716411000336

Ullman, M. T., Corkin, S., Coppola, M., Hickok, G., Growdon, J. H., Koroshetz, W. J., & Pinker, S. (1997). A neural dissociation within language: Evidence that the mental dictionary is part of declarative memory, and that grammatical rules are processed by the procedural system. *Journal of Cognitive Neuroscience, 9*(2), 266–276. https://doi.org/10.1162/jocn.1997.9.2.266

Wright, H. H., Capilouto, G. J., Wagovich, S., Cranfill, T., & Davis, J. (2005). Development and reliability of a quantitative measure of adults' narratives. *Aphasiology, 19*(3–5), 263–273. https://doi.org/10.1080/026870304440 00732

Zanini, S., Tavano, A., & Fabbro, F. (2010). Spontaneous language production in bilingual Parkinson's disease patients: Evidence of greater phonological, morphological and syntactic impairments in native language. *Brain and Language, 113*(2), 84–89. https://doi.org/10.1016/j.bandl.2010.01.005

Zhou, S., Chen, X., Wang, C., Yin, C., Hu, P., & Wang, K. (2012). Selective attention deficits in early and moderate stage Parkinson's disease. *Neuroscience Letters, 509*(1), 50–55. https://doi.org/10.1016/j.neulet.2011.12.049

16 Discourse in ALS: Interplay of Language, Motor, and Executive Factors

Sharon Ash and Sanjana Shellikeri

Introduction

Individuals afflicted with amyotrophic lateral sclerosis (ALS) are characterized first and foremost by their motor system impairments, which affect voluntary muscle movements. These deficits interfere with a person's ability to walk, talk, chew, drink and, eventually, to breathe. However, it is well known that ALS is highly heterogeneous in its manifestations. There is variability in the site of initial symptom onset, which may be bulbar, predominantly affecting the muscles involved in speech, swallowing, and tongue movements; spinal, producing muscle weakness and wasting of the limbs; or mixed. There is also variability in progression to secondary and tertiary sites, rate of disease progression, and relation of lower motor to upper motor neuron involvement.

While the hallmark of ALS is the deterioration of motor function, features of frontotemporal dysfunction are also common in ALS. The current, revised criteria for the diagnostic classification of patients with ALS (Strong et al., 2017) include a variant characterized by behavioral impairment (ALS with Behavioral Impairment; ALSbi) and a variant characterized by cognitive impairment (ALS with Cognitive Impairment; ALSci). Some patients may meet criteria for both behavioral and cognitive impairments (ALSbci). Impairments in behavior in ALS may reach a degree of severity that meets criteria for the behavioral variant of frontotemporal dementia (bvFTD). Impairments in behavior that meet criteria for bvFTD are reported to occur in about 6% to 14% of ALS patients (Consonni et al., 2013; Montuschi et al., 2015; Murphy et al., 2016), while around 30% exhibit executive dysfunction severe enough to be classified as cognitively impaired (Beeldman et al., 2016; Ceslis et al., 2020; Consonni et al., 2013). The diagnosis of cognitive impairment requires evidence of impairment either on measures of executive functioning, including attention, working memory, planning and organization, inhibitory control, initiation and apathy, and mental flexibility, among other skills; or on impairments in language; or a combination of the two.

Speech and Language Characteristics in ALS

Language in ALS is routinely tested for naming, comprehension, and letter and category fluency. However, as noted below, letter and category fluency depend on both executive and language capabilities and are typically considered separately, primarily as an indicator of executive functioning. In recent years, the study of language at a higher level of complexity has attracted the attention of researchers striving to understand the heterogeneous presentations of this multisystem disorder. Indeed, there is evidence that language impairments are more common than executive deficits in ALS (Taylor et al., 2013). Production and comprehension of the connected speech of everyday communication is a major part of the fabric of daily life. It is clearly valuable to advance our understanding of the deficits in language inflicted by neurodegenerative conditions to differentiate among them and to find ways to support individuals living with ALS and their caregivers. An early study of language and executive impairments in ALS concluded that 43% of the patients exhibited a language impairment, compared to 31% with an executive impairment (Taylor et al., 2013). Some 55% of ALS patients are reported to be unimpaired in language and executive functioning (Ceslis et al., 2020).

The predominant areas of language functioning that have been studied include syntactic production and comprehension, verb naming and action verb processing, and semantic and verbal paraphasias (Beeldman et al., 2016; Byrne et al., 2012; Giordana et al., 2011; Kasper et al., 2016; Murphy et al., 2016; Zago et al., 2011). Studies of language at a higher level of complexity than single-word production and comprehension are still relatively rare.

Dysarthria, and speech errors in general, have a major impact on a person's ability to communicate. Subsets of ALS patients with and without dysarthria are important in the evaluation of ALS patients' communicative competence. However, in what follows, we will not examine the manifestations of dysarthria since it is beyond the scope of this chapter; that is a subject for a discussion of phonetics and phonology, rather than discourse.

The question of whether deficits in language in ALS reflect an impairment of language itself or an impairment of other cognitive functions that affect language processing has been of major concern to researchers. Abrahams et al. (2000) studied the deficits in verbal fluency of ALS patients and concluded that they result from deficits in the supervisory attentional system or central executive component of working memory, not from primary linguistic abilities. Abrahams et al. (2004) conducted an fMRI study to determine whether word-retrieval deficits and underlying cerebral abnormalities were specific to letter fluency, implicating executive dysfunction, or were also present in confrontation naming, indicating language dysfunction. In confrontation naming tasks, they found impaired activation in middle and inferior frontal gyri and anterior cingulate, in addition to regions of parietal and temporal lobes for letter fluency, and impaired activation in less extensive prefrontal regions of inferior frontal and regions of the temporal, parietal, and occipital lobes. This provides evidence of cerebral abnormalities in ALS in the network of regions involved in both language and executive functions.

The objective of this chapter is to describe findings on language at the level of discourse and to add recent data that may further illuminate the discourse features pertinent to ALS. We also aim to examine the evidence for the co-occurrence versus independence of language and executive functioning. Language at the level of discourse involves executive, social cognition, and linguistic functions as well as intact articulatory motor function, all of which are commonly impaired in the ALS-FTD spectrum. Thus, the study of discourse may be particularly important in this population, not only clinically for potential markers supporting early detection and tracking of cognitive and motor disease in ALS, but also more generally, contributing to our understanding of the neurobiology of language.

Discourse Studies

Roberts-South and colleagues (2012), in a rare longitudinal study, examined ALS patients without dementia to assess the progression of language impairments using both standardized tests and discourse measures, including discourse productivity (speech output) and discourse content. To evaluate discourse, the authors obtained descriptions of the Cookie Theft scene from the Boston Diagnostic Aphasia Examination (Goodglass & Kaplan, 1972). This drawing is widely used to elicit semistructured samples of spoken or written language. Discourse productivity was assessed for total words, total utterances, and mean length of utterance in words (MLU). Discourse content was evaluated for correct information units (CIUs) (Nicholas & Brookshire, 1993) and content units (CUs) (Yorkston & Beukelman, 1980), the number of different novel concepts used to describe the picture. Discourse efficiency was calculated as the percent of words that met criteria for a CIU out of the total number of words in the sample, and content efficiency was calculated as the proportion of total number of words to

the number of CUs. Discourse measures are summarized in Box 16–1.

> ### BOX 16–1. Discourse Measures Used by Roberts-South et al. (2012)
>
> Discourse Productivity: Total words, total utterances, and mean length of utterance in words (MLU)
>
> Discourse Content: Correct information units (CIU), content units (CU), number of different novel concepts used to describe the picture
>
> Discourse Efficiency: Percent of words that met criteria for a CIU out of the total number of words in the sample
>
> Content Efficiency: Proportion of total number of words to the number of CUs

The standardized language tests yielded a negative result; there were no differences between patients and controls on standardized language tests over a period of 24 months. A similar result was found for discourse productivity; as has been reported by others (Abrahams et al., 2004; Gordon et al., 2010), there was no significant difference between groups on these measures at any time point. However, other measures of discourse revealed an impairment in ALS patients. Discourse efficiency, the proportion of words that contributed to the information conveyed, was significantly lower for patients than for controls at study inception and after 6 months. Testing was repeated at 12 and 18 months after study inception, but there were no significant differences between patients and controls at the later times of testing. Content efficiency, the number of words per CU, also differed between patients and controls at the time of first testing, with patients producing more words per CU than controls, but there were no statistically significant differences between patients and controls at later testing times. This lack of a difference between groups at later testing times may be due in large part to attrition in the number of participants. At the time of first testing, there were 16 patients and 12 controls, but these numbers declined steadily over the course of the study, and at the final time point there were only 3 patients and 4 controls.

Overall, language productivity in ALS patients did not differ systematically from that of controls, but the production of discourse content by patients was less than that of controls. This is consistent with the reports of others who have found reduced content due to lexicosemantic deficits in individuals with neurodegenerative disease (Ash et al., 2006; Bschor et al., 2001; Wilson et al., 2010). These findings imply that discourse measures are a valuable tool in the assessment of communicative competence in individuals with ALS. They reveal impairments that are not evident on standardized language tests and suggest areas for compensatory strategies that may improve quality of life for patients and caregivers.

Tsermentseli et al. (2016) examined the potential of formal standardized language testing and spontaneous speech analysis for the identification of linguistic markers of ALS. They excluded patients with bulbar symptoms and respiratory difficulty, as well as clinically diagnosed frontotemporal dementia and primary progressive aphasia. This enabled them to examine language impairments without interference from respiratory insufficiency, fatigue, and dysarthria affecting speech output. They administered tests of confrontation naming, semantic access, and single-word and syntactic comprehension, and they elicited a speech sample using the Cookie Theft description task. The speech and language samples were assessed for measures of speech production, disruptions to fluency, lexical content, and syntactic structure and complexity.

The ALS patients were impaired relative to controls on frequency of sound distortions, frequency of incomplete sentences, MLU, and frequency of semantic errors. The Revised ALS Functional Rating Scale (ALSFRS-R; Cedarbaum et al., 1999) dysarthria score (the speech subscale) was correlated with duration of the speech sample for the full set of patients, but there were no other significant correlations of speech production measures with the dysarthria score. However, the ALS patients were impaired relative to controls on the Test for Reception of Grammar (TROG; Bishop, 2003) and a modified Token Test, a test of verbal comprehension, working memory, and the ability to follow directions (Coughlan & Warrington, 1978). Using stepwise discriminant analysis, the authors found that 82% of ALS patients and 96% of controls were correctly classified by the combination of MLU, frequency of incomplete sentences, and the score on the modified Token Test. These features all depend on competence in syntactic processing, suggesting that syntax is an important area for the potential identification of ALS patients. Furthermore, by virtue of the inclusion criteria for this study, the patients performed in the normal range on executive measures.

These results support the position that components of language may be separable from executive functioning. They also suggest that the impairments in both production and comprehension of syntax may be specific to ALS and can appear at an early stage of disease. The authors cite the research of Yoshizawa et al. (2014), who found reduced activation in Broca's area in ALS patients with impaired syntactic comprehension. These researchers proposed that in ALS, neurodegeneration may occur in Broca's area without also affecting the prefrontal gyrus. This could explain a syntactic impairment in the absence of a concomitant executive impairment. Collectively, the clinical implications from these two studies are that, while language deficits in ALS may not be obvious in simple tests of naming, they may appear more clearly at the higher levels of linguistic structure, in the areas of syntax and discourse. Such impairments may appear to be subtle, but they have a major effect on the impaired individual's ability to communicate effectively with caregivers and others.

Narrative Discourse: The Frog Story

In a study that examined discourse at the level of a larger speech sample, Ash et al. (2014) elicited narratives by asking participants with ALS to tell a story from a book with no printed words, presented in the children's picture book, *Frog, Where Are You?* (Mayer, 1967). The participants were asked to page through the book to become familiar with the story, then to begin at the beginning and tell the story as if reading the book to a child. The story consists of 24 detailed drawings, which elicit an extended speech sample with a known target and with well-defined structure.

The story was analyzed as comprising seven episodes, each consisting of a sequence of orientation, one or more complicating actions, and a resolution, following the analysis of narrative detailed in Labov and Waletzky (1967). The seven episodes comprise 30 events. The full listing of the

episodes and events established for the analysis of the Frog Story narrative is provided in Appendix 16–1.

The example in Box 16–2 illustrates how the narratives were scored for local and global connectedness and maintenance of the search theme. Local connectedness is the linking of each event to the preceding event, which is accomplished by rhetorical markers such as sequencing adverbials (e.g., *then, next*); pronominal reference to preceding nouns; reference by definite as opposed to indefinite determiners (*They found the frog* versus *They found a frog*); and statements of cause and effect. Global connectedness is a categorical variable that reflects whether the speaker recognizes the point of the story—that the frog found at the end is the frog that escaped from the boy's room at the beginning. Maintenance of the search theme is scored on a 5-point scale by counting points accrued for mentions of the search (Reilly et al., 2004).

The Frog Story narrative in Box 16–2 was produced by an ALS patient with an impairment of the discourse features listed here. Lines that express local connectedness are indicated by LC; lines that express the search theme are indicated by S. In the transcript given below, LC1 corresponds to the first event of the story, and numbering continues for the following events. LC3 is followed by LC8 in this narrative, indicating that LC4 to LC7 were omitted in the narrator's telling. An "-x," such as that given for LC8-x on line 4, means that this event was not connected by rhetorical devices to the previously mentioned event. This patient reported only 17 of the 30 events in the story, two of which did not follow logically from the preceding events. There are three mentions of the search theme, and global connectedness is present. This narration is notable for the elements that are missing: 13 events are missing altogether; in

---

BOX 16–2. Frog Story Narrative

Disease duration = 1 year, Mini-Mental State Exam (MMSE) = 29, Age at test = 58 years

Line	Local connectedness (LC) and search theme (S)	
1	LC1	He, um the boy, and his dog have frog in a bottle
2	LC2	and the frog, he got out, while the boy and the dog were asleep
3	LC3, S	when they woke up, they, went to find the frog.
4	LC8-x[1]	and the dog broke the bottle.
5	LC9, S	so they went, off into the woods, to find the frog.
6	LC11, LC12	and they found bees and a gopher
7	LC17	and, the boy uh climbed a tree
8	LC16-x[1]	and, the bees ran after the dog
9	LC18	and, ah the owl came out of the tree
10	LC20	so the boy climbed the rock
11	LC21	and he fell on a deer
12	LC23	and the deer dropped the boy into the water with his dog.
13	LC27, LC28, LC29, S	and they found a— a log, and found the frog with his wife and their babies.
14	LC30	so they took, a little baby home
15		and . . . that's the end

x[1]Local connectedness is not present

---

two instances, the speaker fails to provide local connectedness to the previous material; and only three out of a possible four or more mentions of the search for the frog are given.

Frog Story Studies: Analysis and Interpretation of Results

Results of the Ash et al. (2014) study were analyzed for the whole group of ALS sub-jects, and then separately for a subset of ALS subjects without executive impairments and for a subset without dysarthria. Results are shown in Table 16–1. These findings imply that local connectedness and maintenance of the search theme depend at least in part on executive functioning. This logically cor-responds to the demands of the task: to con-nect one statement or description of a scene to the previous one calls on the speaker's ability to recognize the sequencing of events in the story, and maintenance of the search

Table 16–1. Correlations of Narrative Discourse Measures With Executive Functioning in ALS

	Letter Fluency (FAS)		
	All ALS **(n = 26)**	**ALS With No Cognitive Deficit** **(n = 22)**	**ALS With No Dysarthria** **(n = 18)[1]**
Local Connectedness	.41*	.61**	.61**
Search Theme	.54**	.49*	.47*
Global Connectedness	NS	NS	NS

Notes: [1]Excludes 2 outliers with low scores on letter fluency but high scores on local connectedness; *p < .05; **p < .01.

theme requires the speaker to keep in mind the purpose of the successive scenes of the story. In contrast, there was no significant correlation of global connectedness with letter fluency for either the total number of ALS patients, the subset with no cognitive impairment, or the subset of patients with no dysarthria. Global connectedness, unlike local connectedness and maintenance of the search theme, is limited to the demand on memory of remembering the frog in the first two scenes and connecting it to the frog in the last three scenes after its absence in the 19 intervening scenes. The absence of a correlation of global connectedness with the executive measure of letter fluency is consistent with the view that memory is the most important factor contributing to global connectedness. For clinicians, these findings imply that difficulty in the planning and organization of a narrative in ALS suggests an underlying executive impairment, even in patients who are not overtly cognitively impaired.

Ash et al. (2014) investigated the possible effect of a motor disorder by examining correlations of local connectedness and maintenance of the search theme with two measures of motor functioning in patients for whom two motor measures were avail-able, the ALSFRS-R and vital capacity (supine). There were no significant correlations of either discourse variable with either of these measures of motor functioning for the entire cohort of ALS patients, the subset with no cognitive deficit, or the subset with no dysarthria. Thus, it appears that the large-scale organizational demands of telling a story are at least in part dependent on executive functioning but are independent of motor functioning. Deficits in the executive domain interfere with a patient's ability to communicate effectively in the recounting of a narrative, a form of discourse that is employed ubiquitously in human interactions. See the companion website for imaging results showing further information about the correlations of discourse measures with brain atrophy.

Another study of the Frog Story narratives in ALS examined discourse at the level of the sentence (Ash et al., 2015). This investigation evaluated the group of all ALS patients, the subsets of ALS patients with and without cognitive impairment, and ALS patients with and without dysarthria. The study focused on features of speech output and grammaticality. The T-unit, as defined by Hunt (1965), was used to designate a syntactic unit. A T-unit consists of an independent clause and all clauses dependent on it. For example, "the frog got out while the boy and the dog were asleep" is one T-unit, containing an independent clause ("the frog got out") and a dependent clause ("while the boy and the dog were asleep"). A statement such as "the boy climbed a tree and the bees ran after the dog" is two T-units: "the boy climbed a tree," which is an independent clause, and "and the bees ran after the dog," which is a second independent clause. For analysis purposes, sentence fragments not connected to any independent clause were considered a syntactic unit and counted as a T-unit. A T-unit that consists of a complete sentence with no grammatical errors is deemed a well-formed sentence. Grammaticality was measured as the percentage of T-units that are well-formed sentences.

The full cohort of ALS patients was impaired relative to controls on speech rate in words per minute (WPM), number of words produced, the frequency of speech articulation errors, the number of T-units produced, and the percent of T-units that were grammatically well-formed sentences. ALS patients without dysarthria were not impaired on speech rate or speech errors but were impaired on the number of words, number of T-units produced, and percent of T-units that were grammatically well-formed sentences. The frequency of well-formed sentences as a measure of grammaticality is perhaps one of the most clinically useful markers of impaired spoken language, as listeners notice grammatical errors more readily than slowed speech rate or other measures of output. Patients with dysarthria were impaired relative both to controls and to patients without dysarthria on speech rate and speech errors, suggesting, as expected, that these two features of speech production are affected by a motor impairment. The dysarthric patients and the subset of patients without an executive impairment were both impaired relative to controls on the same measures as the full cohort of ALS patients.

In this study of speech production, it was observed that impairments in the production of grammatically well-formed sentences did not appear to be related to a motor deficit, since both patients with and without dysarthria were impaired on this measure. In addition, a grammatical deficit was found in patients without executive impairment. As was noted in several of the studies discussed above, this suggests that the grammatical impairment in ALS patients is independent of both their motor impairments and their executive impairments. It appears that grammaticality in ALS depends primarily on linguistic competence and that this is independent of executive resources. The implication of these findings in ALS is that clinicians should attend to the syntax, grammaticality, and completeness of reported content in the spoken language of patients, given thoroughly assessed motor speech and executive functions. Neural imaging from this study and the work of other research teams suggest that white matter disease plays a role in ALS patients' grammatical impairments (see the companion website for additional information).

Expository Discourse: Cookie Theft Picture Description

An alternative task for eliciting connected speech is the description of a single picture, such as the Cookie Theft scene from the Boston Diagnostic Aphasia Examination (Goodglass & Kaplan, 1972). This black-

and-white drawing depicts a scene in a kitchen. Ash et al. (2013) enumerated the events depicted in the scene, as shown in Box 16–3.

> ### BOX 16–3. Key Events in Cookie Theft Picture Description
>
> 1   A woman is washing dishes.
>
> 2   The sink is overflowing.
>
> 3   The woman is standing in a pool of water.
>
> 4   A boy is standing on a stool, trying to get cookies from a high shelf.
>
> 5   The stool is tilting and is about to fall over.
>
> 6   A girl is standing next to the boy and reaching up to get a cookie from him.
>
> 7   The woman does not notice any of the events that are going on in the room.

A measure of the discourse adequacy of a Cookie Theft description is available as a count of the number of reported content items given by the speaker (Ash et al., 2013). A speaker receives a point for each of the seven elements that is mentioned. An additional point is given for any description of the scene outside the window, and a point is given for any description of other details in the kitchen, such as the clothes that the three people are wearing, the curtains on the window, the dishes on the counter, or the cabinets in the room, for a maximum possible score of 9.

The task of describing the Cookie Theft scene differs from that of narrating the Frog Story in several ways. First, there is no obligatory temporal order to the recounting of elements in the Cookie Theft scene, so the speech produced in response to it is expository, not narrative. There is no analog to the local connectedness, search theme, or global connectedness measures that can be assessed in the Frog Story task. In addition, the Frog Story task is untimed and usually takes about 4 minutes for both ALS patients and healthy controls, whereas administration of the Cookie Theft task typically limits the speaker to about 1 minute. Participants describing the Cookie Theft scene sometimes declare, "That's it" after 30 seconds or even less and have to be prompted to continue. Because of the limited duration of the task, the volume of speech and associated semantic and grammatical complexity generated in response to the Cookie Theft scene is much less than that of the Frog Story. It requires correspondingly less time to transcribe and to analyze a Cookie Theft description, and the two tasks yield different measures at the micro- and macrolinguistic levels.

Cookie Theft Picture Description: Results and Analyses

We have studied 102 ALS patients and 47 healthy controls (HCs) who have provided spoken Cookie Theft scene descriptions. The presence of a motor impairment was assessed using the ALSFRS-R. The presence of an executive impairment was evaluated using the Edinburgh Cognitive and Behavioral ALS Screen (ECAS; Abrahams & Bak, 2009–2013), a brief neuropsychological assessment designed to accommodate the physical impairments of patients with ALS, including limitations in the ability to speak or write. Recent work has defined thresholds for cognitive impairment in ALS using quantile regression that takes into account age and education in a North American cohort (McMillan et al., 2020). Out of 102 ALS patients, ECAS scores were available for 93 patients, and these were assigned status as "intact" or "impaired" based on the ALS-Specific ECAS threshold score for the patients' corresponding age and education. For three patients, cognitive status was based on patient records in an online database; six were assigned cognitive status as given in their medical charts; and one had cognitive status identified in an earlier study. Additional demographic, motor, cognitive, and selected neuropsychological characteristics of the participants are summarized on the companion website.

Measures of speech production are summarized in Table 16–2 for controls, the full set of ALS patients, the subsets of ALS patients with and without executive impairment as assessed by the ECAS ALS-specific score, and the subsets of ALS patients with and without dysarthria, as assessed from the ALSFRS-R speech subscale, clinician's notes, and review of the recordings. The features listed relate to quantity of output in the number of words and number of T-units; the rate of output in words per minute; and measures that reflect grammatical competence such as MLU, the frequency of dependent clauses, and the frequency of grammatically well-formed sentences. MLU is a rough measure of syntactic complexity, since a T-unit is lengthened by being made more complex. The frequency of dependent clauses is a more precise measure of discourse complexity, as it reflects the number of clauses that are combined into one syntactic unit. The percent of well-formed

sentences indicates the degree to which a speaker's speech is grammatically correct. We also recorded the duration of silences ≥2.0 sec, a measure of fluency that reflects word-finding or initiation difficulty, apathy, or other deficits. We use the report of content, with a maximum score of 9 as described above, as a summary measure of the discourse competence of the speakers.

The characteristics of speech production in this cohort of ALS patients and controls are similar to the results found in other studies, as shown in Table 16–2. ALS patients overall produce less speech than controls, as reflected in the number of words and T-units produced and the overall speech rate (WPM). ALS patients without an executive impairment exhibit similarly reduced output and speech rate. ALS patients without dysarthria do not differ from controls on the features of speech production examined here. ALS patients with executive impairment have reduced output, like the ALS cohort as a whole, but they also are impaired on all three measures of grammaticality: MLU, dependent clauses, and well-formed sentences. They are impaired not only relative to controls on these measures, but also relative to ALS patients without executive impairment. The patients with an executive impairment also spend significantly more time in long pauses than either controls or ALS patients without executive impairment, and they report significantly less content than controls. Box 16–4 shows a Cookie Theft scene description given by an ALS patient with executive impairment.

In this description of the Cookie Theft scene, the speaker produces 80 words in 11 T-units in a span of 59 seconds. There is only one dependent clause, in line 6. The T-units in lines 7, 8, and 9 are ungrammatical: In lines 7 and 8, the definite article is missing,

Table 16–2. Mean (SD) Speech Production Characteristics of ALS Patients and Controls[1]

Speech Output	Controls (n = 47)	All ALS (n = 102)	ALS Without Executive Impairment (N = 82)	ALS Without Dysarthria (N = 76)	ALS With Executive Impairment (N = 20)	ALS With Dysarthria (N = 26)
Number of words	160 (76)	131 (49)*	135 (48)	139 (49)	114 (49)*	107 (40)**DD
Number of T-Units	15.4 (6.7)	12.8 (4.6)*	12.8 (4.6)*	13.3 (4.7)	12.7 (4.9)	11.2 (4.1)**
Words per Minute	137 (35)	120 (36)**	125 (32)*	129 (33)	101 (45)**E	94 (33)*DD
MLU	10.8 (3.2)	10.5 (2.7)	10.8 (2.3)	10.8 (2.8)	9.3 (3.7)*EE	9.7 (2.2)
Dependent Clauses/ 100 T-Units	42.4 (43.4)	35.5 (23.0)	38.6 (21.5)	38.1 (23.2)	22.8 (25.1)*EE	28.0 (21.1)
% Well-Formed Sentences	90.9 (10.1)	87.9 (13.0)	89.3 (11.9)	90.5 (9.2)	82.0 (16.0)*E	80.2 (18.6)**DD
% Pause Time (for pauses ≥2 sec)	9.5 (14.6)	14.7 (17.7)	11.7 (15.3)	14.5 (17.1)	27.1 (21.7)**EE	15.3 (19.8)
Report of Content (max = 9)	6.9 (1.3)	6.5 (1.5)	6.7 (1.3)	6.9 (1.2)	5.9 (1.9)*	5.7 (1.9)**DD

Notes: [1]ALS differs from controls, *$p < .05$; **$p < .01$; differs from ALS without executive impairment E$p < .05$, EE$p < .01$; differs from ALS without dysarthria D$p < .05$, DD$p < .01$.

BOX 16–4. Cookie Theft Description

Disease duration from onset = 2 years, age at test = 66 years

1   Well the boy is trying to get the cookies out of the cookie jar

2   but he's gonna fall and get hurt

3   the stool is going over

4   the lady is doing the dishes

5   but the sink, is overflowing

6   and, I can't see if anything else is going on in the yard

7   but . . . lady's doing dishes

8   sink is overflowing

9   kids, boy getting cookies

10   the chair is going to fall. [Examiner: Anything else?] (14.5 sec)

11   Well she's standing in the pile of water

Discourse duration = 59 sec, # of words = 80, report of content = 5, WPM = 81, MLU = 7.3, dependent clauses per 100 T-units = 9.1, % of T-units that are well-formed sentences = 72.7

---

and line 9 is missing an article and an auxiliary verb. The speaker mentions five of the nine obligatory items of content: the woman is doing dishes, the sink is overflowing, the woman is standing in water on the floor, the boy is getting cookies, and the stool is falling. There is no mention of four obligatory items: the woman does not notice what is happening, the girl is helping her brother, any description of other features inside the room, and any description of anything outside the room. In sum, this Cookie Theft description is significantly limited in number of words, speech rate, MLU, dependent clauses, well-formed sentences, and report of content.

The results of this analysis are similar to the overall results of the analyses of the Frog Story task with the addition of the variable of report of content. While local connectedness and maintenance of the search theme are related to executive resources, global connectedness is not, and it plausibly depends instead on memory. The report of content in the present cohort was not impaired relative to controls for the group of all ALS patients and the subgroups without executive impairment and without dysarthria. For patients without an executive impairment, the report of content was correlated with measures of motor and executive functioning, the speech subscale of the ALSFRS-R, seated vital capacity, and letter fluency (Table 16–3). This is the same pattern of correlations that is seen for measures of output, WPM, and number of words and T-units. The percent of pause time exhibits a similar pattern: It is correlated with seated vital capacity, letter fluency, and reverse digit span. The relation of report of content to verbal output bears further investigation.

The measures of grammaticality (MLU, the frequency of dependent clauses, and the percent of well-formed sentences) suggest they are independent of both motor functioning and executive functioning. This was found in both discourse samples and has been reported by others (Taylor et al., 2013; Tsermentseli et al., 2016; York et al., 2014). The current data provide further evidence to suggest that grammaticality relies on a domain of language resources that is separate from executive functioning in ALS.

Underlying Neural Mechanisms

Advances in neural imaging have made it possible to learn much more about the neural substrates of ALS variants as well as other neurodegenerative disorders. Some of the discourse studies described in this chapter have included imaging components that contribute to our understanding of the underlying mechanisms of observed cognitive and linguistic deficits associated with discourse in ALS. Interested readers can go to the companion website to see an overview of some of this neural imaging research.

Table 16–3. Correlations of Speech Performance Measures With Motor and Executive Functioning in Cognitively Intact ALS Patients (*N* = 82)[1]

	Motor Functioning		Executive Functioning	
	ALSFRS-R Speech Subscale	Vital Capacity, Seated	Letter Fluency	Reverse Digit Span
Words	.417**	.459**	.411*	.206 (*p* = .063)
T-Units	.359**	.370**	.357**	NS
WPM	.500**	.524**	.448**	NS
MLU	NS	NS	NS	NS
Dependent Clauses/ 100 T-Units	NS	NS	NS	NS
% Well-Formed Sentences	NS	NS	NS	NS
% Pause Time	NS	−.421**	−.288**	−.306**
Report of Content	.329**	.222*	.220*	NS

Notes: 1. *$^*p$* < .05; **$^{**}p$* < .01; NS *p* > .1.

Conclusions

The recurrent theme of studies of discourse in ALS is that ALS is a multisystem disorder with differing consequences for different individuals. A sizeable proportion of ALS patients, likely more than half, possess normal executive functioning, language, and social cognition. Some patients exhibit reduced and slowed speech output, which can be related to their motor deficits and to executive deficits. In patients with grammatical impairments, this deficit appears to be largely an independent feature of language functioning. At a higher level of language production, involving the organization of sentences into an extended discourse such as a narrative or picture description, the executive deficits of ALS patients may interfere with the coherence and completeness of a body of spoken discourse. However, ALS patients are not the only patients with neurodegenerative disease that are afflicted by such impairments (see Chapters 13, 14, and 15).

We have seen that there is overlap in the language impairments of bvFTD with ALS, as can be expected from their shared executive impairments and pathology. There is also overlap with nonfluent/agrammatic Primary Progressive Aphasia (naPPA), as can be expected from their shared grammatical impairments and pathology. ALS is most prominently a motor disorder, but the ramifications of the disease are varied and variable as they affect speech and language. Clinicians working with persons living with ALS are advised to consider the higher levels of language comprehension and production—that is, the levels of the sentence, the paragraph, and the larger message that the speaker wishes to communicate. These levels of speech are critical for the meaningful assessment and possible treatment interventions for the speech of persons afflicted with ALS and their partners in communication.

References

Abrahams, S., & Bak, T. H. (2009–2013). *The Edinburgh Cognitive and Behavioral ALS Screen*. The University Court of the University of Edinburgh.

Abrahams, S., Goldstein, L. H., Simmons, A., Brammer, M., Williams, S. C., Giampietro, V., & Leigh, P. N. (2004). Word retrieval in amyotrophic lateral sclerosis: A functional magnetic resonance imaging study. *Brain, 127* (Pt. 7), 1507–1517. https://doi.org/10.1093/brain/awh170

Abrahams, S., Leigh, P. N., Harvey, A., Vythelingum, G. N., Grisé, D., & Goldstein, L. H. (2000). Verbal fluency and executive dysfunction in amyotrophic lateral sclerosis (ALS). *Neuropsychologia, 38*(6), 734–747. https://doi.org/10.1016/s0028-3932(99)00146-3

Ash, S., Evans, E., O'Shea, J., Powers, J., Boller, A., Weinberg, D., . . . Grossman, M. (2013). Differentiating primary progressive aphasias in a brief sample of connected speech. *Neurology, 81*(4), 329–336. https://doi.org/10.1212/WNL.0b013e31829c5d0e

Ash, S., Menaged, A., Olm, C., McMillan, C. T., Boller, A., Irwin, D. J., . . . Grossman, M. (2014). Narrative discourse deficits in amyotrophic lateral sclerosis. *Neurology, 83*(6), 520–528. https://doi.org/10.1212/wnl.0000000000000670

Ash, S., Moore, P., Antani, S., McCawley, G., Work, M., & Grossman, M. (2006). Trying to tell a tale: Discourse impairments in progressive aphasia and frontotemporal dementia. *Neurology, 66*, 1405–1413. https://doi.org/10.1212/01.wnl.0000210435.72614.38

Ash, S., Olm, C., McMillan, C. T., Boller, A., Irwin, D. J., McCluskey, L., . . . Grossman, M. (2015). Deficits in sentence expression in amyotrophic lateral sclerosis. *Amyotrophic Lateral Sclerosis and Frontotemporal Degen-*

eration, 16(1–2), 31–39. https://doi.org/10
.3109/21678421.2014.974617

Beeldman, E., Raaphorst, J., Klein Twennaar, M.,
de Visser, M., Schmand, B. A., & de Haan, R.
J. (2016). The cognitive profile of ALS: A systematic review and meta-analysis update.
*Journal of Neurology, Neurosurgery, and Psy-
chiatry, 87*(6), 611–619. doi: 10.1136/jnnp
-2015-310734

Bishop, D. V. (2003). *Test for the Reception of
Grammar (TROG-2)*. Harcourt Assessment.

Bschor, T., Kühl, K. P., & Reischies, F. M. (2001).
Spontaneous speech of patients with dementia of the Alzheimer type and mild cognitive
impairment. *International Psychogeriatrics,
13*(3), 289–298. https://doi.org/10.1017/s104
1610201007682

Byrne, S., Elamin, M., Bede, P., Shatunov, A.,
Walsh, C., Corr, B., . . . Hardiman, O. (2012).
Cognitive and clinical characteristics of
patients with amyotrophic lateral sclerosis
carrying a C9orf72 repeat expansion: A population-based cohort study. *Lancet Neurology, 11*(3), 232–240. https://doi.org/10.1016/
s1474-4422(12)70014-5

Cedarbaum, J. M., Stambler, N., Malta, E., Fuller,
C., Hilt, D., Thurmond, B., & Nakanishi, A.
(1999). The ALSFRS-R: A revised ALS functional rating scale that incorporates assessments of respiratory function. BDNF ALS
Study Group (Phase III). *Journal of Neurological Sciences, 169*(1–2), 13–21. https://doi
.org/10.1016/S0022-510X(99)00210-5

Ceslis, A., Argall, R., Henderson, R. D.,
McCombe, P. A., & Robinson, G. A. (2020).
The spectrum of language impairments in
amyotrophic lateral sclerosis. *Cortex, 132*,
349–360. https://doi.org/10.1016/j.cortex
.2020.09.003

Consonni, M., Iannaccone, S., Cerami, C.,
Frasson, P., Lacerenza, M., Lunetta, C., . . .
Cappa, S. F. (2013). The cognitive and behavioral profile of amyotrophic lateral sclerosis:
Application of the consensus criteria. *Behavioral Neurology, 27*(2), 143–153. https://doi
.org/10.3233/ben-2012-110202

Coughlan, A. K., & Warrington, E. K. (1978).
Word comprehension and word retrieval in
patients with localized cerebral lesions. *Brain,
101*(1), 163–185. https://doi.org/10.1093/
brain/101.1.163

Giordana, M. T., Ferrero, P., Grifoni, S., Pel-
lerino, A., Naldi, A., & Montuschi, A. (2011).
Dementia and cognitive impairment in amyotrophic lateral sclerosis: A review. *Neurological Sciences, 32*(1), 9–16. https://doi.org/10
.1007/s10072-010-0439-6

Goodglass, H., & Kaplan, E. (1972). *Boston Diagnostic Aphasia Examination*. SpringerLink.

Gordon, P. H., Goetz, R. R., Rabkin, J. G., Dalton,
K., McElhiney, M., Hays, A. P., . . . Mitsumoto,
H. (2010). A prospective cohort study of neu-
ropsychological test performance in ALS.
Amyotrophic Lateral Sclerosis, 11(3), 312–320.
https://doi.org/10.3109/17482961003622585

Hunt, K. W. (1965). *Grammatical structures written at three grade levels*. National Council of
Teachers of English.

Kasper, E., Zydatiss, K., Schuster, C., Machts, J.,
Bittner, D., Kaufmann, J., . . . Prudlo, J. (2016).
No change in executive performance in ALS
patients: A longitudinal neuropsychological
study. *Neurodegenerative Diseases, 16*(3–4),
184–191. https://doi.org/10.1159/000440957

Labov, W., & Waletzky, J. (1967). Narrative analysis: Oral versions of personal experience. In
J. Helm (Ed.), *Essays on the verbal and visual
arts: Proceedings of the 1966 annual spring
meeting of the American Ethnological Society*
(pp. 12–44). University of Washington Press.

Mayer, M. (1967). *Frog, where are you?* Penguin
Putnam.

McMillan, C. T., Wuu, J., Rascovsky, K., Cosen-
tino, S., Grossman, M., Elman, L., . . . Bena-
tar, M. (2020). An evaluation of empirical
approaches for defining cognitive impairment in amyotrophic lateral sclerosis. *medRxiv*,
2020.2012.2023.20248410. https://doi.org/10
.1101/2020.12.23.20248410

Montuschi, A., Iazzolino, B., Calvo, A., Moglia,
C., Lopiano, L., Restagno, G., . . . Chiò, A.
(2015). Cognitive correlates in amyotrophic
lateral sclerosis: A population-based study in
Italy. *Journal of Neurology, Neurosurgery, and
Psychiatry, 86*(2), 168–173. https://doi.org/10
.1136/jnnp-2013-307223

Murphy, J., Factor-Litvak, P., Goetz, R., Lomen-Hoerth, C., Nagy, P. L., Hupf, J., . . . Mitsumoto, H. (2016). Cognitive-behavioral screening reveals prevalent impairment in a large multicenter ALS cohort. *Neurology, 86*(9), 813–820. https://doi.org/10.1212/wnl.0000000000002305

Nicholas, L. E., & Brookshire, R. H. (1993). A system for quantifying the informativeness and efficiency of the connected speech of adults with aphasia. *Journal of Speech and Hearing Research, 36*(2), 338–350. https://doi.org/10.1044/jshr.3602.338

Reilly, J., Losh, M., Bellugi, U., & Wulfeck, B. (2004). "Frog, where are you?" Narratives in children with specific language impairment, early focal brain injury, and Williams syndrome. *Brain and Language, 88*(2), 229–247. https://doi.org/10.1016/S0093-934X(03)00101-9

Roberts-South, A., Findlater, K., Strong, M. J., & Orange, J. B. (2012). Longitudinal changes in discourse production in amyotrophic lateral sclerosis. *Seminars in Speech Language, 33*(1), 79–94. https://doi.org/10.1055/s-0031-1301165

Strong, M. J., Abrahams, S., Goldstein, L. H., Woolley, S., McLaughlin, P., Snowden, J., . . . Turner, M. R. (2017). Amyotrophic lateral sclerosis—frontotemporal spectrum disorder (ALS-FTSD): Revised diagnostic criteria. *Amyotrophic Lateral Sclerosis and Frontotemporal Degenereration, 18*(3–4), 153–174. https://doi.org/10.1080/21678421.2016.1267768

Taylor, L. J., Brown, R. G., Tsermentseli, S., Al-Chalabi, A., Shaw, C. E., Ellis, C. M., . . . Goldstein, L. H. (2013). Is language impairment more common than executive dysfunction in amyotrophic lateral sclerosis? *Journal of Neurology, Neurosurgery, and Psychiatry, 84*(5), 494–498. https://doi.org/10.1136/jnnp-2012-303526

Tsermentseli, S., Leigh, P. N., Taylor, L. J., Radunovic, A., Catani, M., & Goldstein, L. H. (2016). Syntactic processing as a marker for cognitive impairment in amyotrophic lateral sclerosis. *Amyotrophic Lateral Sclerosis and Frontotemporal Degenereration, 17*(1–2), 69–76. https://doi.org/10.3109/21678421.2015.1071397

Wilson, S. M., Henry, M. L., Besbris, M., Ogar, J. M., Dronkers, N. F., Jarrold, W., . . . Gorno-Tempini, M. L. (2010). Connected speech production in three variants of primary progressive aphasia. *Brain, 133*(Pt. 7), 2069–2088. https://doi.org/10.1093/brain/awq129

York, C., Olm, C., Boller, A., McCluskey, L., Elman, L., Haley, J., . . . Grossman, M. (2014). Action verb comprehension in amyotrophic lateral sclerosis and Parkinson's disease. *Journal of Neurology, 261*(6), 1073–1079. https://doi.org/10.1007/s00415-014-7314-y

Yorkston, K. M., & Beukelman, D. R. (1980). An analysis of connected speech samples of aphasic and normal speakers. *Journal of Speech and Hearing Disorders, 45*(1), 27–36. https://doi.org/1044/jshd.4501.27

Yoshizawa, K., Yasuda, N., Fukuda, M., Yukimoto, Y., Ogino, M., Hata, W., . . . Higashikawa, M. (2014). Syntactic comprehension in patients with amyotrophic lateral sclerosis. *Behavioral Neurology, 2014*, 230578. https://doi.org/10.1155/2014/230578

Zago, S., Poletti, B., Morelli, C., Doretti, A., & Silani, V. (2011). Amyotrophic lateral sclerosis and frontotemporal dementia (ALS-FTD). *Archives Italiennes Biologie, 149*(1), 39–56. https://doi.org/10.4449/aib.v149i1.1263

APPENDIX 16-1

Comprehensive Episodes and Events for Frog Story

Episode	Role	Page	Event	
1	O(rientation)	1	1	A boy and his dog are looking at a frog in a jar in the boy's bedroom. It's nighttime; the moon is seen through the window and the boy is wearing pajamas.
	A(ction)	2	2	The boy and dog are asleep, and the frog climbs out of the jar.
	R(esolution)	3	3	It's morning. The boy and dog wake up and sees that the frog is gone.
2	O	4	4	The boy and dog look for the frog. The boy has gotten dressed and is looking in his boot.
	A	4	5	The dog puts his head in the jar.
	A	5	6	The boy opens the window and calls out. The dog is in the window with his head stuck in the jar, about to fall.
	A	6	7	The dog falls out of the window.
	R	7	8	The jar is broken on ground. The boy is holding the dog and looking angry while the dog licks his face.
3	O	8–9	9	The boy and dog are outside the house near a stand of trees. The boy is calling out.
	A	10	10	The boy peers into a hole in the ground, still calling to the frog.
	R	11	11	The boy recoils from the hole, with his two hands holding his nose, and a groundhog is partway out of the hole (having nipped, licked, or otherwise touched the boy on his nose).
4	O	8–9	12	The boy and dog are outside the house near a stand of trees. The dog is eying a stream of bees forming a line to a hive on a nearby tree.

Episode	Role	Page	Event	
	A	10	13	The dog jumps up toward the beehive.
	A	11	14	The dog is barking at the beehive, with his front feet on the tree.
	A	12–13	15	The beehive has fallen on the ground, and the dog is standing on his hind legs with his two front paws against the tree, while the bees are coming out of the hive toward the dog.
	R	14–15	16	The dog is running away from the bees, which are swarming after him.
5	O	12–13	17	The boy has climbed onto a large tree branch and is peering into a hole in the tree.
	A & R	14–15	18	An owl emerges from the hole in the tree with wings spread, and the startled boy falls backward onto the ground.
6	O	16	19	The boy fends off the owl and begins to climb up onto a large rock.
	A	17	20	The boy stands on top of the big rock, leaning against a branch of a shrub and calling out, while the owl watches from a nearby tree. The dog comes slinking back with its head down and its tail between its legs.
	A	18	21	The boy is lifted up on the head of a large deer; what appeared to be branches were actually the deer's antlers.
	A	19	22	The deer runs toward the edge of a drop-off with the boy on its head, while the dog runs alongside, barking.
	A	20–21	23	The boy and dog fall over the edge of the bank into a pond, while the deer remains at the edge.
	R	22	24	The boy and dog land in the water, with the deer at the edge of the drop-off above looking smug.
7	O	23	25	The boy sits up in the water and cocks his ear; the dog has climbed up onto his shoulders and head.
	A	24	26	The boy approaches the edge of the water next to a large hollow log and shushes the dog.

Episode	Role	Page	Event	
	A	25	27	The boy and dog lean over the log; we see their backs.
	R	26	28	On the other side of the log, the boy and dog find their frog with a lady frog.
	A (Coda)	27	29	The boy and dog see eight baby frogs emerge from the brush next to the log.
	R (Coda)	28–29	30	The boy and dog wave a cheerful goodbye to the frog family as they wade back across the pond, carrying one of the baby frogs.

SECTION V
Discourse Databases for Use With Clinical Populations

Carl A. Coelho, Co-Editor

In this chapter, the authors provide a summary of TalkBank, a large online multimedia database consisting of several categories of spoken language. The goal of TalkBank, as indicated on their website (https://www.talkbank.org/), is to "foster fundamental research in the study of human communication with an emphasis on spoken communication." Included in the database are discourse samples from the clinical populations discussed throughout this book, including normal aging, aphasia, traumatic brain injury (TBI), right hemisphere disorders (RHD), primary progressive aphasia (PPA), and Alzheimer's dementia. In addition to extensive examples of coded discourse, TalkBank includes an array of teaching resources for researchers and clinicians interested in learning more about discourse analysis.

TalkBank has facilitated the documentation of discourse disorders and acted as a catalyst for increasing our understanding of discourse analysis. Data in TalkBank have been contributed by researchers worldwide working in the area of communication and discourse. These data have resulted in hundreds of high-impact publications and presentations.

17 Discourse Databases for Use With Clinical Populations

Davida Fromm and Brian MacWhinney

Introduction

To build a scientific discipline, one cannot overstate the advantages of shared databases and shared resources. The scientific process is built on verification and replication of empirical data. This is particularly true for the study of discourse in clinical populations. Even the best descriptions of language samples, coding systems, reliability procedures, and outcome measures pale in comparison with the ability to see and hear speakers, see coded transcripts, and replicate results. Terms that describe features of language samples (e.g., *nonfluent, fluent, paraphasic, circumlocutory, agrammatic, aprosodic, paragrammatic, tangential*) and severity of impairment (e.g., *mild, moderate*) may mean slightly different things to different people based on their training and experience. Likewise, within a given research or clinical program there may be good reliability on coding correct information units (CIUs) or word-finding problems, but does that reliability extend to other researchers and clinicians? Do we have the raw materials and conditions necessary not only to verify and replicate data, but also to establish psychometric proper-

ties such as test-retest metrics so we can confidently credit treatment for changes in discourse?

The Open Science and Open Data initiatives have stressed the importance of making language data widely available (Chiarcos & Pareja-Lora, 2019), citing both the immense effort of creating resources and the potential gains of sharing and reusing data for purposes of replication, new applications, or novel experiments. Given the time invested in transcription, it makes sense to extend the results beyond single clinics or research laboratories. Data sharing also makes it possible to have online collaborative commentaries (MacWhinney, 2007) and conduct systematic, data-based comparisons to ascertain best practices for discourse measurement and analysis. Large databases allow for more robust statistical treatment of data, avoiding the limitation mentioned so often at the end of research articles about small sample sizes, insufficient power, and risks of Type II errors. More specifically, large normative databases, particularly for aging populations, are necessary to fully appreciate typical performance profiles in otherwise healthy or unimpaired populations. Finally, at the most fundamental level, scientific research, especially that funded by public funding, comes with the responsibility of opening data and results to the public in a fully transparent fashion.

In this chapter, we describe the primary discourse databases currently available for adult populations with and without communication disorders. The meaning of "currently available" is not a trivial matter. Li et al. (2019) published a systematic review of worldwide resources for speech databases and found 10 databases that met these criteria: targeting individuals with neurological disorders, recording audio or video samples, and making their resources available for other researchers. However, some of the database links provided are no longer active, and the review did not specify the actual steps involved in obtaining access to the database. In this chapter, we focus on the TalkBank databases, which are both currently available and readily accessible to authorized professionals. We then examine a few of the other major databases currently being used in published research, although access to other data sets often requires more extensive application, review, and approval procedures.

Discourse Resources Available Through TalkBank Clinical Banks

The goal of the TalkBank project (https://talkbank.org/), funded by the National Institutes of Health and the National Science Foundation, is to support data sharing and direct, communitywide access to naturalistic recordings and transcripts of human and animal communication. TalkBank is the world's largest open-access, integrated repository of data on spoken language, containing shared databases of multimedia interactions for the study of child language,

aphasia, traumatic brain injury (TBI), right hemisphere disorder (RHD), fluency, autism spectrum disorder, and more. This larger project grew from the model created by the original CHild Language Data Exchange System (CHILDES) project (MacWhinney, 2014), which began in 1984 and focused on first-language acquisition in young children. This section will present information about four TalkBank clinical language banks: AphasiaBank, DementiaBank, RHDBank, and TBIBank. Before describing each of the banks, we will highlight some shared features of the TalkBank clinical banks and explain how the Computerized Language ANalysis (CLAN) program (https://talkbank.org/manuals/CLAN.pdf) expedites and improves the process of transcription and discourse analysis.

Shared Features of TalkBank Clinical Banks: Index to Corpora

Each of the clinical language banks in TalkBank has its own webpage with links to valuable resources for researchers, educators, and clinicians. These starting pages are all accessible from https://talkbank.org. Each webpage has a link called "Index to Corpora," which shows a list of all the corpora in that database with relevant information (e.g., age, number of participants, type of discourse tasks, type of media). Clicking on any corpus name in that list brings up a page with more specific information about the corpus, the contributors, and the project from which the discourse data were collected. From those individual corpus pages, there are also links for downloading the language transcripts and media files or going to the Browsable Database, where you can listen to and watch (for video files) the language sample while also following along with the transcript. It should be noted here that these clinical data are password protected and available only to licensed clinicians, educators, and researchers who agree to abide by the TalkBank Ground Rules for data sharing (https://talkbank.org/share/).[1]

Shared Features of TalkBank Clinical Banks: CHAT and CLAN

All transcripts in the TalkBank databases use a single consistent format, called Codes for the Human Analysis of Talk (CHAT) (https://talkbank.org/manuals/CHAT.pdf). This format has been developed over many years to accommodate the needs of a wide range of research communities and disciplines. Transcripts in CHAT format can then make use of an extensive set of analysis programs, called CLAN (https://talkbank.org/manuals/CLAN.pdf). The CLAN program is free to download from the main TalkBank website for Windows, Mac, and Unix. Complete CHAT and CLAN user manuals are available at the website, as is an *SLP's Guide to CLAN*, which provides an abridged and more user-friendly introduction to transcribing and analyzing samples for SLPs. In addition, the website has a link to *Tutorial Screencasts*, with more than 40 short video tutorials on how to transcribe and perform many different CLAN-related functions.

CHAT transcripts start with header tiers that give information about the language and the speakers. As you can see in the example below from DementiaBank, the transcript includes a participant and an investigator; the participant is a 66-year-old male from the Pitt corpus, who was diagnosed with probable Alzheimer's disease and scored 20 on the Mini-Mental Status Exam.

@Begin

@Languages: eng

@Participants: PAR Participant, INV Investigator

@ID: eng|Pitt|PAR|66;|male|ProbableAD||Participant|20||

@ID: eng|Pitt|INV|||||Investigator|||

Most CHAT file transcripts at the shared databases will look like the example below, where the speaker's utterance (transcribed manually) is followed by two lines that get added to the file automatically by running the MOR command. The %mor tier has morphological tagging and part-of-speech categories; the %gra tier shows pairwise grammatical relations between words. The information on these tiers is used for many automatic discourse analysis commands in CLAN. The black dot next to the utterance holds the temporal information, linking that utterance to the audio or video file in milliseconds.

*PAR: I would grab two slices of bread . •

%mor: pro:sub|I mod|will&COND v|grab det:num|two n|slice-PL prep|of n|bread .

%gra: 1|3|SUBJ 2|3|AUX 3|0|ROOT 4|5|QUANT 5|3|OBJ 6|5|NJCT 7|6|POBJ 8|3|PUNCT

---

[1]Passwords are provided to all licensed SLPs, educators, and researchers. They should send an email request for TalkBank membership to Brian MacWhinney (macw@cmu.edu) with contact information, affiliation, and a brief general statement about how they envision using the resources. Students interested in accessing the data should ask their faculty advisors to join as members.

Advantages of transcribing in CHAT and analyzing a transcript with CLAN include:

(a) Smooth transcription. Transcribers can use normal English orthography (e.g., *can't, shoes, girl's*), and the morphological structure of these forms will be analyzed automatically by CLAN's MOR program.

(b) Sound playback. It is simple to time-link utterances in a CHAT file to the audio or video file and then replay the utterances individually to transcribe, add coding, check accuracy, add gestures, measure pauses, and so on.

(c) Faster analysis. Once transcripts are prepared, it takes seconds to run commands on a single transcript or hundreds of transcripts in a single step.

(d) Less demand for expertise and better reliability. Automatic analyses and computations are thoroughly replicable because repeated runs of the same command will always produce the same results. Results will not be dependent on the varying training and linguistic expertise of research and or clinical staff.

Shared Features of TalkBank Clinical Banks: Browsable Database

All TalkBank shared databases include links to the Browsable Database, which opens to a page of simple instructions on how to watch and hear videos (or audio files) while following along with the language transcript. A directory of corpora and files appears in the top left corner of the page in the Browsable Database. To watch, click on the file of interest and then press the play arrow next to the line in the transcript where you want to begin or on the video that appears in the lower left corner.

AphasiaBank

AphasiaBank (https://aphasia.talkbank.org/) is a shared, multimedia database for the study of communication in aphasia (Fromm, Forbes, et al., 2020; MacWhinney et al., 2011). Adults with aphasia often have impairments that affect their ability to communicate successfully at the discourse level. Analyses of discourse in aphasia have received a great deal of attention, with clinicians and researchers working to identify psychometrically sound approaches to discourse assessment and measurement. Since its inception in 2007, this database has grown to contain well over 1,000 videos and transcripts of people with aphasia (PWAs) and controls doing a variety of discourse tasks. A unique feature of this language bank is its standard discourse protocol and elicitation script for gathering language samples, which include free speech, picture descriptions, the *Cinderella* story narrative, and a procedural discourse task. The tasks were selected by a group of aphasiologists to capture a variety of discourse genres that were relevant to the population and used in the existing literature. For example, the protocol includes a free speech stroke story, asking individuals to tell what they remember about when they had their stroke and then about their recovery. Control participants were asked to tell what they remember about any illness or injury they had. Another protocol task is the *Cinderella* story, which has been used in aphasia literature for well over 30 years and is the second-most frequently reported language sampling technique for eliciting narratives in aphasia (Bryant et al., 2016).

The standard discourse protocol is augmented by comprehensive demographic data collection on all participants and a standard test battery that includes the Western Aphasia Battery–Revised (WAB-R) Aphasia Quotient subtests (Kertesz, 2007), the Boston Naming Test (Kaplan et al., 2001), the Verb Naming Test (Cho-Reyes & Thompson, 2012), and a repetition test developed to assess word-level and sentence-level repetition skills. Two tests of comprehension were added to the battery after initial data collection started: Sentence Comprehension, from the Philadelphia Comprehension Battery (Saffran et al., 1988); and Complex Ideational Material–Short Form, from the Boston Diagnostic Aphasia Exam (Goodglass et al., 2001). All this material (e.g., scripted discourse protocol, stimulus pictures, test materials) is available at the AphasiaBank website. The protocol collection includes more than 450 videos and transcripts of PWAs and more than 250 for controls in English. The protocol has been translated into other languages (e.g., Cantonese, Croatian, French, Italian, Mandarin, Spanish) and those corpora have been contributed to the database as well. Researchers and clinicians have also contributed videos and transcripts with media for nonprotocol-based discourse samples such as conversations, story retells, assessment tasks (e.g., Quick Aphasia Battery [Wilson et al., 2018], WAB-R picture descriptions, Grey Oral Reading Test [Wiederhold & Bryant, 2012]), and various types of treatment sessions (e.g., script training, group therapy).

Currently, password-protected access to the AphasiaBank corpora, demographic data, and test results has been granted to more than 1,250 faculty and licensed clinicians from more than 55 countries, all of whom have agreed to abide by the TalkBank data sharing ground rules. They work in a range of fields (e.g., speech-language pathology, linguistics, psychology, neurology, English, computer science, engineering) and use the database for research, teaching, and clinical purposes, examples of which are highlighted below. The database has been used in hundreds of publications, conference presentations, and theses, which can be accessed (without a password) from links at the AphasiaBank website (*Publications, Posters, and Presentations*). Given the amount of work that has been done, a review of what has been learned is beyond the scope of this chapter. However, the main areas of research include the development of new discourse outcome measures and norms, psychometric properties of discourse measures, new automatic discourse analysis tools, comparisons between manual and automatic analyses, comparisons of discourse outcome measures across genres, comparisons of different lexical diversity measures, informativeness and naming, coherence and cohesion, grammar, verb types and verb argument structure, gesture, fluency, paraphasia classification and error analysis, syndrome classification, demographic factors (e.g., race, sex, gender), change over time, and treatment effects.

Teaching Resources

The *Teaching* section of the webpage contains links to material gathered from various database resources. The goal for this section was to curate the vast resources to present cases, examples, and exercises that could be used for a wide range of educational purposes. A particularly complete teaching component is the *Grand Rounds* guided tutorial on aphasia, which focuses on how language differs across aphasia types (e.g., anomic, Broca's, conduction, global, transcortical motor, transcortical sensory, Wernicke's) and language tasks (e.g., free speech, naming, repetition, picture description).

The *Grand Rounds* pages include short case histories and discussion questions built around 40 captioned video segments from dozens of PWAs. Additional "Treatment Focus" questions stimulate thinking and discussions about ways to approach intervention to improve communication for each case presentation.

The *Examples* webpage provides very short, captioned video clips of common features from the connected speech of PWAs at the word level, sentence level, and discourse level. This page is organized by features (e.g., phonemic paraphasia, circumlocution, agrammatism, empty speech), with a description of the feature and links to video examples. Each video link includes basic information about the speaker (e.g., WAB-R AQ, aphasia type).

The *Classroom Activities* link downloads a Word file with ideas for exercises such as clinical assessment and treatment planning, measuring different aspects of discourse (e.g., CIUs, mean length of utterance [MLU]), using the EVAL command from the CLAN program (described below), coding speech errors (e.g., phonemic and semantic paraphasias), examining main concepts in narratives, and comparing across aphasia types as well as across other disorders (e.g., right hemisphere disorder). Several of these exercises were contributed by AphasiaBank members, and we appreciate and encourage this type of resource sharing. Surveys have repeatedly shown that knowledge about discourse analysis (e.g., measurement, sampling methods) is a major barrier to its use (Bryant et al., 2019; Bryant et al., 2017; Stark et al., 2021), making this an important area for continued development.

Discourse Analysis

The AphasiaBank homepage has a link to a webpage that is regularly updated with information about approaches to discourse analysis. The analyses currently featured include coherence (Wright et al., 2013; Wright et al., 2014), core lexicon (Dalton et al., 2020; Kim & Wright, 2020), CIUs (Nicholas & Brookshire, 1993), main concepts (Dalton & Richardson, 2019; Richardson & Dalton, 2020), story grammar (Greenslade et al., 2020; Richardson et al., 2021), and systemic functional linguistics (Groenewold & Armstrong, 2018). The page also describes methods for automated computation of the Northwestern Narrative Language Analysis (Fromm, MacWhinney, et al., 2020; Thompson et al., 1995) and the Quantitative Production Analysis (Fromm et al., 2021; Rochon et al., 2000; Saffran et al., 1989). Clicking on any of those topics brings up a page with descriptions of the analysis, links to relevant references, and tools and instructions for conducting the analyses. Along with the classroom activities, this is another important resource to continue developing and updating to address barriers to discourse analysis use. In conjunction with work underway by the Methodological and Data Quality task force from FOQUSAphasia (http://www.foqusaphasia.com), this *Discourse Analysis* section will add essential information concerning psychometric properties of commonly used discourse metrics to guide best practices in clinical and research settings (Stark et al., 2021).

CLAN Profile Analyses

Although it is beyond the scope of this chapter to discuss in detail, the AphasiaBank shared database has allowed for the development of several automated measurement tools specific to aphasia as well as the specific tasks in the protocol (Fromm, Forbes, et al., 2020). These commands can be used to get fast, reliable, and informative summaries of language performance. For example, the EVAL command produces a language profile in spreadsheet format that includes 34 output measures such as number of utterances, number of words, MLU, type-token ratio, vocD (Malvern et al., 2004), the moving average type-token ratio (MATTR: Covington & McFall, 2010), words per minute, percent or raw number of various parts of speech, noun-verb ratio, and open-class versus closed-class word ratio (Forbes et al., 2012). This command can show how a given individual compares to controls or others in the AphasiaBank database; it can also compare an individual's performance on the same task done at different points in time to evaluate changes following treatment. The CORELEX command uses core lexicon lists for the five AphasiaBank discourse protocol tasks (Dalton et al., 2020) to compute the number of core lexicon words an individual (or group of individuals) used for each task. FLUCALC can be used to analyze fluency, which is both a critical and yet somewhat elusive concept in the classification of aphasia, as it is associated with both grammatical factors and naming impairments, manifesting in a variety of behaviors such as hesitations, fillers, revisions, sound and sentence fragments, limited output, slower speech rate, and agrammatism (Gordon, 1998; Gordon & Clough, 2020). These tools provide automatic and efficient methods for providing key discourse outcome measures for both clinicians and researchers.

DementiaBank

DementiaBank (https://dementia.talkbank .org/) includes transcripts and media from individuals with various types of dementia as well as individuals with primary progressive aphasia and controls. The largest dementia corpus in the collection is the Pitt corpus (Becker et al., 1984), which con-

tains longitudinal data for four language tasks (Cookie Theft picture descriptions, sentence construction, word fluency, and story retell) from more than 300 individuals with probable Alzheimer's disease (AD) and other types of dementia as well as over 200 elderly controls (Cookie Theft picture descriptions only). Another large database that was recently added is a subset of data from the Wisconsin Longitudinal Study (discussed in more depth below), which also contains Cookie Theft picture descriptions (more than 1,300) but no professional dementia diagnostic data (Herd et al., 2014). Other corpora in DementiaBank include conversations, semistructured interviews, and other language tasks from individuals with AD. The database also includes a corpus of discourse data from individuals with primary progressive aphasia, some seen multiple times, who completed *Cinderella* story narratives and other language tasks. In addition to the English data, DementiaBank corpora are available for German, Mandarin, Spanish, and Taiwanese. Pilot work has recently been initiated to create and use a standard discourse protocol to collect data from individuals with neurotypical and mild cognitive impairment and dementia. The DementiaBank webpage includes a *Protocol* section with details on the tasks and tests, selected specifically for these populations; data will be forthcoming (Lanzi, 2021).

Password-protected access to DementiaBank has been granted to more than 600 researchers, clinicians, and educators from over 50 countries, many of whom are computer scientists using DementiaBank data, primarily from the Pitt corpus (Becker et al., 1994), as the main testbed for the construction and benchmarking of language-based predictors of the onset of cognitive impairment. These data have been of particular interest to researchers who are using machine learning and linguistic analyses to automatically identify AD from short narrative samples as well as researchers who are working to improve speech-recognition skills in personal assistive robots trained to work with older adults with AD (e.g., Rudzicz, Wang, et al, 2014). The data set has been used recently by research groups all over the world in the context of the ADReSS Challenge for Interspeech in 2020 and again in 2021 to train classifiers for early automatic detection of dementia (Luz et al., 2020, 2021). A *Bibliography* link at the DementiaBank website includes more than 200 references to work that used DementiaBank data; a *Posters* link includes copies of posters that were presented at conferences.

RDHBank

RHDBank (https://rhd.talkbank.org/) focuses on the study of communication in adults with RHD resulting from brain damage to the right hemisphere (Minga et al., 2021; see Chapter 11). Symptoms of RHD include cognitive-communication deficits that impair pragmatic skills, resulting in difficulties producing and comprehending discourse. Specifically, difficulties with topic maintenance, discourse coherence and cohesion, inference generation, turn taking, question use, and the integration of contextual nuance are commonly seen in people with RHD (Blake, 2018). The cognitive-communication disorder associated with RHD has a negative impact on quality of life and social integration (Hewetson et al., 2021), leading to calls for better assessment and treatment approaches. Existing research about RHD discourse is limited in quantity and difficult to synthesize due to the use of different discourse tasks and outcome measures as well as methodological issues, such as limited descriptions of participants (Minga et al., 2021).

Like AphasiaBank, the RHDBank database includes a standard discourse protocol, demographic data collection, and a set of assessment procedures. The discourse protocol includes free speech, picture descriptions, the *Cinderella* storytelling task, a procedural discourse task, a question production task, and a first-encounter conversation (Kennedy et al., 1994). Overlaps with the AphasiaBank discourse protocol were intentional to allow for cross-disorder comparisons; other tasks (e.g., conversing to get to know a stranger) were included to assess the specific pragmatic and social discourse aspects of language that commonly affect individuals with RHD. The test battery assesses cognitive-linguistic functioning and visuospatial neglect and includes the Cognitive Linguistic Quick Test (Helm-Estabrooks, 2017), the Apples Test (Bickerton et al., 2011), the General Short Form of the Communicative Participation Item Bank (Baylor et al., 2013), and the Indented Paragraph Test (Caplan, 1987). A small number of other nonprotocol corpora (e.g., Cookie Theft picture descriptions from individuals following right hemisphere strokes) have been contributed to the database as well.

The RHDBank website contains links to a *Bibliography* showing references for published or presented work based on RHDBank data; another link also allows users to see conference *Posters*. So far, discourse analyses have focused predominantly on measures of global coherence, main concepts, question use (type and frequency) in conversation and structured tasks, and the relationship between discourse behaviors and cognitive functioning.

As in AphasiaBank, the teaching resources in RHDBank include a *Grand Rounds* tutorial and a *Classroom Activities* page. The RHD *Grand Rounds* is an educational platform that explains and illustrates the communication behaviors typically seen in individuals with RHD through case presentations, video clips, and discussion questions. The extralinguistic impairments (e.g., anosognosia, aprosodia, neglect) that can occur with RHD are explained as well, and key research articles on these topics are linked and briefly summarized. The *Classroom Activities* link downloads a document with ideas for using RHDBank resources to compare language disorders following left and right hemisphere stroke, plan assessment and treatment for two of the RHD cases from the *Grand Rounds*, code an RHD transcript for global coherence and main concepts, compute CIUs in RHD transcripts and compare them with aphasia and control transcripts, and more. These educational resources are important tools to use to increase exposure to and understanding of the subtle but debilitating cognitive-communication disorders that occur in RHD. These individuals often slip through the cracks both in referrals to SLPs and in research on effective diagnostic and treatment approaches.

TBIBank

TBIBank (https://tbi.talkbank.org/) is a shared database of multimedia interactions for the study of communication in people with TBI. TBI can result in cognitive-communication disorders that may affect all aspects of language (e.g., speaking, listening, reading, writing, pragmatics) as well as attention, reasoning, memory, and executive function (see Chapters 9–10). Discourse in TBI has been described as disorganized, inappropriate, tangential, unclear, redundant, and self-focused. This repository includes two sizeable corpora that each used a standard discourse protocol. One has longitudinal data that allow for the study of communication recovery after TBI (Stubbs et al., 2018; Togher et al., 2014). The complete set of media files in the Togher corpus

have been only partially transcribed, but a wealth of data is available for the same 58 individuals at six measurement times ranging from 3 months to 3 years postonset. Discourse tasks in this corpus were similar to those used in the AphasiaBank protocol with two minor changes: substituting what the individual remembers about their brain injury instead of stroke in the free speech segment, and substituting a Vegemite and cheese sandwich (culturally appropriate for the Australian population) instead of peanut butter and jelly for the procedural discourse segment. Test data were also specific to the population and included a variety of TBI-relevant measures such as the Frenchay Dysarthria Assessment (Enderby & Palmer, 2008) and the Functional Assessment of Verbal Reasoning and Executive Functioning (MacDonald, 2005). The other corpus has 55 speakers with closed head injuries and 52 controls who did a variety of discourse tasks including story retelling, story generation, and informal conversation (Coelho et al., 2003). Demographic data and test results are available for these corpora. Several other smaller corpora include samples of conversations and various other discourse tasks.

Two new corpora were collected with the goal of understanding how typed discourse relates to individual differences in temperament and cognitive-linguistic performance among teens and adults with a recent or chronic history of concussion. One includes 231 written narrative and expository samples from 91 individuals (Stockbridge & Newman, 2019). The other includes multiple written expository samples from a separate group of 487 English-speaking, international roller derby players with significant histories of concussion and subconcussive exposure (Stockbridge et al., 2022).

Currently, there are more than 225 TBI-Bank members from more than 15 countries.

The webpage has links to a *Bibliography* and *Posters and Presentations* that have used the shared database. Examples of the research topics that have been investigated include discourse recovery in the first year following severe TBI (Elbourn et al., 2019), social communication assessment (Steel & Togher, 2019), discourse processing (Peach & Hanna, 2021), and conversational topics discussed by individuals with severe TBI and their communication partners (Brassel et al., 2016).

TBIBank *Grand Rounds* is a teaching resource designed to educate users on characteristics of discourse impairments typically seen in this population (Elbourn et al., 2020). Specifically, it includes modules with text, videos, and question-and-answer sections that cover the cognitive-communication impairment typically seen in TBI as well as its variability, assessment, treatment, recovery patterns, and comorbidities. As with RHDBank, tools that promote a more thorough understanding of the impairment and clinical best practices can translate into better overall outcomes for individuals with TBI.

Other Adult Discourse Database Resources

The literature refers to other adult language corpora, but a variety of factors often prevents their use in advancing research and education. For example, some are not publicly available, and some do not include enough demographic or other relevant metadata for meaningful analysis. However, a few of them have been made available to researchers, who must apply for access and demonstrate that their projects meet ethical criteria of institutional review boards (IRBs) and who are able to have their institutions sign data use agreements (DUAs). These databases ensure confidentiality, security, and privacy protection for participants through anonymization and deidentification. We highlight three resources below, with examples of research projects that have made use of their data. For a broader perspective, we refer readers to a recent systematic review of speech databases that include individuals with aphasia, dementia, stuttering, and other neurocognitive disorders (Li et al., 2019).

Carolina Conversations Collection

The Carolina Conversations Collection (CCC; Pope & Davis, 2011) is a corpus of older speakers from diverse ethnic and language groups, talking about health, illness, and their daily lives. The corpus is divided into two cohorts: unimpaired speakers and those with dementia. It includes audio and video files and time-aligned transcripts (in LaBB-CAT format) that can be downloaded by approved users. Access to this database requires a three-step process of developing a proposal explaining why the data are needed, getting IRB approval for the proposal from one's home institution, and then having the Medical University of South Carolina (MUSC) cosponsor the proposal and getting the MUSC's IRB approval for it as well.

Researchers have used this database to study several topics. Boyd Davis, one of the cocreators of the CCC, has published several articles and book chapters on dementia discourse, much of it focused on social-interactional analyses (Davis & Maclagan, 2009, 2010). Stickle and Wanner (2019, 2020) examined syntactic structures, looking at both grammatical accuracy and the range of linguistic complexity in the conversations of persons with dementia. Nasreen et al. (2019a, 2019b) examined questions, responses, and misunderstandings in conversations with people with AD. Guinn and Habash (2012) conducted a discriminative analysis of AD participants' disfluencies to create algorithms for automatic classification of speakers as AD versus non-AD (Guinn et al., 2014). Abdalla et al. (2018) used automatic extraction methods on this corpus as well as the DementiaBank Pitt corpus to study discourse relations according to Rhetorical Structure Theory. Also working with both DementiaBank and CCC data, Rudzicz, Chang Curry, et al. (2014) extracted more than 200 lexical/syntactic and acoustic features to determine which features were indicative of *trouble-indicating behaviors* in the speech of individuals with AD. Green et al. (2012) used the CCC corpus to inform the development of a computational model for a natural language-processing system that can listen to conversation between someone with AD and an unimpaired partner and make suggestions to the partner that would aid in maintaining the conversational flow. Luz et al. (2018) used logistic regression on content-free features (e.g., dialogue duration, turn duration, number of words, speech rate information) extracted from subsets of these CCC interviews to build a predictive model that could differentiate AD and non-AD speech with 86.5% accuracy (de la Fuente Garcia et al., 2020).

The Wisconsin Longitudinal Study

The Wisconsin Longitudinal Study (WLS; Herd et al., 2014) is a large-scale, long-term longitudinal study of a random sample of more than 1,300 men and women who graduated from Wisconsin high schools in 1957. Data on these participants were collected at

five additional time points through 2011 and covered a wide range of areas. Most relevant to this chapter are the Cookie Theft picture descriptions, which were added to the test protocol in 2011. Measures of category and letter fluency data, immediate and delayed word recall, and similarities data allow for some related measures of cognitive abilities. As mentioned earlier, this subset of WLS data has been shared with TalkBank and is available at the DementiaBank website.

Researchers are beginning to use this large data set as an additional resource for discourse studies in aging. Guo et al. (2021) recently reported on machine learning models to improve the performance of deep learning-based methods. The challenge in using this rich resource is that the WLS metadata do not contain dementia diagnoses. However, these authors used results from cognitive tests to establish groups for automatic dementia detection. Noorian et al. (2017) have also tapped this resource to increase the size of normative data for advancing this work on automated detection. The WLS website is clear and informative, the methodology is well-documented, and the staff is responsive to requests for data sharing and collaboration.

Wisconsin Registry for Alzheimer's Prevention (WRAP)

WRAP is a large, longitudinal study that was established in 2001 and designed to identify cognitive features and biomarkers that may predict AD risk. At time of enrollment, participants are late-middle-aged adults with a parental family history of probable AD (Johnson et al., 2018). Detailed visits occur approximately every 2 years and involve a variety of cognitive assessments, anthropometric measures, laboratory tests, and questionnaire ratings. The data include Cookie

Theft picture descriptions that have been used to analyze connected language for early features of cognitive decline (Evans et al., 2021; Mueller et al., 2016; Mueller et al., 2018). Outside researchers can apply for access to this database by completing a detailed request (e.g., NIH formatted biosketch, project summary, specific aims, significance, approach, deliverables) with proof of IRB approval.

smaller academic programs are unlikely to afford students the opportunity to see a full range of disorders. Additionally, the recent COVID-19 pandemic necessitated remote learning, which further limited students' clinical experiences. The rich data sets have provided material for online tutorials and other teaching resources that fill important gaps in access and breadth of clinical exposure and allow students to learn about state-of-the art discourse analysis techniques.

Conclusions

Most of the research that has utilized these shared databases could not have been accomplished without access to the amount and type of data available from these resources. We hope this chapter has provided encouragement to those who collect valuable discourse data to further this effort by contributing their corpora to shared databases for the benefit of the community. To facilitate this process, it is important to obtain full informed consent for data sharing (https://talkbank.org/share). The DementiaBank Pitt corpus is a prime example of a data set that has served a purpose beyond anything the original investigators could have envisioned and, as a result, has had a major impact on the push to develop clinical tools for automatic screening and detection of dementia.

The advantages of shared databases are many. These shared databases have facilitated the development of new discourse evaluation tools for clinicians and researchers in the field, using automated analyses as well as transcription-based and nontranscription-based analyses. Norms and benchmarks have been established for comparing participants' discourse performance to that of controls or others based their age, sex, and diagnosis. Many

Acknowledgments

We are indebted to the many colleagues who have collaborated with us and contributed data, and especially to the thousands of individuals who have participated and consented to share their data. This work was supported by the National Institute on Deafness and other Communication Disorders [Grant R01-DC008524] (2007–2022, awarded to MacWhinney).

References

Abdalla, M., Rudzicz, F., & Hirst, G. (2018). Rhetorical structure and Alzheimer's disease. *Aphasiology, 32*(1), 41–60. https://doi.org/10.1080/02687038.2017.1355439

Baylor, C., Yorkston, K., Eadie, T., Kim, J., Chung, H., & Amtmann, D. (2013). The Communicative Participation Item Bank (CPIB): Item bank calibration and development of a disorder–generic short form. *Journal of Speech, Language, and Hearing Research, 56*(4), 1190–1208. https://doi.org/10.1044/1092-4388(2012/12-0140)

Becker, J. T., Boller, F., Lopez, O. L., Saxton, J., & McGonigle, K. L. (1994). The natural history of Alzheimer's disease: Description of study cohort and accuracy of diagnosis. *Archives of Neurology*, *51*(6), 585–594. https://doi.org/10.1001/archneur.1994.00540180063015

Bickerton, W. L., Samson, D., Williamson, J., & Humphreys, G. W. (2011). Separating forms of neglect using the Apples Test: Validation and functional prediction in chronic and acute stroke. *Neuropsychology*, *25*(5), 567–580. https://doi.org/10.1037/a0023501

Blake, M. L. (2018). *The right hemisphere and disorders of cognition and communication: Theory and clinical practice*. Plural Publishing. https://www.ch-stquentin.fr/sites/stquentin-ch.local/files/webform/pdf-the-right-hemisphere-and-disorders-of-cognition-and-communication-margaret-lehman-blake-pdf-download-free-book-4836432.pdf

Boyle, M. (2015). Stability of word-retrieval errors with the AphasiaBank stimuli. *American Journal of Speech-Language Pathology*, *24*(4), S953–S960. https://doi.org/10.1044/2015_AJSLP-14-0152

Brassel, S., Kenny, B., Power, E., Elbourn, E., McDonald, S., Tate, R., . . . Togher, L. (2016). Conversational topics discussed by individuals with severe traumatic brain injury and their communication partners during subacute recovery. *Brain Injury*, *30*(11), 1329–1342. https://doi.org/10.1080/02699052.2016.1187288

Bryant, L., Ferguson, A., & Spencer, E. (2016). Linguistic analysis of discourse in aphasia: A review of the literature. *Clinical Linguistics and Phonetics, 30*(7), 489–518. https://doi.org/10.3109/02699206.2016.1145740

Bryant, L., Ferguson, A., Valentine, M., & Spencer, E. (2019). Implementation of discourse analysis in aphasia: Investigating the feasibility of a knowledge-to-action intervention. *Aphasiology*, *33*(1), 31–57. https://doi.org/10.1080/02687038.2018.1454886

Bryant, L., Spencer, E., & Ferguson, A. (2017). Clinical use of linguistic discourse analysis for the assessment of language in aphasia. *Aphasiology*, *31*(10), 1105–1126. https://doi.org/10.1080/02687038.2016.1239013

Caplan, B. (1987). Assessment of unilateral neglect: A new reading test. *Journal of Clinical and Experimental Neuropsychology*, *9*(4), 359–364. https://doi.org/10.1080/01688638708405056

Chiarcos, C., & Pareja-Lora, A. (2019). Open data—linked data—linked open data—linguistic linked open data (LLOD): A general introduction. In A. Pareja-Lora, M. Blume, B. C. Lust, & C. Chiarcos (Eds.), *Development of linguistic linked open data resources for collaborative data-intensive research in the language sciences*. The MIT Press. http://library.oapen.org/handle/20.500.12657/23502

Cho-Reyes, S., & Thompson, C. K. (2012). Verb and sentence production and comprehension in aphasia: Northwestern Assessment of Verbs and Sentences (NAVS). *Aphasiology*, *26*(10), 1250–1277. https://doi.org/10.1080/02687038.2012.693584

Coelho, C. A., Youse, K., Lê, K., & Feinn, R. (2003). Narrative and conversational discourse of adults with closed head injuries and non-brain-injured adults: A discriminant analysis. *Aphasiology*, *17*(5), 499–510. https://doi.org/10.1080/02687030344000111

Covington, M. A., & McFall, J. D. (2010). Cutting the Gordian knot: The moving-average type-token ratio (MATTR). *Journal of Quantitative Linguistics*, *17*(2), 94–100. https://doi.org/10.1080/02687038.2012.693584

Dalton, S. G. H., Kim, H., Richardson, J. D., & Wright, H. H. (2020). A compendium of core lexicon checklists. *Seminars in Speech and Language*, *41*(1), 45–60. https://doi.org/10.1055/s-0039-3400972

Dalton, S. G. H., & Richardson, J. (2019). A large-scale comparison of main concept production between persons with aphasia and persons without brain injury. *American Journal of Speech-Language Pathology*, *28*(Suppl. 1), 293–320. https://doi.org/10.1044/2018_AJSLP-17-0166

Davis, B. H., & Maclagan, M. (2009). Examining pauses in Alzheimer's discourse. *American Journal of Alzheimer's Disease and Other Dementias*, *24*(2), 141–154. https://doi.org/10.1177/1533317508328138

Davis, B., & Maclagan, M. (2010). Pauses, fillers, placeholders and formulaicity in Alzheimer's discourse. *Fillers, Pause,s and Placeholders*, *93*, 189–216. https://doi.org/10.1075/tsl.93

de la Fuente Garcia, S., Haider, F., & Luz, S. (2020). Cross-corpus feature learning between spontaneous monologue and dialogue for automatic classification of Alzheimer's dementia speech. In *2020 42nd Annual International Conference of the IEEE Engineering in Medicine and Biology Society (EMBC)* (pp. 5851–5855). IEEE. https://doi.org/10.1109/EMBC44109.2020.9176305

Elbourn, E., Kenny, B., Power, E., Honan, C., McDonald, S., Tate, R., . . . Togher, L. (2019). Discourse recovery after severe traumatic brain injury: Exploring the first year. *Brain Injury, 33*(2), 143–159. https://doi.org/10.1080/02699052.2018.1539246

Elbourn, E., Togher, L., Steel, J., Power, E., Fromm, D., & MacWhinney, B. (2020). *TBIBank Grand Rounds: Online education platform about cognitive-communication disorders resulting from traumatic brain injury.* https://tbi.talkbank.org/education/class-tbi/

Enderby, P., & Palmer, R. (2008). *Frenchay dysarthria assessment (FDA-2)* (2nd ed.). Pro-Ed.

Evans, E., Coley, S. L., Gooding, C., Norris, N., Ramsey, C. M., Green-Harris, G., & Mueller, K. D. (2021). Preliminary assessment of connected speech and language as marker for cognitive change in late-middle-aged Black/African American adults at risk for Alzheimer's disease. *Aphasiology,* 1–24. https://doi.org/ *(FDA-2)* 10.1080/02687038.2021.1931801

Forbes, M., Fromm, D., & MacWhinney, B. (2012). AphasiaBank: A resource for clinicians. *Seminars in Speech and Language, 30*(3), 217–222. https://doi.org/10.1055/s-0032-1320041

Fromm, D., Forbes, M., Holland, A., & MacWhinney, B. (2020). Using AphasiaBank for discourse assessment. *Seminars in Speech and Language, 41*(41), 10–19. https://doi.org/10.1055/s-0039-3399499

Fromm, D., Katta, S., Paccione, M., Hecht, S., Greenhouse, J., MacWhinney, B., & Schnur, T. T. (2021). A comparison of manual versus automated Quantitative Production Analysis of connected speech. *Journal of Speech, Language, and Hearing Research, 64*(4), 1271–1282. https://doi.org/10.1044/2020_JSLHR-20-00561

Fromm, D., MacWhinney, B., & Thompson, C. K. (2020). Automation of the Northwestern Narrative Language Analysis System. *Journal of Speech, Language, and Hearing Research, 63*(6), 1835–1844. https://doi.org/10.1044/2020_JSLHR-19-00267

Goodglass, H., Kaplan, E., & Barresi, B. (2001). *Boston Diagnostic Aphasia Examination* (3rd ed.). Lippincott Williams & Wilkins.

Gordon, J. K. (1998). The fluency dimension in aphasia. *Aphasiology, 12*(7–8), 673–688. https://doi.org/10.1080/02687039808249565

Gordon, J. K., & Clough, S. (2020). How fluent? Part B. Underlying contributors to continuous measures of fluency in aphasia. *Aphasiology, 34*(5), 643–663. https://doi.org/10.1080/02687038.2020.1712586

Green, N., Guinn, C. I., & Smith, R. W. (2012). Assisting social conversation between persons with Alzheimer's disease and their conversational partners. In J. Alexandersson, P. Ljunglöf, K. F. McCoy, B. Roark, & A. Waller (Eds.), *Proceedings of the Third Workshop on Speech and Language Processing for Assistive Technologies* (pp. 37–46). https://aclanthology.org/W12-2906.pdf

Greenslade, K. J., Stuart, J. E., Richardson, J. D., Dalton, S. G., & Ramage, A. E. (2020). Macrostructural analyses of Cinderella narratives in a large nonclinical sample. *American Journal of Speech-Language Pathology, 29*(4), 1923–1936. https://doi.org/10.1044/2020_AJSLP-19-00151

Groenewold, R., & Armstrong, E. (2018). The effects of enactment on communicative competence in aphasic casual conversation: A functional linguistic perspective. *International Journal of Language and Communication Disorders, 53*(4), 836–851. https://doi.org/10.1111/1460-6984.12392

Guinn, C. I., & Habash, A. (2012). Language analysis of speakers with dementia of the Alzheimer's type. In *2012 AAAI Fall Symposium: Artificial Intelligence for Gerontechnology* (pp. 8–13). Arlington.

Guinn, C., Singer, B., & Habash, A. (2014). A comparison of syntax, semantics, and pragmatics in spoken language among residents with Alzheimer's disease in managed-care facilities. In *2014 IEEE Symposium on Computational Intelligence in Healthcare and e-Health (CICARE)* (pp. 98–103). IEEE. https://doi.org/10.1109/CICARE.2014.7007840

Guo, Y., Li, C., Roan, C., Pakhomov, S., & Cohen, T. (2021). Crossing the "Cookie Theft" corpus chasm: Applying what BERT learns from outside data to the ADReSS challenge dementia detection task. *Frontiers in Computer Science, 3,* 26. https://doi.org/10.3389/fcomp.2021.642517

Helm-Estabrooks, N. (2017). *Cognitive linguistic quick test-plus*. Pearson.

Herd, P., Carr, D., & Roan, C. (2014). Cohort profile: Wisconsin Longitudinal (WLS). *International Journal of Epidemiology, 43*(1), 34–41. https://doi.org/10.1093/ije/dys194

Hewetson, R., Cornwell, P., & Shum, D. H. (2021). Relationship and social network change in people with impaired social cognition post right hemisphere stroke. *American Journal of Speech-Language Pathology, 30*(2S), 962–973. https://doi.org/10.1044/2020_AJSLP-20-00047

Johnson, S. C., Koscik, R. L., Jonaitis, E. M., Clark, L. R., Mueller, K. D., Berman, S. E., . . . Sager, M. A. (2018). The Wisconsin Registry for Alzheimer's Prevention: A review of findings and current directions. *Alzheimer's and Dementia: Diagnosis, Assessment and Disease Monitoring, 10,* 130–142. https://doi.org/10.1016/j.dadm.2017.11.007

Kaplan, E., Goodglass, H., & Weintraub, S. (2001). *Boston Naming Test* (2nd ed.). Pro-Ed.

Kennedy, M., Strand, E., Burton, W., & Peterson, C. (1994). Analysis of first-encounter conversations of right-hemisphere damaged participants. *Clinical Aphasiology, 22,* 67–80. http://aphasiology.pitt.edu/159/1/22-05.pdf

Kertesz, A. (2007). *Western Aphasia Battery–Revised*. Pearson.

Kim, H., & Wright, H. H. (2020). A tutorial on core lexicon: Development, use, and application. *Seminars in Speech and Language, 41,* 20–31. https://doi.org/10.1055/s-0039-3400973

Lanzi, M. A. (2021). *DementiaBank: Methods for studying discourse* [Manuscript in preparation]. Department of Communication Sciences and Disorders, University of Delaware.

Li, Y., Lin, Y., Ding, H., & Li, C. (2019). Speech databases for mental disorders: A systematic review. *General Psychiatry, 32*(3) e100022. https://doi.org/10.1136/gpsych-2018-100022

Luz, S., de la Fuente, S., & Albert, P. (2018). A method for analysis of patient speech in dialogue for dementia detection. https://arXiv.org/abs/1811.09919

Luz, S., Haider, F., de la Fuente, S., Fromm, D., & MacWhinney, B. (2020). *Alzheimer's dementia recognition through spontaneous speech: The ADReSS challenge*. https://arXiv.org/abs/2004.06833

Luz, S., Haider, F., de la Fuente, S., Fromm, D., & MacWhinney, B. (2021). *Detecting cognitive decline using speech only: The ADReSS challenge*. https://arXiv.org/abs/2104.09356

MacDonald, S. (2005). *Functional assessment of verbal reasoning and executive strategies*. CCD Publishing. http://www.ccdpublishing.com/favres.aspx

MacWhinney, B. (2007). The TalkBank project. In J. C. Beal, K. P. Corrigan, & H. L. Moisl (Eds.), *Creating and digitizing language corpora* (Vol. 1, pp. 163–180). Palgrave-Macmillan. https://psyling.talkbank.org/years/2007/palgrave.pdf

MacWhinney, B. (2014). *The CHILDES project: Tools for analyzing talk, Volume I: Transcription format and programs*. Psychology Press.

MacWhinney, B., Fromm, D., Forbes, M., & Holland, A. (2011). AphasiaBank: Methods for studying discourse. *Aphasiology, 25,* 1286–1307. https://doi.org/10.1080/02687038.2011.589893

Malvern, D., Richards, B., Chipere, N., & Purán, P. (2004). *Lexical diversity and language development*. Palgrave Macmillan. https://doi.org/10.1057/9780230511804

Minga, J., Johnson, M., Blake, M. L., Fromm, D., & MacWhinney, B. (2021). Making sense of right hemisphere discourse using RHDBank. *Topics in Language Disorders, 41*(1), 99–122. https://doi.org/10.1097/TLD.0000000000000244

Mueller, K. D., Hermann, B., Mecollari, J., & Turkstra, L. S. (2018). Connected speech and language in mild cognitive impairment and Alzheimer's disease: A review of picture description tasks. *Journal of Clinical and Experimental Neuropsychology*, *40*(9), 917–939. https://doi.org/10.1080/13803395.2018.1446513

Mueller, K. D., Koscik, R. L., Turkstra, L. S., Riedeman, S. K., LaRue, A., Clark, L. R., . . . Johnson, S. C. (2016). Connected language in late-middle-aged adults at risk for Alzheimer's disease. *Journal of Alzheimer's Disease*, *54*(4), 1539–1550. https://doi.org/10.3233/JAD-160252

Nasreen, S., Purver, M., & Hough, J. (2019a). A corpus study on questions, responses and misunderstanding signals in conversations with Alzheimer's patients. *Proceedings of the 23rd Workshop on the Semantics and Pragmatics of Dialogue—Full Papers (SEMDIAL)* (Vol. 13). London, United Kingdom. http://semdial.org/anthology/Z19-Nasreen_semdial_0013.pdf

Nasreen, S., Purver, M., & Hough, J. (2019b). Interaction patterns in conversations with Alzheimer's patients [Poster presentation and abstract]. In C. Martin-Vide, M. Purver, & S. Pollak (Eds.), *Proceedings: Seventh International Conference on Statistical Language and Speech Processing*. Ljubljana, Slovenia. http://www.eecs.qmul.ac.uk/~jhough/papers/NasreenEtAl2019SLSP.pdf

Nicholas, L. E., & Brookshire, R. H. (1993). A system for quantifying the informativeness and efficiency of the connected speech of adults with aphasia. *Journal of Speech, Language, and Hearing Research, 36*(2), 338–350. https://doi.org/10.1044/jshr.3602.338

Noorian, Z., Pou-Prom, C., & Rudzicz, F. (2017). On the importance of normative data in speech-based assessment. *arXiv preprint arXiv:1712.0069*. https://arxiv.org/pdf/1712.00069.pdf

Peach, R. K., & Hanna, L. E. (2021). Sentence-level processing predicts narrative coherence following traumatic brain injury: Evidence in support of a resource model of discourse processing. *Language, Cognition and Neuroscience, 36*(6), 1–17. https://doi.org/10.1080/23273798.2021.1894346

Pope, C., & Davis, B. (2011). Finding a balance: The CCC corpus. *Corpus Linguistics and Linguistic Theory*, *7*(1),143–161. https://doi.org/10.1515/CLLT.2011.007

Richardson, J. D., & Dalton, S. G. H. (2020). Main concepts for two picture description tasks: An addition to Richardson and Dalton, 2016. *Aphasiology, 34*(1), 119–136. https://doi.org/10.1080/02687038.2018.1561417

Richardson, J. D., Dalton, S. G., Greenslade, K. J., Jacks, A., Haley, K. L., & Adams, J. (2021). Main concept, sequencing, and story grammar analyses of Cinderella narratives in a large sample of persons with aphasia. *Brain Sciences, 11*(1), 110. https://doi.org/10.3390/brainsci11010110

Rochon, E., Saffran, E. M., Berndt, R. S., & Schwartz, M. F. (2000). Quantitative analysis of aphasic sentence production: Further development and new data. *Brain and Language, 72*(3), 193–218. https://doi.org/10.1006/brln.1999.2285

Rudzicz, F., Chan Currie, L., Danks, A., Mehta, T., & Zhao, S. (2014). Automatically identifying trouble-indicating speech behaviors in Alzheimer's disease. In *Proceedings of the 16th International ACM SIGACCESS Conference on Computers and Accessibility* (pp. 241–242). http://dx.doi.org/10.1145/2661334.2661382

Rudzicz, F., Wang, R., Begum, M., & Mihailidis, A. (2014). Speech recognition in Alzheimer's disease with personal assistive robots. In J. Alexandersson, D. Anastasiou, C. Jian, A. Nenkova, R. Patel, F. Rudzicz, . . . D. Zhekova, (Eds.), *Proceedings of the Fifth Workshop on Speech and Language Processing for Assistive Technologies* (pp. 20–28). https://aclanthology.org/W14-1904.pdf

Saffran, E. M., Berndt, R. S., & Schwartz, M. F. (1989). The quantitative analysis of agrammatic production: Procedure and data. *Brain and Language, 37*(3), 440–479. https://doi.org/10.1016/0093-934X(89)90030-8

Saffran, E. M., Schwartz, M. F., Linebarger, M. C., Martin, N., & Bochetto, P. (1998). *Philadelphia Comprehension Battery* [Unpublished manuscript].

Stark, B. C., Dutta, M., Murray, L. L., Fromm, D., Bryant, L., Harmon, T. G., . . . Roberts, A. C. (2021). Spoken discourse assessment and analysis in aphasia: An international survey of current practices. *Journal of Speech, Language, and Hearing Research, 64*(11), 4366–4389. https://doi.org/10.1044/2021_JSLHR-20-00708

Steel, J., & Togher, L. (2019). Social communication assessment after traumatic brain injury: A narrative review of innovations in pragmatic and discourse assessment methods. *Brain Injury, 33*(1), 48–61. https://doi.org/10.1080/02699052.2018.1531304

Stickle, T., & Wanner, A. (2019). Transitivity patterns exhibited by persons with dementia in conversation. *Applied Linguistics, 40*(1), 43–63. https://doi.org/10.1093/applin/amx001

Stickle, T., & Wanner, A. (2020). Making sense of syntactic error in conversations between persons with dementia and their non-impaired coparticipants. In T. Stickle (Ed.), *Learning from the talk of persons with dementia* (pp. 85–109). Palgrave Macmillan. https://doi.org/10.1007/978-3-030-43977-4_6

Stockbridge, M. D., Keser, Z., & Newman, R. S. (2022). Concussion in women's flat-track roller derby. *Frontiers in Neurology, 65.* https://www.frontiersin.org/articles/10.3389/fneur.2022.809939/full

Stockbridge, M. D., & Newman, R. (2019). Enduring cognitive and linguistic deficits in individuals with a history of concussion. *American Journal of Speech-Language Pathology, 28*(4), 1554–1570. https://doi.org/10.1044/2019_AJSLP-18-0196

Stubbs, E., Togher, L., Kenny, B., Fromm, D., Forbes, M., MacWhinney, B., . . . Power, E. (2018). Procedural discourse performance in adults with severe traumatic brain injury at 3 and 6 months postinjury. *Brain Injury, 32*(2), 167–181. https://doi.org/10.1080/02699052.2017.1291989

Thompson, C. K., Shapiro, L. P., Tait, M. E., Jacobs, B., Schneider, S., & Ballard, K. (1995). A system for the linguistic analysis of agrammatic language production. *Brain and Language, 51*(1), 124–129. https://doi.org/10.1006/brln.1995.1057

Togher, L., Elbourn, E., Kenny, B., Power, E., McDonald, S., Tate, R., . . . MacWhinney, B. (2014). TBIBank is a feasible assessment protocol to evaluate the cognitive communication skills of with people with severe TBI during the subacute stage of recovery. *Brain Injury, 28*(5–6), 723–723. https://doi.org/10.3109/02699052.2014.892379

Wiederholt, J. L., & Bryant, B. R. (2012). *Gray Oral Reading Tests–Fifth Edition: Examiner's manual.* Pro-Ed.

Wilson, S. M., Eriksson, D. K., Schneck, S. M., & Lucanie, J. M. (2018). A quick aphasia battery for efficient, reliable, and multidimensional assessment of language function. *PLOS ONE, 13*(2), e0192773. https://doi.org/10.1371/journal.pone.0199469

Wright, H. H., Capilouto, G. J., & Koutsoftas, A. (2013). Evaluating measures of global coherence ability in stories in adults. *International Journal of Language and Communication Disorders, 48*(3), 249–256. https://doi.org/10.1111/1460-6984.12000

Wright, H. H., Koutsoftas, A., Capilouto, G. J., & Fergadiotis, G. (2014). Global coherence in younger and older adults: Influence of cognitive processes and discourse type. *Aging, Neuropsychology, and Cognition, 21*(2), 174–196. https://doi.org/10.1080/13825585.2013.794894

Index

Note: Page numbers in **bold** reference non-text material.

A

AAC. *See* Alternative augmentative communication
ABCD–2. *See* Arizona Battery for Cognitive-Communication Disorders
Aboriginal culture, aphasia study and treatment in, 138–145
Aboriginal English. *See* Australian Aboriginal English
Adapted Kagan rating scales, 167, **175**, 179, 214
Adapted Measure of Participation in Conversation (Adapted MPC), 179
Adapted Measure of Support in Conversation (Adapted MSC), 179
ADAS-Cog. *See* Alzheimer's Disease Assessment Scale-Cognitive Subscale
Adjacency pair, 110
Adjuncts, 99
ADReSS Challenge for Interspeech, 318
Affectiva (software), 221
Aging
    about, 4, 9–12
    attention and, 22, 25–26
    bilingualism and, 55, **55**
    cognitive changes in, 54–55
    coherence and, 22–23, 33, 43–45, **45**, **46**
    cohesion and, 11, 22, 41–43, **42**, **43**, 45–46, **46**
    conversation and, **40**, 51–61, **53**, **59**
    discourse elicitation tasks, 33–46
    expository tasks, **40**, **43**, 44–45, **45**
    grammatical skills and, 25–26
    healthy aging, 15–27
    hearing loss and, 53–54
    interactional behaviors and, 58, **59**
    lexical diversity and, 36–39, **38**, **39**, 43, **46**
    lexical retrieval and, 24–25, 59–60, **59**
    macrolinguistic skills and, 22–24
    memory decline and, 21
    microlinguistic skills and, 24–26
    narrative discourse and, 10
    off-topic verbosity, 23
    procedural discourse and, 40, **43**, **44**
    productivity measures and, 56, **59**
    sentence generation and, 25
    single-picture descriptions and, 39, **40**, 44
    storytelling and, 56
    syntax and, 39, **40**, 41, **46**, 56, **59**
    tip of the tongue (ToT) phenomena and, 24, 25, 55–56, 59
    topic content and, 57–58, **59**
    verbosity and, 57, **59**
    visual impairment and, 53–54
    vocabulary and, 55–56, **59**
    word retrieval ability, 54
Agrammatic aphasia, 82, 120
ALSFRS-R. *See* Revised ALS Functional Rating Scale
Alternative augmentative communication (AAC), 247, 248
Alzheimer's disease. *See* Dementia of the Alzheimer's type
Alzheimer's Disease Assessment Scale-Cognitive Subscale (ADAS-Cog), 254
Amyotrophic lateral sclerosis (ALS), 289–302
    about, 230, 231–232, 302
    cognitive impairment in, 289
    language and, 290

Amyotrophic lateral sclerosis (ALS)
(Continued)
neural imaging research, 301
variants, 289, 301
Analyzing Discourse in Communicatively Impaired Adults (Cherney, Shadden, & Coelho), 1, 5
Annotation software, 221
Anomia, LUNA framework used in, 103
Aphasia
about, 4, 67–70, 73–74, 315
agrammatic aphasia, 82, 120
anomia, 103
assessment, 74
Australia First Nations context, 131–145
Australian Aboriginal English setting, 138–145
Boston Diagnostic Aphasia Examination (BDAE), 199
Broca's aphasia, 82, 83, 104
Cinderella story retelling, 77, **77**, **80–82**, 82–85, **85**, 112, 314, 317
Computerized Language ANalysis (CLAN), 220, 316–317
conversation analysis, 70, 113–120, **114**, 129, **130**, 131–145
conversation sampling in, 115
cross-cultural perspective, 4, 70, 131–145
cultural differences and, 68–69
defined, 121
described, 121
as disability, 121
discourse sampling, 84–87, **85**, **86**, 115
fluent aphasia, 67
lexical analysis, 77
linguistic analysis, 69, 73–88, 82
LUNA framework, 93–107
macrolinguistic analysis, 82–84
mean length of utterances (MLU), 79
microlinguistic analysis, 75–80
multilingual speakers and, 68
multimodal communication, 123, **124**
nonfluent aphasia, 79, 302
nonverbal aspects of communication, 115, 117
personal narrative, 69–70, 93–107
repair of conversation trouble spots, 111, 122–123
role of speaking partners, 112, 121–122, 125, 139–140
spoken personal narratives, 93–107
test questions, 125
topic management, 124
turn management, 124–125
Wernicke's aphasia, 83
See also Primary progressive aphasia
AphasiaBank, 86, 214, 221, 237, 314–316, 318, 319
Apples Test, 318
Appraisal analysis, 184
Aprosodia, 218
Arguments, 99
Arizona Battery for Cognitive-Communication Disorders (ABCD–2), 254, 255
Articulation, **19**
Assessment Battery for Communication, 167
Attention
aging and, 22, 25–26
discourse production and, 16, **17–19**, 19, 20
Audience design, 58
Australia
Aboriginal languages, 135
aphasia in First Nations context, 131–145
First Nations peoples, 135–136
Australian Aboriginal English (AAE)
aphasia analysis and treatment, 138–145
features of, 136–137, **137**, **138**

B

Back-channeling, aging and, 58
BAIS model. *See* Bilateral Activation, Inhibition, and Selection (BAIS) model
BDAE. *See* Boston Diagnostic Aphasia Examination
Behaviorally Referenced Rating of Intermediate Social Skills-Revised (BRISS-R), **175**, 177–178
Bilateral Activation, Inhibition, and Selection (BAIS) model, 152, 194–195

Bilingualism, 55, **55**, 276
Boston Diagnostic Aphasia Examination
    (BDAE), 199, 254, 291, 296, 315
Boston Naming Test, 315
BRISS-R. *See* Behaviorally Referenced Rating
    of Intermediate Social Skills-Revised
Broca's aphasia, 82, 83, 104
Broken Window picture, 239, 243, **244**

C

C-units (complete utterances), 60, 78, **78**, 79,
    87, 98, 276
CADL3. *See* Communication Activities of
    Daily Living Assessment
CAPPA. *See* Conversation Analysis Profile
    for People With Aphasia
Carolina Conversations Collection (CCC),
    320–321
CAs *See* Conversation agents
CDA. *See* Clinical discourse analysis
CDR-SOB. *See* Clinical Dementia Rating
    Scale
CHAT. *See* Codes for the Human Analysis
    of Talk
Chatbots, 221
CHild Language Data Exchange System
    (CHILDES) project, 312
Cinderella story retelling
    in aphasia, 77, **77**, **80–82**, 82–85, **85**, 112,
        314, 317
    Core Lexicon analysis, 77, **77**
    Main Concept analysis, 238
    in right hemisphere disorders, 199
    in traumatic brain injuries, **158**, 164,
        164–166, 167
CIUs. *See* Correct information units
CLAN. *See* Computerized Language
    ANalysis
Clauses, 98, 99
Clinical Dementia Rating Scale (CDR-SOB),
    254
Clinical discourse analysis (CDA), **176**, 182
Codes for the Human Analysis of Talk
    (CHAT), 313–314
Cognition, 150, **203**
Cognitive communication disorders
    L(CCDs)

about, 5, 149–153
defined, 150
right hemisphere disorders, 149, 151–152,
    193–204
technology and telepractice use, 152,
    211–222, 227, **228**
traumatic brain injuries (TBI), 149, 151,
    155–169, 173–186, 211–222, 227,
    228
Cognitive-language disorder, 149–150
Cognitive Linguistic Quick Test, **203**, 318
Cognitive skills
    aging and, 21, 54–55
    in discourse production, 16, **17–19**, 19,
        20, 21
    disorganization, 150
Coherence
    aging and, 22–23, 33, 43–45, **45**, **46**
    defined, 43, 196–197
    discourse production and, 3, 9, 11
    Global Coherence Scale, 60
    measures of, 43, **44**, 197
    in right hemisphere disorders, 196–197,
        196
    types, 43
Coherence errors analysis, 43, **44**
Cohesion
    about, 41, 45
    aging and, 11, 22, 41–43, **42**, **43**, 45–46,
        46
    cohesive categories, 41, **42**
    defined, 41, 80
    linguistic analysis of, 80–82, **81**, **82**
    in Parkinson's disease, 277–278
    right hemisphere disorders, 197
Cohesion analysis, 75
Collaborative referencing, 58
Collocation, **81**
Communication
    about, 149
    cognition and, 150
    cross-cultural issues, 132–133
    dementia, deficits in, 254–256
    group talk, 140
    language of confusion, 160
    schemas, 43, **44**, 256–257
    scripts, 247, 257
    See also Linguistic analysis

Communication Activities of Daily Living
Assessment (CADL3), 132
Communication Participation Item Bank,
183, 318
Communication partners
in aphasia, 112, 121–122, 125, 139–140
training, 139–140, 167, 179
in traumatic brain injuries, 163, 167
Communication Performance Scale (CPS),
175, 177, **178**
Communication Rating Scale (CRS), **175**,
177
Communicative transaction, 73
Complete reference chains, 100
Complete utterances (C-units), 60, 78, **78**,
79, 87, 98, 276
Complex Ideational Material-Short Form,
315
Computerized Language ANalysis (CLAN),
76, **168**, 220–221, 312, 313, 316–317
Concept, 101, 101*n*
Conceptual preparation, 19–20
Conjunction, **42**, **81**
Constructs, 101, 101*n*, 102–103
Content efficiency, 291–292
Content units (CUs), 82–83, 291
Context, 111–112
Contextual constraint treatment, 152,
195
Conversation
about, 11, 34–35, 41, 51, 109–113
adjacency pair, 110
aging and, **40**, 51–61, **53**, **59**
bilingualism and, 55, **55**, 276
co-construction, 112
cognition and, 54–55
context, 111–112
contextual context, 173–174
culture and, 70, 131–145
defined, 9, 34, **34**, 109, 150
dual sensory loss and, 54
economy, 111
elements of, 110, **110**
face, 110–111
fronting, 120–121
hearing loss and, 53–54
interactional behaviors, 58
measures for, 60

participation of speaking partners, 112,
121–122, 125, 139–140, 163, 167
politeness strategies, 111
preference organization, 110
productivity measures, 56
progressivity, 111
repair of trouble spots, 111, 122–123
research, 52–53, **53**
sampling of. *See* Conversation sampling
sequential organization, 110
syntax and, 56
topic content and, 57–58
topic management, 124
turn management, 58, 124–125, 201, 220
visual impairment and, 53–54
yarning, 140–142, **142**, 154
Conversation agents (CAs), 221
Conversation analysis (CA)
about, 118–119, 182–183
annotation software, 221
in aphasia, 70, 113–120, **114**, 129, **130**,
131–145
application, 120–122
appraisal analysis, 184
Australian First Nations context,
131–145
cross-cultural context, 131–145
culture and, 70, 131–145
Electronic Goal Attainment Scaling
(eGAS), 185
family involvement in, 139
Goal Attainment Scaling (GAS), 184–185,
184, **185**
in healthy aging, 51–61
identifying behaviors of interest, 118
Interactional Network Tool (INT),
180–181, **180**, **181**
limited transcription analysis, 119
modality analysis, 183–184
quantitative vs. qualitative outcomes,
122–126
in right hemisphere disorders, 198,
201–205
samples, 114–115, **114**
speech act analysis (example), 122, 129,
130
transcriptionless analysis, 119–120
transitivity analysis, 184

in traumatic brain injuries (TBI), 157–169, **159**, 173–186, 211–222, 227, **228**
variety of speech acts, 122, 129, **130**
See also Discourse analysis; Rating scales; Technology; Transcription
Conversation Analysis Profile for People With Aphasia (CAPPA), 122
Conversation Sample Procedures, 60
Conversation sampling
about, 60, 114–115, **114**
in aphasia, 84–87, **85**, **86**, 115
technology use supporting, 220–222
in traumatic brain injury, 158, 160
video recording, 115, 182, 219, 221
Conversational breakdown, repair, 111, 122–123
Cookie Theft picture description
about, 37, 82, **83**, 297, 317, 321–322
in ALS, 291, 296–298, **297**, **299–301**, 300–301
in right hemisphere disorders, **196**, 201–202, **202**, 318
Core Lexicon (CoreLex)
about, 230, 237
in aphasia, 76, **77**, 317
in primary progressive aphasia (PPA), 237, 247
CORELEX command, 317
Correct Information Unit in Conversation (CIUconv), 60
Correct information units (CIUs)
in ALS, 291
in aphasia, 84, 95–96, 97, 102
defined, 84
CPS. *See* Communication Performance Scale
Cross-cultural perspective, aphasia and, 4, 131–145
CRS. *See* Communication Rating Scale
Cultural identity, language and, 135, 138
Cultural linguistics, 134–135
Cultural security, 142–143
Culture
about, 4, 131–135
aphasia in Australia First Nations context, 131–145
conversation analysis and, 70, 132–145
language and, 134–135

CUs. *See* Content units

D

Dementia
automatic detection of, 318
communication deficits in, 254–255
Dementia of the Alzheimer's type (DAT), 253–265
about, 231, 253–255
conversational interactions with Flo, 231, 258–263
perseveration, 258
scripts and schemas, 257–258
Wisconsin Registry for Alzheimer's Prevention (WRAP), 321–322
DementiaBank, 279, 317–318, 322
Diagnostic yarn, 141
Dialect, cultural identity, 138
Disagreements, 111
Discourse
about, 33
coherence, 3, 9
defined, 2, 9, 33, 73, 150
genres and types, 34–36, **34–36**, 84, 150
group talk, 140
multimodal communication, 123, **124**
personal narrative, 93–94
planning of, 16, **17–18**, 19–20
production of, 16, **17–19**, 100, **101**, 105
right hemisphere and, 194–198
types, 9
written discourse, 218–219
See also Conversation; Expository discourse; Narrative discourse; Procedural discourse
Discourse analysis
about, 1–6, 33–34
aging and. *See* Aging
annotation software, 221
in aphasia. *See* Aphasia
challenges and barriers to, 248
clinical discourse analysis (CDA), **176**, 182
in cognitive communication disorders (CCDs). *See* Cognitive communication disorders
cross-cultural perspective, 131–145

Discourse analysis *(Continued)*
  discourse profiles, 157, **157**
  Exchange Structure Analysis (ESA),
    183
  Interactional Network Tool (INT),
    180–181, **180**, **181**
  La Trobe Communication Questionnaire
    (LCQ), 182, **183**, 214
  LUNA, 69–70, 93–107
  macro-/microstructural, 3
  modality analysis, 183–184
  models, 10
  multilevel model approach, **280**, 279–281
  in neurodegenerative disorders. *See*
    Neurodegenerative disorders
  primary progressive aphasia (PPA),
    245–248
  Systemic Functional Linguistics (SFL),
    183–184
  theoretical framework, 100–104
  Topic Analysis, **176**, 181–182
  See also Conversation analysis; Discourse
    databases; Macrolinguistic analysis;
    Microlinguistic analysis; Rating scales;
    Technology
Discourse Contribution Measure, 201
Discourse databases
  about, 311–312, 320, 322
  AphasiaBank, 86, 214, 221, 237, 314–316,
    318, 319
  Carolina Conversations Collection (CCC),
    320–321
  DementiaBank, 279, 317–318, 322
  RDHBank, 60, 203, 318–319
  TalkBank, 5, 309, 312–320
  TBIBank, 158, **158**, 186, 319–320
  Wisconsin Longitudinal Study (WLS),
    317, 321
  Wisconsin Registry for Alzheimer's
    Prevention (WRAP), 321–322
Discourse efficiency, 291
Discourse profiles, 157, **157**
Disfluency, in Parkinson's disease, 274–275
Divergent information, in right hemisphere
    disorders, 195–196
Divided attention, discourse production and,
    16, **17–19**, 19, 20, 22
Dyad Conversation Protocol, 60

E

EBP. *See* Evidence-based practice
Edinburgh Cognitive and Behavioral ALS
    Screen (ECAS), 297–298
Elderly adults. *See* Aging
Electronic Goal Attainment Scaling (eGAS),
    185
Elicitation
  aging and, 33–46
  right hemisphere disorders, 199, **200**
Ellipsis, **42**, **81**
Emotion perception, technology use and,
    217
Episodic buffer, **17**
EQclinic (software), 221
ESA. *See* Exchange Structure Analysis
Evidence-based practice (EBP), 94
Exchange Structure Analysis (ESA), 183
Executive function, discourse production
    and, 16, **17–19**, 19, 20
Expository discourse
  about, 35, 52
  aging and, **40**, **43**, 44–45, **45**
  defined, 9, **34**, 150
  task probes, **35**
Extranarrative content, 97
Eye contact, cross-cultural considerations,
    139

F

Face, 110–111
False starts, 97
Family involvement, 139, 163, 167
FCLI-3. *See* Functional Linguistic-
    Communication Inventory
Feature Summary scale (FSS), 178–179
First Nations people
  aphasia analysis and treatment in,
    138–145
  in Australia, 135
  cultural security, 142–143
Flowerpot Incident test, 161–162, **161**, **162**
FLUCALC command, 317
Fluency
  in ALS, 290
  in Parkinson's disease, 274
Fluent aphasia, 67

FOQUSAphasia, 316
Formalist perspective, 74
Frenchay Dysarthria Assessment, 319
Friedman's test, 185
Frog, Where Are You?, 293–296, **294, 295, 305–307**
Fronting, 120–121
Frontotemporal dementia (FTD), 253
FSS. *See* Feature Summary scale
Functional Assessment of Verbal Reasoning and Executive Functioning, 319
Functional Linguistic-Communication Inventory (FCLI–3), 255

G

GAS. *See* Goal Attainment Scaling
Genres, 84, 150
Gestures, 115, 117, 123, 124, **124**, 183
Global Coherence Scale, 60
Global connectedness, 293, 295
Global Impression scales, **175**, 179, 214
Goal Attainment Scaling (GAS), 184–185, **184, 185**
Grammar, in Parkinson's disease, 276
Grammatical processing, **18**, 25–26
"Green Book" (Cherney, Shadden, & Coelho), 1, 230
Grey Oral Reading Test, 315
Group talk, 140
Group video conferencing, 217
Gumerri assessment, 141

H

Hearing loss, aging and, 53–54
Hemispatial neglect, assessment, **203**
Home Language. *See* Australian Aboriginal English

I

INCOG, 155, 157–158, **157**
Incomplete reference chains, 100
Incomplete utterances, 98
Indented Paragraph Test, 318
Indigenism, 135
Information content
in Parkinson's disease, 275
in right hemisphere disorders, 198
story grammar, 99–100, 197–198
Informative discourse, **34**, 35
Inhibition, discourse production and, 21–22
Inhibition deficit hypothesis, 23
Inhibitory control
aging and, 21, 23
discourse production and, **17–19**
Inhibitory partner behavior, 125
INT, **176**
Integrative discourse models, 10
Interactional behaviors, aging and, 58, **59**
Interactional Network Tool (INT), 180–181, **180, 181**
Interpersonal Process Recall, 219
Interviews, 52
Intonation, 217–218

J

Jeffersonian Transcription System, 115, **116**, 117–118

K

Kagan rating scales, 167, **175**, 179, 214
Kriol (language), 136

L

La Trobe Communication Questionnaire (LCQ), 182, **183**, 214
Language
Australian Aboriginal languages, 135
bilingualism, 55, **55**, 276
cross-cultural issues, 132–133
cultural identity, 135, 138, 144
development of in childhood, 15–16
multilingualism, 68
schemas, 43, **44**, 256–257
scripts, 247, 257
See also Linguistic analysis
Language of confusion, 160
Language Underpins Narrative in Aphasia (LUNA), 93–107
Clinical DAP, 94–95, **95**
codesign process, 96

Language Underpins Narrative in Aphasia
(LUNA) *(Continued)*
creation, 94
decision making, 96–100
examples of use, 103–105
measurement in, 104
Research DAP, 94, 95, **95**
research knowledge base, 95–96
theoretical framework, 100–104
treatment using, 104–107
Latent semantic analysis (LSA), 45
LBSD. *See* Lewy body spectrum disorders
LCQ. *See* La Trobe Communication
Questionnaire
Lemma, **18**, 20
Lewy body spectrum disorders (LBSD), 269,
273
Lexical access, 2, **18–19**, 21–22
Lexical analysis, 75–78
Lexical content and diversity, 75–78, **76, 77**
Lexical diversity (LD)
aging and, 36–39, **38, 39**, 43, **46**
defined, 36
measures of, 36, **37**, 75–77, **76, 77**, 97
nonpictorial discourse, 45
Lexical processing, 16, 24
Lexical retrieval, aging and, 24–25, 59–60, **59**
Lexical selection
aging and, 24–25
discourse production and, **17–18**, 19–20
Lexicalization, defined, **42**
Life Participation Approach to Aphasia
(LPAA), 68
Likert-based rating scale, 43, 44, **44**, 178, 179
Limited transcription analysis, 119
Linguistic analysis
aphasia and, 69, 73–88, 82
of cohesion, 80–82, **81, 82**
discourse sampling and, 60, 84–87, **85,
86**
interpreting meaning from, 84
software for, 76
Linguistic component
in discourse production, **101**, 106
in LUNA, 102–105
Linguistic decline, aging and, 16
Linguistic fillers, 97
Local connectedness, 295

Logopenic variant PPA (lvPPA), 237,
242–245, **242, 245**, 246
Long-term declarative memory, 16, **17–19**,
19, 21
Long-term nondeclarative memory, **18, 19**,
25
LPAA. *See* Life Participation Approach to
Aphasia
LSA. *See* Latent semantic analysis
LUNA. *See* Language Underpins Narrative in
Aphasia
LUNA framework, 93–107

M

Macrolinguistic analysis, 75, 82–84, **83**, 247
Macrolinguistic processes, 16, 22–24
Macrostructural analysis, 3
Macrostructure, 19–20
Macrostructure planning, **101**, 102–103, 106
Main Concept analysis (MCA)
about, 43, 230–231, 237
in aphasia, 83
defined, **44**, 83
in primary progressive aphasia (PPA),
237–238, 241–245, **241**, 247
in right hemisphere disorders, 195–196
in traumatic brain injury (TBI), 163–164
Main Concept, Sequencing, and Story
Grammar (MSSG), 238
Main event analyses, 278
Management yarn, 141
MATTR. *See* Moving average type-token
ratio
MCA. *See* Main concept analysis
Mean length of utterance (MLU)
in ALS, 291, 292, 298
in aphasia, 79
defined, 78
in Parkinson's disease, 275
Measures of textual lexical diversity
(MTLD), 36, **37**
Mediated Discourse Elicitation Procedure,
60
Memory, 16, **17–19**, 19, 20, 21, 26
Mental lexicon, 20, 24
Merge operation, 16, 20
Microlinguistic analysis

aphasia, 75–80, 246–247
    lexical content and diversity, 75–78, **76**, **77**
    morphosyntactic structure, 78–79, **78**, **80**
Microlinguistic processes, 16, 24–26
Microproposition, 10
Microstructural analysis, 3, 230
Microstructure, 20
Mild cognitive impairment, 230
Mini-Mental State Examination (MMSE), 254
Mixed multilevel analyses, 185
MLU. *See* Mean length of utterance
Modality analysis, 183–184
Morphosyntactic structure, 78–79, **78**, **80**
Moving average type-token ratio (MATTR), 36, **37**, 75–76, **76**
MSSG. *See* Main Concept, Sequencing, and Story Grammar
MTLD. *See* Measures of textual lexical diversity
Multiclause utterances, 98
Multicultural world. *See* Cross-cultural perspective; Cultural linguistics; Culture
Multilingualism
    aphasia and, 68
    See also Bilingualism

N

Naming performance, aging and, 24, 25
NARNIA (treatment mode), 247
Narrative discourse
    about, 33, 35–36, 52
    aging and, 10, 15–27
    defined, 9, **34**, 150
    personal narrative in aphasia, 69–70, 93–107
    probes, **36**
    See also Conversation; Conversation analysis
Narrative recounts, **34**, 35, 36, 46
Narrative words, 97
NDW. *See* Number of different words
Neurodegenerative disorders
    about, 5, 229–232
    amyotrophic lateral sclerosis (ALS), 230, 231–232, 289–302, **305–307**

dementia of the Alzheimer's type (DAT), 231, 253–265
mild cognitive impairment, 230
Parkinson's disease (PD), 231, 269–282
primary progressive aphasia (PPA), 230–231, 235–248
Nonarguments, 99
Nonfluent/agrammatic primary progressive aphasia (nvfPPA), 240–242, **240**, **241**, 246, 302
Nonfluent aphasia, 79
Nonlinguistic fillers, 97
Nonverbal communication, 115, 117, 124, **124**, 183
Northwestern Narrative Language Analysis, 316
Number of different words (NDW), 36, **37**

O

Off-topic language. *See* Verbosity
Older adults. *See* Aging
ONDRI study, 278
Open Data initiative, 311
Open Science initiative, 311

P

Paraphasias, 123
Parkinson's disease (PD), 231, 269–282
    about, 269–271, **271**
    conversation and, 271–278, **272**, 273, **273**
    macrostructural changes in speech, 278
    microstructural changes in speech, 274–278
Partners in communication. *See* Communication partners
PAS. *See* Predicate-argument structure
Perseveration, 258
Person-Directed Behavior Scale (PDBS), 178
Personal Conversational Style Scale (PCSS), 178
Personal narrative. *See* Narrative
Persuasive discourse, **34**, 35
Philadelphia Comprehension Battery, 315
Phonological working memory, **18**, **19**, 20 21, 26
Pictorial stimuli, 43, 44

Pictorial stimuli *(Continued)*
　See also Sequential-picture descriptions;
　　Single-picture descriptions
Pigeon: Impossible retelling, 199
Pitch, 217–218
Pitt corpus, 317, 322
Politeness markers, 215, **216**
Politeness strategies, 111
Post-traumatic amnesia (PTA), 155–156,
　156, 160
POWERS. *See* Profile of Word Errors and
　Retrieval in Speech
PPIC. *See* Profile of Pragmatic Impairment
　in Communication
Pragmatic Protocol, 174, **176**, 177
Pragmatic Rating Scale (PRS), **176**, 179–180
Pragmatics, **101**, 103
Predicate-argument structure (PAS), 99, 102
Predicates, 99
Preference organization, 110
Primary progressive aphasia (PPA), 235–248
　about, 230–231, 235–236
　case histories, 236–237, 239–240,
　　242–245, **244**, 247
　change over time, 246–247
　Core Lexicon analysis, 237, 247
　differential diagnosis of variants, 245–246
　logopenic variant (lvPPA), 237, 242–245,
　　242, **245**, 246
　Main Concept analysis, 237–238, 241–245,
　　241, 247
　nonfluent/agrammatic variant (nvfPPA),
　　240–242, **240**, **241**, 246, 302
　planning for future, 247–248
　progression, 247
　semantic variant (svPPA), 238–240, **238**,
　　246
　speech language pathologists and,
　　235–236
　treatment response, 247
　variants, 235, 238–246
Procedural discourse
　about, 33, 52
　aging and, **40**, **43**, 44
　defined, 9, **34**, **36**, 150
　probes, 36, **36**
Procedural memory, **19**
Productivity measures

aging and, 56, **59**
ALS and, 291, 292
Parkinson's disease and, 274
Profile of Pragmatic Impairment in
　Communication (PPIC), **175**, 178–179,
　178
Profile of Word Errors and Retrieval in
　Speech (POWERS), 60, 122
Progressivity, 111
Project Euphonia, 220
Propositions, **101**, 102, 105–106
Prosody, technology use and, 217–218
Prototype theory, 257
PRS. *See* Pragmatic Rating Scale

Q

Quantitative Production Analysis, 316
Quick Aphasia Battery, 315

R

Ranchos Los Amigos Scale-Revised (RLAS-
　R), 155, **156**
Rating scales, **44**, 167, 174, **175–176**,
　177–180
　Adapted Measure of Participation in
　　Conversation (Adapted MPC), 179
　Adapted Measure of Support in
　　Conversation (Adapted MSC), 179
　Behaviorally Referenced Rating of
　　Intermediate Social Skills-Revised
　　(BRISS-R), **175**, 177–178
　Boston Diagnostic Aphasia Examination
　　(BDAE), 199, 254, 291, 296, 315
　clinical discourse analysis (CDA), **176**,
　　182
　Communication Participation Item Bank,
　　183, 318
　Communication Performance Scale
　　(CPS), **175**, 177, **178**
　Communication Rating Scale (CRS), **175**,
　　177
　Discourse Contribution Measure, 201
　Electronic Goal Attainment Scaling
　　(eGAS), 185
　Exchange Structure Analysis (ESA), 183
　Feature Summary scale (FSS), 178–179

Global Impression scales, **175**, 179, 214
INT, **176**
Kagan rating scales, 167, **175**, 179, 214
La Trobe Communication Questionnaire
    (LCQ), 182, **183**, 214
Likert-based rating scale, 43, 44, **44**, 178,
    179
Person-Directed Behavior Scale (PDBS),
    178
Personal Conversational Style Scale
    (PCSS), 178
Pragmatic Protocol, 174, **176**, 177
Pragmatic Rating Scale (PRS), **176**,
    179–180
Profile of Pragmatic Impairment in
    Communication (PPIC), **175**, 178–179,
    178
Profile of Word Errors and Retrieval in
    Speech (POWERS), 60, 122
Ranchos Los Amigos Scale-Revised
    (RLAS-R), 155, **156**
Social Communication Skills
    Questionnaire-Adapted (SCSQ-A),
    183
Social Skills Questionnaire-Traumatic
    Brain Injury (SSQ-TBI), **183**
Systemic Functional Linguistics (SFL),
    183–184
Topic Analysis, **176**, 181–182
RCI. *See* Reliable Change Index
RDHBank, 60, 203, 318–319
Recipient design, storytelling, 113
Recounts, **34**, 35, **36**, 46
Reference, **42**, 81–82, **81**
Reference chains, 100
Referential targets, renaming, 197
Reiteration, **81**
Reliable Change Index (RCI), 158, 160, **160**
Repair of conversation, 111, 122–123
Repetitions, 97
Retelling tasks. *See* Story retelling
Revised ALS Functional Rating Scale
    (ALSFRS-R), 292, 295
Rhetorical structure theory, 321
Right hemisphere, discourse and, 194–198
Right hemisphere disorders, 149, 151–152,
    193–204
    about, 193–194

Bilateral Activation, Inhibition, and
    Selection (BAIS) model, 194–195
coherence, 196–197, **196**
cohesion, 197
comprehension deficits, 195
contextual constraint treatment, 195
conversation, 198
discourse analysis, 199–204
divergent information, 195–196
elicitation techniques, 199, **200**
RDHBank, 60, 203, 318–319
story grammar, 197–198
Structure Building Framework, 152,
    195
weight-based suppression of information,
    195
Rigney's Indigenism, 135
RLAS-R. *See* Ranchos Los Amigos
    Scale-Revised

S

SALT. *See* Systematic Analysis of Language
    Transcripts
Sampling. *See* Conversation sampling
Schemas, 43, **44**, 256–257
Scripts, 247, 257
SCSQ-A. *See* Social Communication Skills
    Questionnaire-Adapted
Segmentation conventions, in Parkinson's
    disease, 276–277, **277**
Selective attention, discourse production
    and, 16, **17–19**, 19, 20, 22
Semantic paraphasias, aging and, 24–25
Semantic variant PPA (svPPA), 238–240,
    238, 246
Sentence generation, **17**, 20, 25, 26
Sentence-level decision making, 97–99
Sentences, defined, 79
Sequential organization, 110
Sequential-picture descriptions, **34**, 35, 39,
    40, 43, 75
SFL. *See* Systemic Functional Linguistics
Single-picture descriptions, **34**, 35, 39, **40**,
    43, 44
Situational discourse, 10
Social Communication Skills Questionnaire-
    Adapted (SCSQ-A), **183**

Social Conversation Collection Protocol, 60
Social Skills Questionnaire-Traumatic Brain
    Injury (SSQ-TBI), **183**
Social yarn, 141
Software, for linguistic analysis, 76
Speech act analysis (example), 122, 129, **130**
Speech act theory, 177
Speech rate, in Parkinson's disease, 274
Story grammar, 99–100, 197–198, 199
Story Retell Procedure, 214
Story retelling, **34**, 36
    Broken Window picture, 239, 243, **244**
    Cookie Theft picture description, 37, 82,
        83, 201–202, **202**, 291, 296–298, **297**,
        299–301, 300–301, 317, 318, 321–322
    Frog, Where Are You?, 293–296, **294**, **295**,
        305–307
    Pigeon: Impossible retelling, 199
    in right hemisphere disorders, 199, **200**
    See also Cinderella story retelling
Storytelling
    about, **34**, 35–36, 112–113
    aging and, 56
    recipient design, 113
    in right hemisphere disorders, 199, **200**
Structural organization, 10
Structure Building Framework, 152, 195
Substitution, **42**, **81**
Superstructure-level decision making, 99–100
Surface-level impairment, 10
Sustained attention, 16, **17–19**, 20, 22
svPPA. *See* Semantic variant PPA
Syllabification, 21
Syntactic analysis, 78, **78**
Syntactic complexity, 39, **40**, 41, 45, **46**
Syntax
    aging and, 56, **59**
    in Parkinson's disease, 275–277
Systematic Analysis of Language Transcripts
    (SALT), 76, **168**, 276
Systemic Functional Linguistics (SFL), 183–184

T

T-scores, 185
T-units, 78, **78**, 84, 276–277, 295–296, 298
TalkBank, 312–320
    about, 5, 309

AphasiaBank, 86, 214, 221, 237, 314–316,
    318, 319
Codes for the Human Analysis of Talk
    (CHAT), 313–314
Computerized Language ANalysis
    (CLAN), 76, **168**, 220–221, 312, 313,
    316–317
DementiaBank, 279, 317–318, 322
index to corpora, 312–313
RDHBank, 60, 203, 318–319
TBIBank, 158, **158**, 186, 319–320
TBIBank, 158, **158**, 186, 319–320
Technology
    annotation software, 221
    automation, 316
    chatbots, 221
    Computerized Language ANalysis
        (CLAN), 76, **168**, 220–221, 312, 313,
        316–317
    conversation agents (CAs), 221
    for discourse sampling, 220–222
    emotion perception, 217
    group videoconferencing, 217
    to monitor changes in discourse, 219
    overview, 152, 186
    Project Euphonia, 220
    prosody and, 217–218
    sample analysis supported by, 220–222
    Theory of Mind, 217
    in traumatic brain injury, 211–222
    video recording, 115, 182, 219, 221
    virtual reality, 222
    Voicemail Elicitation Task (VET), 152,
        215–217, **215**, 219, 227, **228**
    Work-Related Communication (WoRC),
        19
    written discourse evaluation, 218–219
Telepractice
    with dementia patients, 264
    guidelines, 212–214, **213**
    overview, 152
    planning, 152
    with traumatic brain injury patients,
        211–222, **213**
    validated assessment methods, 214
Test for Reception of Grammar (TROG), 292
Test questions, 125
Theory of Mind, **17**, 19, 217

Thinking out loud tasks, 201
Tip of the tongue (ToT) phenomenon, aging and, 24, 25, 55–56, 59
Token Test, 292
Tokens, 75
Topic Analysis, **176**, 181–182
Topic content, aging and, 57–58, **59**
Topic initiation and maintenance, aging and, 56–57, **59**
Topic management, in aphasia, 124
Torres Strait Islander people, 136
    See also Australian Aboriginal English
Transcription
    CHAT transcripts, 313–314
    conversation sampling, 115, **116**, 117–120, 129, **130**
    Jeffersonian Transcription System, 115, **116**, 117–118
    multilevel model approach, 279–281, **280**
Transcriptionless analysis, 119–120
Transitivity analysis, 184
Traumatic brain injuries (TBI)
    about, 149, 151, 173
    Cinderella story retelling, **158**, 164, **164–166**, 167
    conversation assessment, 157–169, **159**, 173–186, 211–222, 227, **228**
    cross-cultural considerations, 139
    early recovery, 160–163, **160–162**
    facial expression analysis, 221
    language of confusion, 160
    later recovery, 167
    mid-recovery, 163–164, **164–166**
    outcomes, 151
    post-traumatic amnesia (PTA), 155–156, **156**, 160
    recovery continuum, 155–169
    technology and telepractice use, 152, 186, 211–222, 227, **228**
    tips for the SLP, 167–168, **168**
    turn taking, 220
TROG. *See* Test for Reception of Grammar
Trouble-Source Repair analysis (TSR), 271
TTR. *See* Type-token ratio
Turn management, 124–125
Topic management, 124
Turn-taking skills, 58, 124–125, 201, 220
Type-token ratio (TTR), 36, **37**, 75, 97

Types, 75

U

Utterances, 78, **78**, 86, 98

V

Verb Naming Test, 315
Verb Network Strengthening Treatment (VNeST), 79
Verbosity, aging and, 23, 57, **59**
Verbs, aphasia and, 79, **80**, 82, 86
VET. *See* Voicemail Elicitation Task
Video recording, 115, 182, 219, 221
Videoconferencing, 217, 263
Virtual reality (VR), 222
Visual cues, 43, 44
Visual impairment, aging and, 53–54
VNeST. *See* Verb Network Strengthening Treatment
Vocabulary, 55–56, 134
Vocabulary analysis, 75
Voice banking, 247, 248
Voicemail Elicitation Task (VET), 152, 215–217, **215**, 219, 227, **228**

W

Wangi talking project, 142, **142**
Wernicke's aphasia, 83
Western Aphasia Battery-Revised (WAB-R), 132, 254, 315
Wisconsin Longitudinal Study (WLS), 317, 321
Wisconsin Registry for Alzheimer's Prevention (WRAP), 321–322
Word class, 97
Word-level decision making, 96–97
Word retrieval, aging and, 54–55
Work-Related Communication (WoRC), 19
Working memory, 16, **17–19**, 19, 20, 21
WRAP. *See* Wisconsin Registry for Alzheimer's Prevention
Written discourse, technology to evaluate, 218–219

Y

Yarning, 140–142, **142**, 143